COMMUNICATION SKILLS AND CLASSROOM SUCCESS

D0018809

COMMUNICATION SKILLS AND CLASSROOM SUCCESS

Assessment of Language-Learning Disabled Students

Edited by
CHARLANN S. SIMON

Speech-Language Pathologist
Tempe, Arizona

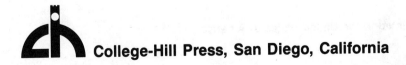
College-Hill Press, San Diego, California

College-Hill Press
4284 41st Street
San Diego, California 92105

Library of Congress Cataloging in Publication Data
Main entry under title:
Assessment of language-learning disabled students.

    (Communication skills and classroom success)
    Bibliography: p.
    1. Language disorders in children—Diagnosis.
2. Learning disabilities—Diagnosis. I. Simon, Charlann S. II. Series.
RJ496.L35A87   1984   618.92'89   84-26344

ISBN 0-933014-31-7

Printed in the United States of America

DEDICATION

This book is dedicated to my mother, Catherine E. Scheid. As a keen observer of situations and individuals, this spunky lady has always sought improvement and even perfection. She is the type of person who is responsible for progress and achievement because she will not settle for less than *justice* or *attainment of potential.* Although she emphasized the importance of being a good student during my school years, it was never a point upon which she perseverated. Instead, she provided multiple opportunities for me to develop creative skills in drama, dance and music. It was through these avenues that I first developed self-confidence. The professional achievements I have attained are either the direct or indirect result of the principles she instilled. I treasure her love and support; and I respect and admire her strength of character.

CONTENTS

CONTRIBUTORS

Lorian Baker, PhD, Research Psycholinguist, Neuropsychiatric Institute, University of California at Los Angeles, Los Angeles, California 90024

Mary Balfour Calvert, MA (CCC), Speech-Language Pathologist, Naples, Italy (formerly with Children's Hearing and Speech Center, Children's Hospital National Medical Center, Washington, DC)

Arthur G. Blouin, PhD, Adjunct Professor, Carleton University, Neuropsychologist, Ottawa Civic Hospital, Ottawa, Ontario, Canada

Dennis P. Cantwell, MD, Joseph Campbell Professor of Child Psychology, Neuropsychiatric Institute, University of California at Los Angeles, Los Angeles, California 90024

Gerald E. Chappell, PhD, Professor, Center for Communicative Disorders, University of Wisconsin at Stevens Point, Stevens Point, Wisconsin 54481

Nancy A. Creaghead, PhD, Associate Professor, Department of Communication, Speech, and Theater; Speech and Hearing Laboratory, University of Cincinnati, Cincinnati, Ohio 45221

Jack S. Damico, PhD, Department of Speech Communication, Theatre, and Communication Disorders, LSU Speech and Hearing Center, Louisiana State University, Baton Rouge, Louisiana 70803

Craig Dougherty, PhD, Dougherty Associates, Fulton, NY 13069

Carl B. Feinstein, MD, Associate Professor, Department of Psychiatry, George Washington University School of Medicine and Health Sciences; Director, Out-Patient Services, Department of Psychiatry, Children's Hospital National Medical Center, Washington, DC 20010

M. Suzanne Hasenstab, PhD, Associate Professor, Director of Hearing Impairment, Department of Speech Pathology and Audiology, University of Virginia, Charlottesville, Virginia 22903

Cynthia L. Holway, MA (CCC), Speech-Language Pathologist, Scottsdale, Arizona

Stephen Isaacson, MS, Doctoral Fellow, Department of Special Education, Arizona State University, Tempe, Arizona 85283

Sharon L. Murray, PhD, Assistant Professor, Department of Child Health and Development, George Washington University School of Medicine and Health Sciences, Supervisor, Speech-Language Pathology, Children's Hearing and Speech Center, Children's Hospital National Medical Center, Washington, DC 20010

Nickola Wolf Nelson, PhD, Associate Professor, Department of Speech Pathology and Audiology, Western Michigan University, Kalamazoo, Michigan 49008

Diane J. Sawyer, PhD, Associate Professor, Director of Clinical Services, Reading Clinic, Reading and Language Arts Center, Syracuse University, Syracuse, New York 13210

M. Shelly, PhD, Reading and Language Arts Center, Syracuse University, Syracuse, New York 13210

Charlann S. Simon, MA (CCC), Speech-Language Pathologist, Tempe Elementary Schools, and Adjunct Faculty Member in Speech and Hearing Sciences, Arizona State University, Tempe, Arizona 85283

L. Spaanenburg, PhD, Reading and Language Arts Center, Syracuse University, Syracuse, New York 13210

Sandra S. Tattershall, PhD, Director, Language and Learning Clinic, Florence, Kentucky 41042

CONSULTING EDITOR: Carolyn Ausberger Wiener, MA (CCC), Speech-Language Pathologist, Syndactics, Inc. Phoenix, Arizona 85064

PREFACE

In Latin, *communicatus* means to impart, share, and make common. The ability to communicate and to participate in communication focuses on the giving and receiving of information. Fortunately, for most individuals communication skills develop normally. As events are experienced and attitudes are formed, they can be shared with others through communication. Through this means, learning takes place as we refine perceptions and viewpoints and seek new knowledge or clarification of current knowledge by engaging in inquiry. For a sizable number—with estimates ranging between 3% and 15% of the school-age population—inferior communication skills inhibit learning and contribute to feelings of failure in "the student role." It is this population—the children who have difficulties within the academic setting—that is the focus of this volume and its companion volume.

In January, 1983, College-Hill Press contacted me about writing a book on the relationships between communications skills and classroom success. I was honored; I was also realistic about the depth and complexity of the topic. For this reason, I suggested an edited volume. With the understanding that I would provide "transitional sections" between each of the chapters that would be designed to unite the content, the project was under way. What began as a single book turned into a two-volume set: *Communication Skills and Classroom Success: Assessment of Language-Learning Disabled Students* and *Communication Skills and Classroom Success: Therapy Methodologies for Language-Learning Disabled Students.*

A major goal of these volumes is to provide educators and special educators with information about children who have deficits in skills or strategies that are required for school success, to provide suggestions for the assessment of these skills and strategies as well as suggest that it is equally necessary to reflect on the quality of instruction and instructional materials, and to provide some specific suggestions for helping students develop the cognitive strategies and communication skills needed so that they will be able to become more adept in "playing the school game." The two volumes are equally useful to the professional currently in the field and to university students studying speech-language pathology, learning disabilities, educational counseling and guidance, and classroom teaching.

In this volume on Assessment, the chapters by Simon, Cantwell, Nelson, and Tattershall provide descriptive information about the school-age child with communication and classroom problems. In addition, the reader is asked to consider the interactive variables of instructional style, instructional content, and student behavior. Communication assessment strategies are presented by Calvert and Murray, Damico, and Chappell;

Murray comments on the descriptive value of one popular standardized test. Simon and Holway address the question of how communication assessment data should be organized and presented during staffing conferences, as well as how to write reports, so that educators better understand how an individual's communication skills and cognitive strategies can affect classroom performance. While Sawyer presents descriptive information about the relationship between communication behavior and reading performance, Hasenstab offers suggestions for the evaluation of reading skills from a communcation-based theoretical position. Sawyer, Dougherty, Shelly, and Spaanenburg elaborate on the evaluation of auditory segmenting ability. The assessment of written language is addressed by Isaacson. Between each of these chapters, the reader will find "transitional notes" that bridge the content from the earlier chapter to the following chapter as well as provide some synthesis of additional material available on the topic from other sources.

I want to thank College-Hill Press for providing the opportunity to organize the theoretical and clinical perspectives of educators and clinicians who are working on methods to better understand what can be done to help children enjoy success during their school years. In this volume, there are 17 participating authors; in both volumes, a total of 33 authors. Their enthusiasm for the project and professional commitment to deadlines have made it possible to have these books on the market within 18 months after work was initiated. I cannot thank each of them sufficiently for their time, their sterling work, and their cooperative attitudes. Next, to Carolyn Ausberger Weiner, I am greatly indebted! At the publisher's final review of the volumes, I was asked to reduce the length of each; I was, however, too close to the project to make any further deletions. I called upon my friend and colleague of the past decade for assistance. Within one week she engaged in skillful trimming of both volumes without losing the essence of each author's contribution. Lastly, I want to extend special thank you's to my husband, Sheldon, and son, Alex, for being supportive while taking telephone messages from participating authors and wading through stacks of papers and books in our home office for the past 18 months while my organization of this project, writing, and editing have been in progress. It has been team work from the beginning—and I thank everyone involved!

Charlann S. Simon, MA (CCC)
Speech-Language Pathologist
Tempe, Arizona

CHAPTER 1

The Language-Learning Disabled Student: Description and Assessment Implications

Charlann S. Simon

"Oh, please God! Don't make me *normal!*" It would be to the psychological credit of many language-learning disabled students if they could have this ego-strength displayed by the heroine from *The Fantastics*. Unfortunately, in our culture, to be different is not infrequently equated with being disabled. If someone looks at a task in a new way—with fresh perspective, perhaps, and an unusual interpretation—the result is evaluated as being "wrong" or "weird."

When school-age children are referred to special educators or medical facilities for evaluation, it is usually because they do not seem to be "normal" in the classroom, in terms of completing the objectives of the curriculum or interaction with peers and teachers, or both. According to Rosenthal (1984), a parent's greatest concern regarding a child's school entrance is whether or not the child will learn to read. Whether it is parent concern or teacher suggestion that prompts a psychoeducational evaluation, it is important that the resulting assessment be composed of procedures that evaluate the child's strengths as well as weaknesses. In addition, it is important for the evaluator not only to focus on the child as the subject of study, but also to be equally interested in investigating how the learning and cultural environment are contributing to opportunities for the child to show inherent potential. The dynamics of the environment, educational content, the child's cognitive-linguistic and motor-perceptual skills, and instructional language should be dissected (Anastasiow, Hanes, and Hanes, 1982; Gruenewald and Pollak, 1984; O'Brien, 1983).

The assessment process itself is worthy of reflection. There has been an emphasis in the past on focusing on the product of the evaluation to the exclusion of looking at the process and the student's reaction to it. It is important for the evaluator to analyze *why* a student has reacted to certain assessment probes in the manner observed. This means that innovative strategies are frequently required or there needs to be a fresh look at popular standardized procedures to see how a score can be "milked" for descriptive information. For example, the Peabody Picture Vocabulary Test (Dunn and Dunn, 1981) is often administered as a measure of receptive vocabulary. The scores obtained upon completion of the test are really rather sterile. It is more important to analyze the errors. This might mean any of the following:

1. Observing the age range in which most errors occurred.

2. Noting specific words that the student missed so that these can be shared with the classroom teacher during the multidisciplinary staffing conference.

3. Asking the student at a subsequent point to define several of the words missed.

Let's say, for example, that the student responded incorrectly when asked to show you "sorting." At a later time, the student can be asked, "What does the word 'sorting' mean to you?" If the student says "Looking through things," you know that the concept is only partially understood. This becomes especially apparent as you refer back to the choice of four stimulus pictures and you notice that the student chose the picture of children looking through books in a library rather than the postal employee placing letters in pigeonhole slots. Therefore, it is reasonable to assume that the student has an *incomplete* conceptualization rather than a *wrong* conceptualization of the word "sorting." The student has not refined the conceptualization of "looking through things" to include the reason for or result of looking through things—that is categorization.

The problem for many of the students who are labeled "language-learning disabled" is that they themselves equate "disabled" with "retarded." They are sensitive to being categorized as "handicapped" when they know that they are not unintelligent; yet, they feel unintelligent when confronted with the types of tasks that are stressed and valued in the academic setting—such as segmenting words in phonics or solving multiple-step story problems in mathematics. They realize that the student sitting next to them in class, getting A's in all the tests and responding rapidly to memory-based comprehension questions from the teacher, may get lost going home from school and could never figure out how to open a complicated gate fastener through analysis of its working parts. The language-learning disabled child knows he has skills, but it just so happens they are not the skills valued by the educational setting. There is, therefore, little opportunity to show his or her special talents or be rewarded for them with a good grade. This point is addressed particularly well by McCarthy (1980) with her development of "The 4-Mat System" of teaching content, which allows opportunities for different learning styles to be rewarded within any unit of study.

The educational system sometimes contributes to the language-learning disabled student's image as a "passive learner" or "inactive learner" (Bransford, 1979; Wong, 1982). Kevin, a 20 year old college student interviewed by Altwerger and Bird (1982) was quoted as saying, "I often wonder if it would have been better if I would have been forced to conform to the system—to expend a little energy" (p. 75). I wonder how Kevin and other language-learning disabled students have felt when they were asked to attend an end-of-the-year conference and heard recommendations for future placement such as, "I think he would be more comfortable in basic math because standard math is too high. The lower group would be better." Although these are well-meaning educators, such comments contribute to "negative programming" (Knepflar and Laguaite, 1985).

Perhaps it is with too great a visceral reaction that the author of this chapter approaches the topic of language-learning disability. I am grateful that the term "learning disability" was not in vogue in 1946 when I started elementary school. Considering my behavioral profile, I have few reservations about concluding that I would have been labeled "disabled." I used mirror writing in first grade, and in addition I was not able to learn to read through a "new phonics-based program" that was being tried in the one first grade room in which I was placed. Only when I reached second grade and followed a more traditional (at that time) "look-say" approach to reading did I learn to read. Prolonged difficulties with segmentation and repeating phonemic sequences produced many moments of discomfort in the classroom as I was unable to pronounce a new multisyllabic vocabulary word. "But *why* can't you say 'transoceanic'? After all, you wrote the class Christmas play!" Mathematics has been (and continues to be) the thorn in my existence! My parents were told annually that I was not achieving at the level of my potential. To counterbalance curricular demands that were not compatible with my learning style, the Dewey-based educational system I was in provided a supportive grading procedure. Students were allowed to do extra-credit assignments, and these were integrated with regular assignments at grading time. Those of us who did more and different types (usually more of the creative, imaginative kinds of projects), were graded on par with the students who did only what was expected but did the work at a high achievement level. There was, then, some flexibility in the system that permitted students with different learning styles to avoid being labeled "disabled." By the time I attended Northwestern University as an undergraduate, it was becoming increasingly apparent that my study habits were not conducive to "efficient learning." Was it possible that in all of the time that I had attended school, I had not learned how to learn? To escape academic probation and impress my fiance, a doctoral student, I made a concerted effort to survey the study habits of my sorority sisters who were on the Dean's List. During my senior year, I received better positive reinforcement than M&M's—a 4.0 grade point average.

For students who do not naturally "fit in," mandatory school attendance in an inflexible system that assumes study skills that are not there can be a demeaning experience. These students are in a twilight zone where a lot of events do not seem to fit together, and they feel out of step to the beat of the academic drummer. Instead of viewing this difference as an alternative (or perhaps even a desirable state, as did the heroine in *The Fantastics)*, they frequently develop attitudes characterized by helplessness (Dweck and Licht, 1980; Hagen, Barclay, and Newman, 1982) or defiance (Compton, 1975; Wilgosh and Paitich, 1982). Assessment, then, should be broad-based enough to include observation of the student, the context, the content, and the interacting peers and teachers. Only through such a comprehensive observational procedure can "mismatches" be determined and modifications made or learning strategies developed. Assessment should be, by definition, description of interacting variables.

WHO IS THE POPULATION?

Estimates of the incidence of learning disability range from 3% to 15% of the school-age population (Sheridan, 1983). This figure usually includes students with reading problems. In the United States, initial research in the psychological characteristics and needs of learning disabled children began in Michigan with Dr. Heinz Werner, a comparative psychologist, and Dr. Alfred A. Strauss, neuropsychiatrist, in approximately 1940 (Cruickshank, 1977; Hallahan and Kauffman, 1976). The term "learning disabilities" was suggested by Samuel Kirk in 1963 in an address to a parent group in Chicago (Hallahan and Kauffman, 1976).

Hallahan and Kauffman (1976) observe "There are five major points that almost universally are present in any definition of learning disability. The learning disabled child:

1. has academic retardation
2. has an uneven pattern of development
3. may or may not have central nervous system dysfunctioning
4. does not owe his learning problems to environmental disadvantage
5. does not owe his learning problems to mental retardation or emotional disturbance." (p. 20)

Kinsbourne (1983) offers a succinct description of the various explanatory models of learning disabilities:

1. *Individual difference model.* This is a normal variation.

2. *Deficit model.* In this instance malfunction is due to adverse influences outside the bounds of normal variation; there has been actual disruption of the developing brain.

3. *Delay model.* Damage has occurred at the neural level, which influences behavior of younger children.

4. *Brain organization model.* Although there are several variations, the simplest explanation proposes a deficiency with the language area of the left hemisphere in which there is compensatory function by the right hemisphere; Samuel Orton's hypothesis of a failure to lateralize language has also been pursued.

In an excellent overview of the literature on the etiology of reading disability, Vellutino (1977) organizes the variety of explanations offered into four basic types. These explanations are based on

1. deficiencies in visual processing
2. deficiencies in intersensory integration
3. dysfunction in temporal order perception
4. deficiencies in verbal processing

Vellutino (1979) says that language deficits are a recurrent theme in the literature on dyslexia.

A variation on the basic theme of a medical versus behavioral explanation for learning problems has been termed the "strategy versus deficit controversy" (Swanson, 1982). The controversy revolves around the question, "Have learning disabled children not learned how to learn or do they have neurological limitations and constraints?" A basic assumption of those who support a strategy explanation is that the rules and specific strategies employed by learning disabled children do not appear to tap or exhaust their intellectual capabilities. Hiscock (1983) reminds us that "researchers now recognize what special classroom teachers have known all along, viz., that learning disabled children are a diverse group with various academic characteristics" (p.18). According to Kinsbourne (1983), the major factors, as isolated in factor analysis studies, that might impinge on learning to read and generally succeeding within a classroom are verbal ability, perceptual organization, and freedom from distractibility.

Ames (1983) addresses the "readiness factor" as being a crucial determinant in being "learning disabled." She says, "Our clinical finding [at the Gesell Institute of Human Development, New Haven, Connecticut] over the years since the term learning disability has come into vogue is that a large percentage of the boys and girls referred to our own clinical service as learning disabled have been children of apparently quite normal academic potential who were simply overplaced in school. In our opinion, these children are having trouble in school chiefly because they were started too soon—on the basis of their chronological age rather than their behavioral age" (p. 19). According to Hasenstab and Laughton (1982), readiness factors are certainly not new hypotheses, but they are crucial considerations. These authors define readiness from various perspectives: "Readiness is seen to be a time in which various skills are consolidated or interrelated. . . .Readiness can also be considered to be the time in which a child is mastering prerequisite knowledge and experiences that will permit the emergence of new or further developmental behaviors. . . .Readiness is a summation of previous and current experience and knowledge of the time at which the child is able to accomplish a new task or master a more sophisticated process. . . .Readiness is not confined to the prereading period. . . .It is a dynamic process. . .a time of awareness" (Hasenstab and Laughton, 1982, pp. 42–44).

Assessment guidelines are frequently necessitated by definitions, regardless of the underlying philosophical biases of the individual evaluator. In the public schools, the bottom line is called "eligibility criteria." The definitions currently being used are as follows:

1. From the U.S. Office of Education, appearing in the Federal Register, 1977 (Donahue, Pearl, and Bryan 1982), "Children with learning disabilities are defined as those with normal intelligence, intact sensory and emotional functioning, but who still exhibit a disorder in one or more of the basic psychological processes involved in understanding or using language, spoken or written."

2. From the National Joint Committee for Learning Disabilities, 1981 (Kirk and Kirk, 1983), "Learning disability is a generic term that refers to a heterogeneous group of disorders manifested by significant difficulties in the acquisition and use of listening, speaking, reading, writing, reasoning, or mathematical abilities. These disorders are intrinsic to the individual and presumed to be due to central nervous system dysfunction. Even though the learning disability may occur concomitantly with other handicapping conditions (e.g., sensory impairment, mental retardation, social and emotional disturbances) or environmental influences (e.g., cultural differences, insufficient or inappropriate instruction, psychogenic factors), it is not the direct result of those conditions or influences."

Although eligibility criteria determine ultimately who will and who will not be included in a special education program, readiness factors frequently prompt educators to request a psychoeducational assessment of a student.

If educators can be taught to be informal evaluators of communication and classroom skills, they can be a critical link in a child's chain of educational experiences. Anastasiow and colleagues (1982), Gruenewald and Pollack (1984), Hasenstab and Laughton (1982), and Vetter (1982) all present guidelines for spotting "the high-risk child." Monroe (1965) emphasized many years earlier how important general language development is to success in reading and suggested that a language sample should be part of the evaluation of reading readiness skills. It is surprising, and somewhat horrifying, that a child can still enter the door of a first grade classroom in September and say to his teacher, "Hi! My name Wandy. I six year old," and to have this indication of his linguistic sophistication be ignored. Instead, Randy is plugged into the reading program adopted by his school district, which is usually phonics-based. In other words, Randy is asked to segment the linguistic code before he has even learned to *use* it for communication. It is not fair to a child to begin his school experience with such weak links that he is programmed for disability. The major purpose of this book is to provide guidelines for educators so that the dynamic interactions of readiness, the curriculum, the child's learning style, and the teacher's pedagological style can be systematically subjected to observation for the educational benefit of the student.

CHILDREN WHO HAVE TROUBLE IN SCHOOL: AN OVERVIEW OF THE LITERATURE

Two research areas in particular have provided descriptive information on the types of children who have difficulty in the school setting: sociolinguistics and special education. Each of these areas will be reviewed separately, with an emphasis on the research from special education.

Sociolinguistics

Sociolinguistics, as a discipline, utilizes concepts of sociology and linguistics in the study of the functioning of language in a society. Research on the relationships between cultural patterns and the preparation for cognitive-linguistic skills required in school has shed light on why children from middle-class homes—regardless of ethnicity—do better in school than children of lower socioeconomic backgrounds (Anastasiow et al., 1982). According to the synthesis of the research conducted by Moore (1971) and later by Anastasiow and associates (1982), there are predictable patterns of school behavior that can be associated with the nature of child-rearing practices. To be specific, according to Martin (1975), the set of variables that seem to be most facilitating consists of verbal stimulation, moderate warmth and emotional support, responsiveness, low use of physical punishment, and push toward achievement.

Bernstein (1964, 1970) says that language is controlled by social structure and that the social structure is maintained and transmitted through language. Bernstein isolated four basic socializing systems (family, peer group, school, and work) and within each system, the individual occupies certain roles. The nature of the socializing system somewhat determines the range of behavioral opportunities available to the child and, consequently, the different types of communication opportunities that occur. Halliday (1978), operating on Bernsteins's basic description of the social system and its relationship to communication opportunities, states: "Suppose that the [language] functions that are relatively stressed by one group are positive with respect to school. They are favored and extended in the educational process, whereas those that are relatively stressed by another group are largely irrelevant or even negative in the educational context. We have, then, a plausible interpretation of the role of language in educational failure" (p. 106).

One of the environments that seems to promote the type of interactional and linguistic skills that are rewarded in the classroom is referred to by Bernstein (1970) as a "person-oriented decision-making milieu." In a family setting in which hierarchical power is not stressed, family members have greater opportunity to interact and express opinions that might not be those of the "ranking family member." Individual differences are expressed verbally and reinforced. A role system like this promotes communication and orientation toward the motives and dispositions of others. To this, Bernstein contrasts the "position-oriented" family system. Verbal exploration of individual intentions and motives is not encouraged, and the child responds to status requirements. Because there are prescribed roles for the various family members, an atmosphere is created in which there is a smaller range of alternative behaviors and verbal strategies available for use and practice. "The greater the range of alternatives permitted by the role system, the more individualized the verbal meanings, the higher the order (of thinking) and the more flexible the syntactic and vocabulary selection.." (Bernstein, 1970, p. 34).

Luria (1976) and Vygotsky (1978) found in their research that the educational level of the adults had a significant effect on the acquisition of logical thinking, moral reasoning, perceptual illusions, and depth of knowledge of self. Reinforcing these findings is research by Broman, Nicholas, and Kennedy (cited by Anastasiow et al., 1982), who studied 55,000 women and their children and found that among all the variables measured, years of mother's education was the best predictor of a child's

IQ at age 4 years. Anastasiow and colleagues also state that, in their opinion, IQ scores are measures that predict whether a child will have success or difficulty in middle-class-type schools, in which verbal ability and comprehension are dominant skills. "Most lower SES [socioeconomic status] children learn to communicate, but not in the ways that are prized by the dominant culture and that are related to school success. [At the same time], some lower class children do quite well in school as a product of the stimulation received in their homes. The IQ test is constructed to measure skills that are related to school success. Poverty children tend to do less well on these measures due to the preferred styles of the culture in which these children are reared and, in some cases, due to the outmoded and debilitating childrearing practices of the homes into which these children have been born or placed" (Anastasiow et al., 1982, p. 26).

Tough's (1977) study in England found similar discrepancies between middle-class and lower-class children's preparation for school. She found that while the middle-class children tended to use language to predict, work together, and imagine creatively, lower-class children used language to get attention and service their needs. Moore (1971) observed that "fragmentary evidence suggests that the lower-class child enters school with a hesitancy to question, to initiate verbal interactions with adults and, in general, to gain important information through verbal means" (p. 26). As Ogbu (1974) points out, it is a vicious circle for these children, because their failure to use language and logic as well as middle-class children is perceived as a lack of ability rather than a lack of training. Teachers expect less of them and rate them lower on academic measures of performance.

When it comes to the assessment of communication and classroom skills of lower-class children, Anastasiow and colleagues (1982) caution that educators should examine whether a child's assumed lower verbal talents are due to value preferences of the caregiver or to the caregiver's lack of knowledge of how to enhance the infant's language development so that the child can succeed in the middle-class–dominated culture of the schools. Once again, then, it is emphasized that we must always include in our evaluation procedures not only the *child* but also the *variables* that interact with and affect the child's potential. This includes cultural pressures and practices, lowered teacher expectations, and reduced stimulation as a result of lack of caregiver education.

Special Education

From the field of special education, we have observations on "the learning disabled child" and "dysteachia." Fortunately, there has always been a nucleus of special educators who began their professional lives with the intuition or the training that made them ask two questions, not just one:

1. What is the child doing wrong?
2. What is the educator doing wrong?

This balance has produced individualized programs for students and task analysis of educational objectives. This section will include two subsections, dealing with the student and the teacher. Each will attempt to pinpoint specific behaviors that seem to enhance or inhibit student performance in the classroom.

Learning Disabilities

The "learning disabled" population is marked by one characteristic: diversity. A second shared characteristic seems to be ADD (attention deficit disorder) (Hagerman, 1984). In an attempt to synthesize and yet organize the literature on the nature of learning disabilities, research notations will be grouped into the following categories: cerebral involvement, psychodynamic variables, linguistic-pragmatic deficits, information processing problems, and differences in cognitive style.

Cerebral Involvement. Cruickshank (1977) conceptualizes learning disabilities as being the *result* of something. In particular, he isolates "perceptual processing deficit" to be the underlying reason for learning problems. "The term 'perceptual' as used here relates to those mental [neurological] processes through which the child acquires his basic alphabets of sounds and forms" (Cruickshank, 1977, p. 9). The neurophysiological involvement he specifies is summarized in five major characteristics:

1. Sensorimotor hyperactivity: Response to irrelevant stimuli and in a constant state of physical alertness, which is characterized by wiggling and squirming or seemingly never to be in a relaxed state.
2. Dissociation: The inability to see things as a whole or "seeing the trees but not the forest."
3. Figure-background reversal: A perceptual focus on the total immediate environment (such as a book page) rather than the crucial stimulus (a particular word).
4. Perseveration: a prolonged after-effect of a stimulus on subsequent activities.
5. Motor immaturity: A lack of coordination in gross and fine motor skills, similar to that seen in a younger child.

Rosenthal (1973) suggests that in the learning disabled child there is "differential brain function" rather than "minimal brain disfunction" (MBD). Rosenthal views the learning disabled child as one who evidences educational, psychological, medical, social, economical, and political difficulties. As Hagerman (1984) points out, a neurodevelopmental assessment of the learning disabled child usually yields normal results. More important, she says, are the observations a physician can make about the manner in which the child takes in information from the environment. In other words, the child may pass the test to meet normal limits, but the process or strategy used may be suspect—such as rate of processing directions during the examination.

Another area of research that tends to support *some* kind of brain involvement in *some* learning disabled children stems from the effects of medication used to control ADD and improve attention to classroom tasks. Levine, Busch, and Aufseer (1982) compared ADD children with other learning disabled children. The ADD group often had more perceptual and academic deficiencies than the non-ADD learning disabled child. For example, the classic symptoms of ADD are hyperactivity, inattentiveness, impulsivity, distractibility, inconsistency, impaired selectivity in focusing on stimuli, disinhibition, insatiability, frequency of occurrence of soft neurological signs (such as fine motor dyspraxia, visual motor incoordination, and motor impersistence) (Hagerman, 1984). Hagerman goes on to cite research that documents how medication (stimulants) work at the level of the brain stem to correct the imbalance of neurotransmitters, which serve the function of reducing attention deficit disorders. If the brain were not involved in this aspect of learning disability, why would the medication make a difference in classroom and interpersonal performance? Hagerman mentions that medication for ADD improves not only attention but also accuracy and vigilance, reaction time, fine motor coordination (as used in handwriting), and central auditory processing, and it reduces soft neurological signs and overactivity.

Brain involvement in learning disability seems to be substantiated more empirically in some areas than in others. Whereas ADD seems to be associated with learning disability more than any other single characteristic (Rosenthal, 1984), there are other "brain involvements" that are more tenuous. For example, Hiscock (1983) says that investigation of handedness, eyedness, and mixed dominance as correlates of learning disability have failed to produce a consistent set of results, and that one needs to seriously question the relevance of measuring a child's handedness, for example, in an attempt to discern the lateralization of that child's language. "Perhaps because deviant humans [who are the 10% who do not show right-hand dominance] constitute a rather small minority, educators tend to view left-handed and bilateral children with some suspicion. . . .Speculations about fundamental differences between the cerebral hemispheres in cognitive or personality style run far ahead of scientists' actual knowledge about hemispheric differences. . . . Two recent large-scale studies of children failed to reveal any trace of cognitive deficit among left-handed children relative to their right-handed peers" (Hiscock, 1983, pp. 14–25).

Whereas Hiscock suggests indirectly that there is a difference rather than a deviance in individuals who show a "right brain profile," Gordon (1983) states directly that it cannot be assumed that everyone with a right-brain processing problems will have classroom problems. "Perhaps the difference is that some people are locked into a right-brain processing mode even when it is not conducive to the task at hand. For example, math, reading, spelling, and grammar call upon left-brain functioning. If one tries to use a right mode of thought for these tasks, it is not difficult to see how deficits may occur" (Gordon, 1983, p. 35). Hunter (1976) noted that traditional educational methods tend to focus on the rational, unemotional, and analytical learning style of the left hemisphere and ignore the intuitive, emotional, and imaginative skills and style of the right hemisphere. As Gordon quips, "Those who cannot draw, sing, or solve jigsaw puzzles are excused for their disability" in school (Gordon, 1983, p. 37).

Psychodynamic Variables. Research since the 1940s has shown clear links between an individual's judgment of his or her ability and competence and actual performance on school-related tasks, which Hagen, Barclay, and Newman (1982) mention is currently referred to as a person's "self-schemata." An individual's self-perceptions of social and cognitive features affect motivation as well as task persistence. These self-perceptions may be associated with poor motivation and low self-esteem, which, in turn, lead to inactive learning and continued suppressed academic performance. The term "learned helplessness" was used by Dweck and Goetz (1978) and Dweck and Licht (1980) to describe the child who, after experiencing failure or being labeled by the school system as "disabled," engages in nonproductive thoughts about his ability.

With lower self-esteem frequently comes depression. As Wertz (1963) has pointed out, depression results in less psychic energy for learning and increases difficulty in concentration. Wertz feels that isolation of this type of student into special classes and resource rooms might even contribute to a worsening of the child's already poor self-concept; this is especially evident in the adolescent population Wertz studied.

Do learning problems and the resulting school placement result in psychological problems or do psychological problems appear as learning problems? Hollon (1970) and Colbert, Newman, Ney, and Young (1982) see disruption of a household as a predictable cause for depression, which in turn affects the quality of concentration needed for classroom performance. In fact, 71% of the 111 depressed children studied by Colbert and associates (1982) were in regular classrooms (in Canada) but were significantly underachieving by one or more grade levels in one or more academic areas in relation to expectations based on their intelligence and grade placement.

Depression can be the underlying factor in withdrawal, which in its most extreme state takes the form of suicide (Hollinger, 1979). Depressed children also frequently "act out." They can be irritable and quarrelsome, and their aggressive behavior is one of the most frequent causes for referral to a psychologist or other special educators (Pozanski and Zrull, 1970). According to Phillips (1979), a depressed child complains of being bored, is restless, and may even become involved in antisocial behavior in an attempt to get excited and dispel a gloomy affect. Such children also have a variety of somatic complaints, such as headaches and stomachaches, and show disrupted sleep patterns.

When studying incarcerated juvenile delinquents, who were classified as "learning disabled," Wilgosh and Paitich (1982) noted that 89% of their juvenile delinquent subjects were experiencing academic performance at one or more grades below age expectation. These data compare favorably with those from Compton (1975), who found that 90% of the delinquents studied could be described as "learning disabled." Other sources (Anderson, 1970; Kratoville, 1974; Kronick, 1975; Ramos, 1978) have addressed the relationship between juvenile delinquency and learning problems. A law enforcement officer quoted in Ramos (1978) made the following statement about this population:

"[The learning disabled child] is at a complete disadvantage, particularly from the moment he enters school. Frustrated by his inability to learn, his self-concept becomes poorer and poorer. To cope with feelings of rejection and sense of isolation, he begins 'acting out' by fighting, clowning around and defying authority figures. As he gets older, he becomes more and more of a problem at school and is eventually expelled, suspended, or just drops out. He becomes instilled with a sense of failure, he is a very likely candidate for delinquency and his self-concept is even more damaged by contact with the juvenile justice system" (Ramos, 1978, p. 12).

Looking at juvenile delinquents' performance profiles in terms of academic component skills, Zinkus and Gottlieb (1983) focused on the degree to which auditory processing problems played a role in academic failure. They found that the delinquent subjects with more severe degrees of underachievement academically were also those with the most severe processing deficits. "It was hypothesized that the problems in academic competence were more closely linked to perceptual disorders than to delinquency, per se" (Zinkus and Gottlieb, 1983, pp. 39–40).

Cantwell and Carlson (1983) have addressed the problem of a variety of affective disorders in children and adolescents, including results of a study on the interrelationships of communication, learning, and psychological status. They found that intervention in only one area, speech-language, did not prevent problems in related areas. Cantwell and Baker (1980) found that in 74% of their subjects, improvements occurred in communication skills but not in learning disorders or psychiatric problems. To a basic research question that these authors posed ("Are learning disorders and psychiatric disorders associated in children who show communication disorders?"), they had to answer "yes." Cantwell and Baker discuss this research in Chapter 2.

Linguistic-Pragmatic and Metalinguistic Deficits. In her 1973 article, Potter reminded us that speech-language pathologists have worked for over 50 years with individuals who have faulty language processes. Because the U.S. Office of Education's definition of learning disability (cited earlier in this chapter) contains a focus on poor receptive and expressive language skills as correlate behaviors, Potter suggests that educators should keep in mind the speech-language pathologist's expertise in this area. Hallahan and Kauffman (1976) note that it was Samuel Kirk, using the communications model of C. E. Osgood, who shifted emphasis from perceptual-motor deficits underlying learning disabilities to the underlying factors of language disabilities. Considerable research on cognitive-linguistic problems has followed throughout the 1970s to the present time, with a general consensus that there is a significant relationship between a student's cognitive-communication skills and classroom performance. This section of the chapter will deal with expressive (social-interactive) language and metalinguistic deficits associated with maladaptive school performance. Receptive language variables will be discussed later in this chapter under "Information Processing Problems."

Prutting (1982) presents a chronology of research interests in the area of language development and use. She notes that prior to a pragmatic approach—or an interest in the *use* of language for communicative purposes—the bulk of research in the 1960s and 1970s was directed first to the structural forms used by a child and later to the underlying semantic intent. Snyder (1980) suggests that paying attention to meaning made researchers look more closely at the communication context and aspects of cognitive and social development that preceded or accompanied communication growth. "Research into the functional or pragmatic aspects of child language extended the view of language development beyond the static components of syntactic form and semantic content to the dynamic mobilization of form and meaning for communication. . . .The language disordered child is now evaluated in terms of his ability to manipulate the linguistic code to achieve his communicative goals or purposes" (Snyder, 1980, pp. 31–32). Prutting adds that "[Another] area of research interest has to do with the organization of conversational rules. . .[where] it is necessary to examine both the linguistic or verbal behavior as well as the nonlinguistic or paralinguistic/nonverbal context in order to determine the range of conversational rules used by children" (Prutting, 1980, pp. 128).

A relatively new area of interest is the degree of development evidenced in a student's metalinguistic skills—i.e., the ability to think and talk about language in contrast to the functional use of language for communication (Flood and Salus, 1982). Hakes (1980) states, "Metalinguistic abilities are different from and emerge later than the abilities involved in producing and understanding language. It is proposed that metalinguistic abilities show their greatest development during middle childhood, the period between roughly four and eight years. Their emergence is the linguistic manifestation of the cognitive developmental changes which Piaget has characterized as the emergence of concrete operational thought" (p. 2).

Metalinguistic abilities should be of observational interest to educators from the earliest years of education. When a child is asked, "What is the first letter of this word?," the educator has entered the realm of metalinguistics. Not until school entrance are most children exposed to the concept that a word is something that can be dissected; prior to school entrance, "word" has been synonymous with "concept label." Words, then, are meaningful representations of people, objects, and events in the child's environment and not the focus of analysis in their own right.

Linguistic and Pragmatic Variables. What has research uncovered with respect to a description of linguistic and pragmatic deficits in the language-learning disabled population? Simon (1979) synthesized the observations of a number of researchers investigating aspects of communicative competence versus incompetence. A summary of this synthesis appears in Chapter 9 of this book. Wiig and Semel (1976, 1980) have utilized Guilford's (1967) Structure of the Intellect model as the basis for organizing their observations of cognitive-linguistic deficits in children and adolescents. Some of the specific behaviors Wiig and Semel note as being typical of the school-age language-learning disabled student include the following: word finding and retrieval deficits; use of a large number of words in an attempt to describe a concept because the name of the concept eludes them (such as "the thing you cut bread with" to indicate "knife"); use of grammatically incorrect and incomplete sentences; overuse of limited vocabulary and basic syntactic structures (compared with the use of combining and embedding ideas into more complex constructions); use of a number of fillers, such as "and the," "um," "let's see;" difficulty defining words, recalling names of items in classes (such as animals or foods), and retrieving verbal opposites. Wiig and Semel note that language-learning disabled students often show greater divergent cognitive-linguistic skills than convergent skills. Chappell, in Chapter 7 of this book, takes an analytical point of view similar to that of Wiig and Semel.

Observation of linguistic structures relied upon by language-learning disabled students indicates that there is greater reliance on basic sentence types, with little creativity in the use of more interesting sentence constructions. For example, Bryan and Pflaum (1978) found that in their spontaneous speech with peers, school-identified learning disabled children used less complex syntax. Wiig and Semel (1980) noted that in a 1975 study, the longest phrases used by the learning disabled adolescents they studied contained an average of five words, which were stated in a simple, declarative manner. They found, in contrast to this the academic achieving control group used structurally varied sentences, and their longest phrases contained an average of 11 words.

Bryen (1981) observed that when learning disabled youngsters were given sentences that required particular transformational operations (such as the use of passive rules) during a sentence imitation task, they tended to delete these and imitate the sentence in a reduced style. They tended to use the fewest number of transformational operations necessary during their imitation, which is a strategy observed in younger normal children. Bryen concludes that the productive language problems associated with learning disabilities can be described as reflecting reduced cognitive and linguistic abilities. She said that she observed use of the following strategies:

1. Use of those morphemes and rules of grammar that require the least amount of abstraction and yet express the most meaning.

2. Use of those syntactic and pragmatic structures that require the smallest number of mental operations.

3. Use of more words rather than fewer and more complex structures (Bryen, 1981, p. 54).

Wiig and Semel (1976) say that 75% to 85% of learning disabled youngsters may experience significant delays in the acquisition of syntax and morphological markers, and that these delays may continue well into adulthood. Loban (1976) also documents the persisting oral language difficulties of children who were identified in kindergarten as being less proficient communicators. Teachers' ratings of the 211 students whom Loban studied for 13 years remained remarkably similar from year to year as the students were rated on their speaking, listening, reading, and writing skills. Aram and Nation (1980) found that, when they did follow-up research on preschool language disordered children, many of these children later had difficulties with reading and writing when they entered school.

Bennett and Runyan (1982) conducted a survey of classrooom teachers to determine whether communication skill deficit was considered to be an educational handicap. The results of their survey of 282 educators indicated that 66% of them believed that communication disorders did have an adverse effect on educational performance. Knight (1974) notes that sometimes the first formal indicator of possible language disability in students is when the school psychologist finds a wide gap between scores on the verbal and performance scales of the WISC. Freeman (1970) indicates that informal observation by educators, however, might uncover problems much earlier: "The preschool child with limited verbal abilities more often than not matures into a prime candidate for a classroom of mentally handicapped, neurologically impaired or emotionally disturbed children. Lack of development in verbal skills, in fact, is symptomatic of learning problems which have broad and long-term educational implications" (Freeman, 1970, p. 23). A list of "high-risk behaviors" to which educators should become sensitive is presented by Hasenstab in Chapter 11 of this book.

Donahue and colleagues (1982) noted that teachers seem to identify children as learning disabled more readily by the students' written language performance than by their use of oral language. In order to identify these linguistically impaired students at an earlier age, these authors suggested observational guidelines. The student shows the following traits:

1. Difficulty in social interaction with peers.

2. Difficulty internalizing pragmatic rules for varying contexts (such as shifting style when talking with a peer compared with the school principal).

3. Inept referential descriptions, which are not very useful to the listener because not enough detail is given.

4. Rare—if any—use of clarification questions when ambiguous messages or directions are received.

5. Less assertive and effective conversational skills with peers.

6. Less adept skills at expressing and eliciting opinions as well as maintaining proper control in conversations.

7. Less adequate vocabulary development, word retrieval, and comprehension or production of various grammatical morphemes and syntactic structures.

8. Use of syntactically simple sentences and lack of complex usage as well as reliance upon a few subject-verb-object types of structural coding.

As Blue (1975) reminds us, some students with language disabilities go unnoticed because they are "marginal communicators." Although these students are not truly competent communicators, their communication problems are not blatant. More often than not, this type of student ceases to practice communication and never really advances to more than minimal responses. "It may lie in the failure of the child to develop the necessary motivation to use and acquire reward from socially interactive speech. A child's repeated failure to participate in class is a problem that demands direct attention. We can't 'wait until he grows out of it' for the result is, too often, a young adult with reduced skills who fails to communicate satisfactorily with his employer and fellow workers" (Blue, 1975, pp. 33–36).

In looking at pragmatic behaviors observed in language-learning disabled students, both verbal and nonverbal deficits surface. Cruickshank (1977) notes obvious personal and social interactional problems observable in this population, which he attributes to perceptual processing problems. Specific characteristics Cruickshank mentions are the individual's difficulty in restraining himself or herself from reacting to all external stimuli, often in desperate and thoughtless ways; lack of insight into cause and effect relationships or the intellectual desire to modify a situation that prompts action; failure to perceive socially appropriate responses to a given situation, which may result in behaviors such as exaggeration, "storytelling," boasting, or reporting an observed event inaccurately. Soenksen, Flagg, and Schmits (1981) also observe that learning disabled students seem to lack social perceptiveness or sensitivity to the feelings expressed by others. Axelrod (1982) found that learning disabled adolescents in grades 8 and 9 appeared to have significantly lower nonverbal social perception skills than the control subjects. Excellent guidelines for the observation of social prerequisites to communication are available in Dukes (1981).

Pullis and Smith (1981) have reviewed the literature on factors of social competence in learning disabled students and discuss the findings in terms of cognitive development, role-taking behavior, development of moral reasoning, and communicative competence. Additional studies that discuss social-pragmatic competence in this population include those of Donahue and co-authors (1982), who observed problems in formulating ideas and opinions and in comprehending the intentions of others, and Prinz and Ferrier (1983), who looked at the quality of requesting behavior in relationship to syntactic complexity and cognitive development. Prinz and Ferrier found that whereas some of the less socially able children may have recognized the need to interact more politely, they lacked the linguistic means to produce more indirect forms appropriate to the age of the listener.

**Metalinguistic Variables.** Grieve, Tunmer, and Pratt (1980), in a review of metalinguistic skill development and classroom performance, note that many children who have difficulty with reading, abstract thought, and adjusting to school seem to encounter a number of these problems through a lack of awareness of language and the nature of the communication process. In some cases, when the type of task a student is being asked to address is examined relative to developmental data on requisite cognitive-linguistic skills to complete such a task, the difficulty experienced is not surprising.

Hakes (1980) notes that "One aspect of the development common to metalinguistic abilities and concrete operational [cognitive] abilities is an increasing ability to act and think deliberately and concomitantly to place one's self mentally at a distance from a situation and to reflect upon it. . . .There are, then, sufficient parallels between the cognitive abilities required for engaging in metalinguistic activities and those required for concrete operational functioning to suggest that the emergence of a common set of abilities underlies both kinds of development" (pp. 38–39).

Specific developmental notations include the following:

1. Aspects of language awareness that appear between age two and six are self-corrections in on-going speech, comments on the speech of others, explicit questions about speech and language, comments on the child's own speech and language and response to direct questions about language (Slobin, 1978).

2. Metalinguistic skills that develop after age four include the ability to detect ambiguity, acceptability, synonymy of two sentences that have the same semantic intent but different syntactic coding), grammaticality, meaningfulness, playing with language (as in riddles and puns), and understanding figurative language (Hakes, 1980).

3. In a study by Berthoud-Papandroupoulou (1978), children's concepts of spoken words were examined. The researchers noted that when asked to name a "long word," a typical answer from four and five year old children was "train," a short word that names a long object. Whereas younger children seem to focus on the ways things are named linguistically, by middle childhood there is an increasing ability to evaluate the properties of language.

4. Comprehension of the term "word" begins about age five for content words (such as nouns) but not functors (such as articles). By ages six and one half to eight, children view words as units or "bits of a story," and between ages six to eight the ability to analyze words into their constituent phonemes develops. By ages eight to ten, children are able to define the term "word" with a phrase such as "something that means something; it's written with letters" (Grieve et al., 1980).

Reiterating the importance of these metalinguistic skills to successful classroom performance, the educator cannot assume that all children between ages four and eight have made the same significant gains that are seen in research populations. Flood and Salus (1982), in a synthesis of research on the role of metalinguistic skills and academic performance, say that relationships between certain oral language abilities (such as morphophonological abilities) and reading performance have been established in a number of studies. Their review indicates that studies also show that the ability to segment written words into their phonological components can predict reading performance during early grades. The ability to map letter sequences into sound sequences was found to be of equal importance. Therefore, it appears that both awareness of the relationship between the printed and spoken word and awareness of word segmentation seem to be correlated with beginning reading achievement.

All one needs to do is to reflect upon the directions that are printed in phonics textbooks, workbooks, or manuals to become immediately aware of how the child is bombarded with requests for display of metalinguistic skill. For learning to read, a child must acquire a technical, metalinguistic vocabulary: "Sound out the letters"; "What does this word say?" (Nelson, 1983). Phonics instruction requires the student to reflect upon the isolated sounds of the language, an ability that is expected to be seen in advance of when this metalinguistic skill can be developmentally and conceptually expected (Sheridan, 1983).

Research with children who have learning disabilities has shown that this population lacks metalinguistic awareness—or the ability to reflect on the phonemic, syntactic, and semantic aspects of language (Baker, 1982). To be more specific, Hook and Johnson (1978) have noted that in work with their students the lack of syntactic and semantic awareness affects comprehension, and deficiency in phonemic awareness manifests itself in difficulty with segmenting spoken words into their component parts, thus affecting decoding skills. In addition, the results of a study by Nippold and Fey (1983) document the difficulty that older children, who were previously enrolled in language therapy as preschoolers, have with metaphorical language. While these preadolescent students (with a mean age of 10.7) performed on certain tasks that involved literal aspects of language at a level commensurate with that of the control group, they were deficient in their understanding of metaphorical sentences. "This suggests that children who as preschoolers exhibit difficulty in acquiring language may at a later time have difficulty dealing with figurative aspects of language" (Nippold and Fey, 1983, p. 176). Research also indicates that children with language-learning disorders are less able to make grammatical judgments than linguistically normal children (Shulman and Liles, 1979).

The research findings reviewed in this section all indicate a significant relationship between success in the classroom and the degree of development that can be observed in a student's cognitive-linguistic, pragmatic, and metalinguistic skills. Obviously, evaluation of these skills should be included in any psychoeducational battery. Suggestions for informal teacher observation and clinical evaluation of communication skills are provided in Chapters 3, 4, 5, 6, 7, and 8 in this book. Chapter 10 addresses deficit communication problems observed in poor readers, and Chapters 11, 12, and 13 demonstrate a language-based approach to the analysis of reading and writing skills.

In general, when confronted with the task of evaluating a student's communication skills, we can draw upon syntactical evaluation models (Hannah, 1977; Lee, 1974; Tyack and Gottsleben, 1974) to systematically observe structural skills, and we can draw upon pragmatic theoretical models (Dore, 1973; Grice, 1975; Halliday, 1973; Tough, 1977; Wells, 1973) to observe the degree of flexibility with which a student can use the linguistic code for varying communicative purposes. Additional observations can be made on the basis of skills that have been isolated as being crucial for classroom success or adaptation within life. For example, Bereiter and Engelmann (1966) isolated the "cognitive uses of language" as being the most critical for school achievement, while Bassett, Whittington, and Staton-Spicer (1978) have summarized basic listening and speaking skills that high school graduates should demonstrate in daily maintenance, community interactions, and on the job. Some discussion of the application of pragmatic models and the "cognitive uses of language" for assessment appear in Chapter 6 and 9 of this book; for greater detail, see Simon (1984a, b).

It behooves educators to engage in pretesting of cognitive-linguistic skills that provide the supportive superstructure for learning how to read, write, spell, and solve mathematics story problems or understand basic concepts of seriation and class inclusion (Carlson, Gruenewald, and Nyberg, 1980). No readiness skills should be *assumed.* As Flood and Salus (1982) remind us, school demands that children approach language in a new way. Not only are they asked to comprehend and follow directions that may be stated in unfamiliar terms ("Center your name") or complex embedding ("After you complete the math assignment that we didn't finish yesterday, read the first three paragraphs in the orange literature book in Chapter 5"), but in addition instruction focuses on the *word* as an object of study, not in terms of meaning but in terms of its phonological composition. Observation of interacting variables is crucial for necessary monitoring to occur.

Information Processing Problems. Interest in using an information processing model to explain academic difficulties of children labeled as "learning disabled" dates from the mid-1970s (Torgesen, 1982). Bauer (1982) provides a succinct chronology of the evolving interest in using this model as the basis of research into how the methods of processing information used by academically achieving students differed from the methods used by students showing academic difficulties, despite their having normal potential.

The four stages of the information processing model are encoding, manipulation, response selection, and response execution. It is a computer-based model of learning and memory that looks at the flow of information between successive stages, which are thought to be serial. Each stage has underlying processes. When using this model to analyze learning difficulties in nonachieving students, researchers are concerned with trying to determine "(1) the stage or stages that are deficient, (2) whether the deficit at each stage is due to an ineffective strategy, capacity or allocation of processing time among stages, and/or (3) retrieval" (Bauer, 1982, p. 34).

Torgesen and Greenstein (1982) tell us that information processing theory suggests that individuals may differ from one another in two broad areas of competence:

1. Cognitive structure, which relates to elements rather impervious to change (such as the capacity of short-term memory and speed of processing).

2. Information learned from experience (which includes the content of long-term memory), which can be altered by direct instruction.

Memory problems appear to be a pervasive characteristic of students who have classroom difficulties (Wiig and Semel, 1976). Locke (1969) investigated the ability of first grade children to imitate accurately three German syllables tape-recorded by a native German speaker. Basic auditory memory was tested through digit span retention. The group with high scores on auditory memory for digits was significantly better at imitating the German syllables than those with low auditory memory score. An additional notation that Locke shared was that, although the study group was 55% male, 90% of those in the low memory group were male. The type of information gathered in this study seems to be particularly important as we try to understand why some students have such difficulty with the phonemic sequencing needed to repeat new vocabulary words.

Short-term memory (STM) tasks have been defined by Torgesen and Greenstein (1982) as those that require brief storage of relatively small amounts of information after a single presentation. To be specific, storage intervals are usually greater than 1 second but usually less than 10 to 15 seconds. Various studies have documented the role that short-term memory plays in the successful execution of educational tasks (Baddeley, 1979; Daneman and Carpenter, 1980). Torgesen (1978) found that learning disabled students performed deficiently on STM tasks. Studies reviewed by Torgesen and Greenstein (1982) indicated that one source of performance problems experienced by learning disabled children on STM tasks is their frequent failure to adapt to task requirements by employing efficient strategic processing behaviors. The heterogeneity of the learning disabled population, however, was once again evident in the Torgesen and Greenstein literature review; some subgroups of this population do appear to have "more enduring processing deficits related to their poor performance on STM tasks (1982, p. 57).

Distractibility is another characteristic of nonachieving students. Sometimes there are built-in distractions to auditory attention (such as the ambient noise found in a open-school setting). Generally, over the past 20 years, the classroom and its ambience have changed. More things are happening, with children working in multiple small groups and more direct interaction occurring between peers (Smyth, 1979). These types of environmental changes seem to place an extra burden on many learning disabled students, who find it difficult to select and focus on only a sample of all available stimuli. The ability to engage in this type of auditory focus is called "selective auditory attention" (Cherry and Kruger, 1983). "What matters more with respect to noise is the signal-to-noise ratio rather than absolute noise. This is particularly true of younger children who are still acquiring linguistic rules and cannot rely upon sophisticated knowledge of the rule system to generate contextual inferences about sections of the speech stream that have been over-powered by noise. It is also an appropriate consideration regarding the mainstreamed language-delayed child. Such a child may have difficulty using auditorily based decision-making processes necessary for functional language because of inadequate language experience" (Smyth, 1979, p. 229).

Processing rate is another major factor to consider in uncovering reasons why information processing problems are occurring. Lupert (1981) and Tallal (1983) present convincing evidence about the "rate specific" problems observable in language-learning disabled students when they are attempting to decode acoustic information. Learning disabled children are slower at processing information than are normal achievers (Maisto and Sipe, 1980). Berry and Erickson (1973) showed that reducing presentation rate during the administration of test items improved performance in normal and language-learning impaired populations. "Rate of presentation can be altered by slowing the total rate of words per second presented in the message or by inserting pauses between the noun phrase and verb phrase of a sentence, within the verb phrase or between the verb and the following noun phrase" (Lasky and Chapandy, 1976, p. 166). Data from studies by Curtis (1980) and Hess and Radtke (1981) showed that processing rate is also an important determinant of reading skill.

Yet another information processing variable is syntactic complexity. Syntactic complexity is defined by Lasky and Chapandy (1976) as the number of transformations necessary to get from deep structure to surface structure. They found that there was little consideration of the relationship between syntactic complexity and linguistic sophistication of the target student population when textbook instructions that accompany the texts were analyzed. For example, in a preprimer they found that the writer had suggested the teacher ask the following comprehension question, "How do you think Betty and Tom feel about what Father is doing for Susan?" Lasky and Chapandy point out that the syntactic complexity of this question is almost three times the complexity of utterances expected from normal six year old children. This topic is discussed at length in Chapter 3 of this book, in terms of fostering a better match between teacher-talk and child-listening skill. It is crucial that educators capitalize on the knowledge that there is a predictable relationship between the complexity evident in a child's oral language and the degree of syntactic complexity the child is able to accurately process and comprehend. This "match-mismatch" can be informally assessed by classroom teachers, and the results of their observation can serve as guidelines for their monitoring syntactic complexity when interacting with students who have language deficits.

When teachers do not monitor the complexity of directions or give ambiguous directions, it is necessary for students to engage in auditory evaluation. The student needs to monitor whether or not the direction has been understood, and if it has not been understood, a clarification question needs to be formulated. Kotsonis and Patterson (1980) report that there seems to be a difference in comprehension monitoring or question asking skill between academically achieving and learning disabled students. When these two types of ten year old students were asked to judge when they had sufficient information or rules to play a particular game, the learning disabled children requested fewer rules and were also less able to actually play the game. The authors concluded that the learning disabled students did not actively evaluate their understanding of the rules during their listening performance.

Other parameters of auditory functioning that affect the quality of classroom performance are auditory identification, localization, discrimination, sequencing, and association (Gruenwald and Pollak, 1973). Lupert (1981) mentions difficulties that language-learning impaired students have in processing language at the syllable level during speech sound discrimination tasks because some speech sounds are not perceived in terms of their essential features. Sawyer (1981) found in her study that when four factors (IQ, auditory discrimination, blending, and segmentation) were combined, relatively high levels of predictability on reading achievement could be computed. She emphasizes the apparent interrelationships among these factors: "Success in beginning reading among the subsample of 21 boys appears most related to the effective application of the auditory abilities of discrimination, blending and segmentation in consort rather than the mastery of any *one* of these abilities in isolation" (p. 98). Sawyer and associates address this topic in Chapter 12 of this book.

Clark (1980) states, "Classroom survival does not come easily for all children. For the children with central auditory processing dysfunction, survival is even more difficult" (p. 208). The learning disabled child with a processing disorder has difficulty in the reception and interpretation of auditory information, in the absence of any concomitant loss of hearing acuity. If presentation rate and syntactic complexity of the teacher's instructions are not monitored and the signal-to-noise ratio is not considered when comprehension does not occur, then the student's inherent processing difficulties are exacerbated. "As the result of the processing difficulties these children experience, they are often labeled as slow, unmotivated, indifferent, anti-social, hearing impaired or misbehaved" (Clark, 1980, p. 208).

Differences in Cognitive Style. Cognitive style (or cognitive tempo) has been viewed in terms of active versus inactive style and reflective versus impulsive style. Investigation of cognitive style can be linked with work on information processing. Bransford (1979) noted that research on the active role of the information processor strongly suggests that failure to take on an active role in learning is a major source of performance problems in the learning disabled population.

Taking a look at reflective versus impulsive cognitive styles, Siegelman (1969) reported that reflective children make more comparisons between alternatives before making a decision. This difference in strategy is particularly important when faced with difficult or subtle recognition discriminations for general comprehension or decoding. Kagan (1965) has defined cognitive tempo as a decision-time variable that describes a child's consistent tendency to display slow or fast response times in problem situations with high response uncertainty. Kagan has gathered both reliability and validity data on this dimension. In separate studies, he has reported that reflective children score better on reading and serial learning tasks as well as on inductive reasoning tasks.

Consideration of cognitive style is important during the interpretation of diagnostic data as well as the observation of classroom performance. Haynes and McCallion (1981) note that cognitive tempo can have a significant impact on the quality of observable comprehension. They cite a study in which children who were rated as using a reflective cognitive style on one test instrument performed with greater facility when confronted with a comprehension task. "We believe that when we administer a formal comprehension test, we have evaluated comprehension. . . .We must be aware of what we are really testing and of the variables that affect test performance. Cognitive tempo may be such a variable" (Haynes and McCallion, 1981, p. 79). With language-learning disabled students, an evaluator will sometimes notice a delay in response as the student is thinking about what has been heard. Frequently, this type of response characteristic is not viewed favorably in a classroom. "The child is 'slow.' " It has always been my practice to share with teachers the observation that a student I have just seen for an evaluation appears to have a "slow response rate." This extra time gives the student time to deliberate on what has been heard. Teachers are encouraged to allow this student extra time to respond and discourage other students from interrupting this reflective process. It has been my experience that some learning disabled students get in a habit of impulsively providing *any* answer before they can be interrupted by peers or just as implusively say "I don't know." When we find a reflective style, we should encourage it. On informal auditory probes, such as listening to three clues and solving a riddle (I have two hands and a face. I have numbers. I measure time), when I see a student taking time to reflect upon and integrate the information heard, I will say, "Good for you! You thought about what you heard. You put all of the information together before you answered the riddle."

When we consider cognitive style as a variable in learning disability, we are entering the strategy versus deficit debate. "Most traditional views of learning disabilities have included the assumption of perceptual or neurological deficits. The alternative view of learning disabilities presented [by these researchers] considers that the problem may lie within the child's approach to problem solving. [Learning disabled children's] deficits may, in fact, have become excuses sometimes reinforced by diagnosticians or teachers for not pursuing tasks well within their capabilities" (Hagen et al., 1982, p. 23). While some children clearly have a diagnosed structural deficit, metacognitive approaches might be useful ways of viewing children with functional deficiencies.

"Metacognitive skills" refers to an individual's understanding of how the mind works, of what is easy to do and what is difficult, or how to go about solving particular problems and why some problem-solving attempts tend to be more promising than others (Ryan, Ledger, Short, and Weed, 1982). Wong (1982) describes metacognition as an individual's deliberate, conscious control of his or her cognitive actions in keeping with his or her goals. She says that both metacognitive and elaboration skills are critical in effective learning, a topic also addressed by Bauer (1982). To differentiate the metacognitive and elaboration skills, Wong (1982) says that metacognitive skills involve self-monitoring, predicting, reality testing, and control over deliberate attempts to engage in study, learning, or solving problems. Elaboration skills refer to clarifying and thinking about relationships and implications of acts in the "text," and it provides a richness or embellishment in an individual's encoding of input. This is, also, the way by which connections among sentences are integrated. These connections, in turn, enable the individual to draw inferences. An additional role played by elaboration is the individual's use of his or her own past experience to understand a current situation. A person's general knowledge can be expected to facilitate comprehension.

Wong (1982) says that research in metacognition and elaboration is particularly relevant in explaining some learning problems if the learning disabled student is viewed (and views his or her self) as "an inactive learner." It is suggested, then, that these students are not involved in their learning and are not aware of their cognitive processes or of the task demands. Hence, they fail to generate appropriate, successful strategies to aid their learning. Indications are that learning disabled students are not *lacking* these skills as much as they are not *aware* they have them. Although not all academic problems can be traced to the inhibition of metacognitive ability, inactive metacognitive ability can be viewed as a variable in educational labors. Torgesen (1982) reviewed a 1981 study by McKinney and Feagans that showed, apart from general average IQ and poor achievement, the only common characteristic in the sample of learning disabled children studied was their generally poor level of task-oriented behavior, which included poor attention, concentration, effort, and persistence.

Ryan and associates (1982) review some earlier research that describes metacognitive differences between good and poor readers. Poor readers are less able to judge task difficulty, identify possible strategies, and evaluate reading strategies. They are also less aware that the purpose of reading is to extract meaning and mentally integrate new information with knowledge already available. Cambourne and Rousch (1982) concluded that "groups classified as suffering from a condition known as reading disability and having a pseudomedically based condition, might instead have a very confused idea of how reading works" (p. 67). Wong (1982) additionally observes that "understanding instructions is a matter of comprehension, while knowing that one has or has not understood the instructions is a matter of metacomprehension. . . .With regard to reading, understanding the content of the text illustrates reading comprehension while understanding that one has understood the text illustrates metacomprehension" (p. 45). Related to this is research by Owings, Petersen, Bransford, Morris, and Stein (1980) on spontaneous monitoring and regulation of learning. Their results indicate that less successful students appear to lack metacomprehension (or the awareness that they have or have not understood what has been read) and were not spontaneously monitoring their state of reading comprehension. The less successful students did not realize that one of two stories they were asked to read did not make sense when detail" were added together until the examiner pointed out this possibility. They were asked to reread it and then found the absurdities.

During assessment, we should be alert to a student's cognitive style. We should notice whether or not, after a certain point in the testing, the student begins to get a rather blank stare and just starts guessing, or whether there is an adherence to the task demands. In addition, we need to observe whether or not a student makes use of his or her past experience to make inferences and "educated guesses." Let me cite an example. A student is given this instruction: "You will be hearing the names of three things that belong together. You tell me why they all belong together. For example, why do grape, strawberry, and orange belong together?" A subsequent task is to provide the classification label for franc, yen, and peso. This student lived in Mexico for the first six years of his life, and he visits relatives at least once a year in his Mexican village. If the student says, "I don't know," you might consider that he has forgotten the original directions or that he is not thinking of the directions relative to his experience. Since he has been answering the preceding questions, however, you can probably assume that he remembers the instructions about the nature of the task. What he is not doing is engaging in elaboration, or inferring from the one word that he undoubtedly knows (peso) that you are seeking the response "money." This inference can be made because he knows that all three stimuli have something in common; since he knows the nature of the one item, he could take an "educated guess" about what all three have in common.

This example is given to be juxtaposed to Wong's (1982) comment that a substantial percentage of research on information processing has shown that whether or not learners believe they can affect or control their own learning outcomes, environments, and future appears to be a good predictor of their academic performance. After observing the performance of a student such as the one described earlier, it is possible for an educator to begin teaching the student metacognitive and elaboration skills that permit him or her to gain more self-confidence in the student role.

"Dysteachia"

In an article title "Disabled—the Learner or the Curriculum?" Alterwerger and Bird (1982) base their discussion of this topic on five principles:

1. Reading and writing are whole-language communication processes.
2. Written communication is both meaningful and functional.
3. Children learn language by using language.

4. Language develops in a secure and supportive environment.

5. Written language is the medium through which one learns.

Examples are provided that demonstrate that the curriculum commonly adopted by public school violates these principles. In doing so, the stage is set for greater failure among students than would be otherwise occur. "Failures are usually the result of programs and instructions, not students" (Gruenewald and Pollak, 1973). These authors cite the following as examples: tasks may require functioning at a conceptual level while the child is still at a perceptual level; the child does not understand the basic concept being taught; competing stimuli (both auditory and visual) tax auditory discrimination and memory and serve as distractors; too many task components are presented at one time; and no one has taught the child his or her responsibilities as a listener. Suggestions for systematically observing a mismatch between the teacher and student or the curriculum and student are presented in Chapters 3 and 4.

Lasky and Chapandy (1976) and Nelson (1983) address the contribution of poor classroom directives and textbook instructions (which teachers are told should be read verbatim to students) to learning failures. As Nelson points out with the following example, owing to a lack of focus within a lesson, students are demanded to make rapid cognitive shifts back and forth from content to structural analysis and application:

"What kind of animal do you see at the very top? And where is the rabbit? He's sitting on a radio. Did you ever see a real rabbit sit on a radio? What does rabbit begin with? 'R', all right. And what about the thing he's sitting on? Say the word. Radio. Radio and rabbit both begin with the letter 'r'. OK, can you see how that letter is made? The capital 'R' is how many spaces? Two spaces tall. And the small 'r'? After your name is made at the space at the top, will you make a capital 'R' and a small 'r' on the lines that are shown right beside the rabbit?" (Nelson, 1983)

Lasky and Chapandy (1976), in analyzing directions in textbooks and teacher's manuals, have found equally appalling directions that "professional educators" and publishers have actually *planned* for teachers to say. For example, in a first grade mathematics textbook and manual they analyzed for syntactic and semantic complexity, one of the directions was, "We are going to pick a card from each set and write a number sentence to tell the number of circles on the cards we have chosen." Creaghead and Donnelly (1982) note, "Assuming that school-age children comprehend all types of linguistic forms, classroom teachers and writers of elementary school readers have not paid much attention to controlling linguistic complexity" (p. 177).

Brown and Payne (1979) criticize the strategies for learning used by some teachers. "Students who have not learned as much as other students are automatically labeled in some negative fashion. Many psychoeducational labels are used in schools; and unfortunately, most of the labels are applied to students. No one considers the possibility that some teachers have less success in teaching because they are using inferior instructional procedures" (Brown and Payne, 1979, pp. 11–13).

One instructional practice that is detrimental to many students is lack of direct teaching. Students are not told what is expected of them (Brown and Payne, 1979); they are expected to figure out the objectives of a lesson. This attitude, say Brown and Payne, produces " 'dysteachia' and other pedagological diseases." With regard to why some children do poorly on reading comprehension, Baker (1982) notes, "Children are much better at monitoring their comprehension when they are given very specific instructions as to the standards they should use to evaluate their understanding. That young children (ages 5–10) are clearly capable of monitoring their understanding, but do not spontaneously do so is a strong indication of the need for changes in instructional practice. Children typically are not taught the skills of evaluating their understanding and of taking appropriate measures to deal with failures to understand. Good readers eventually develop these skills on their own, whereas poor readers may not" (pp. 31–32). Durkin (1978–79) observed that very little time was spent in grades 1 through 6 on assisting children through probing questions to understand what was read; "comprehension development" did not seem to be part of the curriculum. Excessive time, on the other hand, was spent giving comprehension *assignments* and assessing comprehension of facts.

With many learning disabled children, we seem to be faced with an intelligent population that "learns the hard way." They do not have a tendency to learn adaptive strategies intuitively. Instead, they seem to be sensitive individuals who look around and see they are not doing things as well as others and infer (or are told) "There's something wrong with me." That these students are thought of as being "inactive" or "passive" learners could be a self-fulfilling prophecy. Van Etten (1978) and Weaver (1978) noted that even students who have been identified as learning disabled receive comprehension training that is inadequate in both quantity and quality. Augmenting this observation, Altwerger and Bird (1982) comment that frequently a prescribed hierarchy of skills and subskills is taught to the student who is not adapting to the mainstream educational program. What the system fails to convey to the student is a concept that is fundamental to successful written language development: reading and writing are communication processes. "The reason many learning disabled students never develop this concept can be found in phonics kits, contrived reading texts and meaningless drills that keep them at their seats. Education's preoccupation with tasks and exercises—sometimes only remotely related to the communication process—alienates the student who is unwilling or unable to cope with meaninglessness" (Altwerger and Bird, 1982, pp. 71–72).

Research is still being conducted on normal development of metacognitive skills, but data available indicate that while these are not used spontaneously, quite young children can develop an awareness of metacognitive skills through training and use these to their advantage (Baker, 1982). If continued research can document that ineffective cognitive monitoring is a cause of poor comprehension, then "perhaps the need for intervention could be eliminated if educators recognized cognitive monitoring as one component skill of comprehension—one that can most be developed through instruction and practice in parallel with other comprehension skills" (Baker, 1982, p. 34). Although knowledge of metacognition as an integral component of reading has been discussed since early in the twentieth century, this knowledge has had little impact on instructional practices (Durkin, 1981). The manner in which reading is currently approached in school may actually retard developmental metacognitive skills that could aid comprehension. In other words, students spend so much time in early reading instruction on decoding that comprehension is not stressed; perhaps the inferred definition of reading becomes "decoding" rather than "comprehension." It is difficult to infer that comprehension is the major goal of reading when material such as this is given to beginning readers:

A bug cannot run with a gun.
A bump on the pump made a lump.
A goat in a boat had a coat.
Eat a bun not a gun.
(Altwerger and Bird, 1982)

We cannot expect students to modify the definition of reading on their own to include "comprehension" when reading has been presented as "decoding" nonsense.

Lack of "automatization of skill" has been suggested as the underlying factor of continued learning problems (Sternberg and Wagner, 1982). "Processing resources that in others have been freed and used to master new tasks are in the disabled person devoted to tasks that others have already mastered. . . .Individuals with such disabilities seem to learn slowly and often incompletely tasks that others have mastered. The use of phonetic codes is a highly automatized skill for normal readers. . . .The reading disabled encounter the difficulties with their first language that many of us encounter learning a second language" as we concentrate on making phonetic sense out of a string of words at the expense of comprehension (Sternberg and Wagner, 1982). Some evidence suggests that incomplete semantic automatization (naming speed) in part underlies impaired effortful semantic processing (memory span and reading comprehension) (Ackerman and Dykman, 1982). These authors note, "It may well be that learning disabled children need to overlearn more than normal students to retain (and learn how to comprehend) information. However, they rarely get this extra practice or drill because they are behind in so many areas that teachers feel the need to push on at the first sign of mastery" (Ackerman and Dykman, 1982, p. 21).

Other researchers have also addressed the topic of how "the system" does not or cannot accommodate the needs of students who learn differently from most. For example, Wiig and Semel (1980) note several instructional characteristics that may tend to inadvertently exacerbate the problems of learning disabled students: long silent reading periods; verbal or written questions that emphasize recall of facts (which necessitates immediate and sequential auditory memory, internal rehearsal, input organization, word finding or retrieval skills); use of a formal language style; reliance on a lecture-type approach to teaching content (in which the lecture content may jump in space and time to make a related point and therefore demands cognitive reorganization of main from secondary ideas); need for note-taking (which requires a greater speed of processing and taxes memory for content and retrieval of graphemes in words to the point that the meaning of the content is lost); emphasis on volume of information transmitted; vocabulary and sentence length being uncontrolled for complexity. Snyder (1980) suggests that part of communication therapy for language-involved students should be aimed at getting them ready to meet school demands.

Blue (1981) suggests that classroom teachers working with language-impaired students should avoid certain types of utterances when communicating with these children. He mentions, in particular, sarcasm ("You're such a hard worker") idiomatic expressions ("Bear down and get it!"), ambiguous statements ("We don't put things in our mouths"), indirect requests ("Must you tap your pencil?"), and words with multiple meanings ("He's a cold person"). When a student is not comprehending message content, Blue suggests that the teacher analyze the content to determine the presence of these types of utterances that cause confusion for many language-learning disabled children. At the same time, such a reaction can be viewed as a diagnostic observation. The teacher or clinician needs to increase the student's awareness of these types of utterances and teach the student to become more comfortable processing them.

Sheridan (1983) takes some of the blame off instructional practices and their curriculum. She examined three non-Latin–based orthographies

(Chinese, Japanese, and Korean) to see how they facilitated or impeded learning to read relative to English orthography. The following findings were shared:

1. Remedial reading classes and dyslexia are virtually nonexistent in Japan.

2. Koreans report a high literacy rate and low incidence of reading disability (which is probably related to the easy 24 symbol, one sound relationship in their orthographic system).

3. Reports from China are not as easy to obtain, but one 1980 report stated that about 12% of the young people were considered illiterate.

In the English language for every rule or generalization in phonics, there are many exceptions, which often confuse or completely escape the learner.

A second factor that is sometimes beyond the teacher's control (such as in open classroom settings) is the level of ambient noise. Smyth (1979) examined the auditory efficiency of school children in the presence of classroom noise while they participated in a reading class. The subjects were between five and twelve years of age and were enrolled in grades 1 through 7. They were asked to identify one of six pictures by listening to its label when (1) the room was quiet, (2) there was classroom noise (as recorded during an open reading class). Of the total sample of 300 children, 45% made errors under noisy conditions when they did not make errors under quiet conditions. The percentage of children making errors when classroom noise was introduced decreased with age. "This study indicates that classroom noise competes for the child's attention and forces speech reception errors which otherwise would not occur" (Smyth, 1979, p. 229). Smyth defines optimal speech reception conditions as when the signal-to-noise ratio existing between the teacher's voice and the ambient classroom noise permits the teacher's voice to be heard without difficulty. Again, while control of the situation is not always possible, monitoring the degree of classroom noise when comprehension difficulties occur permits the educator to look at causal factors other than the child's "disability."

Brown and Payne (1979) offer the following guideline to teachers: "The behavioral viewpoint suggests that the use of [psychoeducational] labels can be avoided and instead, clear statements should be made about the specific behaviors observed. Using a label assumes that you know the behavior present is a result of something being wrong with the student" (pp. 12–13). These authors say that the behavioral approach to analyzing classroom difficulties avoids labeling and encourages the educator to look at the educational *situation;* that makes the child's ability only one variable in classroom success or failure.

SUMMARY

This chapter has considered the characteristics of the student who has difficulties in a school setting, has supplied instructional procedures that seem to help or hinder learning, and has suggested that observational analysis should be directed at the gestalt, not just dissecting the student's differences or deficits. In addition, an introduction to the chapters that follow has been provided through indicating how the contributing authors address the dynamic variables involved in the assessment of a student's communication skills and classroom success.

REFERENCES

Ackerman, P. T., and Dykman, R. A. (1982). Automatic and effortful information-processing deficits in children with learning and attention disorders. *Topics in Learning and Learning Disabilities, 2* (2), 12–22.

Altwerger, B., and Bird, L. (1982). Disabled: the learner or the curriculum? *Topics in Learning and Learning Disabilities, 1* (4), 69–78.

Ames, L. B. (1983). Learning disability: Truth or trap? *Journal of Learning Disabilities, 16* (1), 19–20.

Anastasiow, N. J., Hanes, M. L., and Hanes, M. L. (1982). *Language and reading strategies for poverty children.* Baltimore: University Park Press.

Anderson, L. E. (Ed.). (1970). *Helping the adolescent with the hidden handicap.* San Rafael, CA: Academic Therapy Publications.

Aram, D., and Nation, J. (1980). Preschool language disorders and subsequent language and academic difficulties. *Journal of Communication Disorders, 13,* 159–170.

Axelrod, L. (1982). Social perception in learning disabled adolescents. *Journal of Learning Disabilities, 15* (10), 610–613.

Baddeley, A. D. (1979). Working memory and reading, in P. Kolers, M. Wrolstad, and H. Bouma (Eds.), *Processing of visual language.* New York: Plenum Press.

Baker, L. (1982). An evaluation of the role of metacognitive deficits in learning disabilities. *Topics in Learning and Learning Disabilities, 2* (1), 27–35.

Bassett, R. E., Whittington, N., and Staton-Spicer, A. (1978). The basics in speaking and listening for high school graduates: What should be assessed? *Communication Education, 27,* 300–307.

Bauer, R. H. (1982). Information processing as a way of understanding and diagnosing learning disabilities. *Topics in Learning and Learning Disabilities, 2* (2), 46–53.

Bennett, C. W., and Runyan, C. M. (1982). Educators' perceptions of the effects of communication disorders upon educational performance. *Language, Speech and Hearing Services in Schools, 13* (4), 260–263.

Bereiter, B., and Engelmann, S. 1966. *Teaching disadvantaged children in the preschool.* Englewood Cliffs, NJ: Prentice-Hall.

Bernstein, B. (1964). Elaborated and restricted codes: Their social origins and some consequences. *American Anthropologist, 66,* 55–69.

Bernstein, B. (1970). A socio-linguistic approach to socialization: With some reference to educability, in J. P. de Cecco (Ed.), *The psychology of language, thought and instruction.* New York: Holt, Rinehart, and Winston.

Berry, M. D., and Erickson, R. L. (1973). Speaking rate: Effects on children's comprehension of normal speech. *Journal of Speech and Hearing Research, 16* (3), 367–374.

Berthoud-Papandroupoulou, I. (1978). An experimental study of children's ideas about language, in A. Sinclair, R. J. Jarvella, and W. J. M. Levelt (Eds.), *The child's conception of language.* Berlin: Springer-Verlag.

Blue, C. M. (1975). The marginal communicator. *Language, Speech and Hearing Services in Schools, 6* (1), 32–38.

Blue, C. M. (1981). Types of utterances to avoid when speaking to language-delayed children. *Language, Speech and Hearing Services in Schools, 12* (2), 120–124.

Bransford, J. A. (1979). *Human cognition: Learning, understanding and remembering.* Belmont, CA: Wadsworth Press.

Brown, W. E., and Payne, T. (1979). *Strategies for learning: Prevention and cure of "dysteachia" and other pedagological diseases.* Novato, CA: Academic Therapy Publications.

Bryan, T., and Pflaum, S. W. (1978). Social interactions of learning disabled children: A linguistic, social and cognitive analysis. *Learning Disabilities Quarterly, 1,* 70–79.

Bryen, D. N. (1981). Language and language problems, in A. Gerber and D. N. Bryen (Eds.), *Language and learning disabilites.* Baltimore: University Park Press.

Cambourne, B. L., and Rousch, P. D. (1982). How do learning disabled children read? *Topics in Learning and Learning Disabilities, 1* (4), 59–68.

Cantwell, D. P., and Baker, L. (1980). Academic failures in children with communication disorders. *Journal of the American Academy of Child Pyschiatry, 19,* 579–591.

Cantwell, D. P., and Carlson, G. A. (1983). *Affective disorders in childhood and adolescence.* New York: Spectrum Publications.

Carlson, J., Gruenewald, L. J.., and Nyberg, B. (1980). Everyday math in a story problem: The language of the curriculum. *Topics in Language Disorders, 1* (1), 59–70.

Cherry, R. S., and Kruger, B. (1983). Selective auditory attention abilities of learning disabled and normal achieving children. *Journal of Learning Disabilities, 16* (4), 202–205.

Clark, J. G. (1980). Central auditory dysfunction in school children: A compilation of management suggestions. *Language, Speech and Hearing Services in Schools, 10 (4),* 208–213.

Colbert, P., Newman, B., Ney, P., and Young. J. (1982). Learning disabilities as a symptom of depression in children. *Journal of Learning Disabilities, 15* (6), 321–384.

Compton, R. (1975). Diagnostic evaluation of committed delinquents, in H. Myklebust (Eds.), *Progress in learning disabilities (Vol. III).* New York: Grune and Stratton.

Creaghead, N. A., and Donnelly, K. G. (1982). Comprehension of superordinate and subordinate information by good and poor readers. *Language, Speech and Hearing Services in Schools, 13* (3), 177–186.

Cruickshank, W. M. (1977). *Learning disabilities in home, school and community.* Syracuse, NY: Syracuse University Press.

Curtis, M. E. (1980). Development of components of reading skill. *Journal of Educational Psychology, 72,* 656–699.

Daneman, M., and Carpenter, P. (1980). Individual differences in working memory and reading. *Journal of Verbal Learning and Verbal Behavior, 19,* 450–466.

Donahue, M., Pearl, R., and Bryan, T. (1982). Learning disabled children's syntactic proficiency on a communicative task. *Journal of Speech and Hearing Disorders, 47* (4), 397–403.

Dore, J. A. (1974). A pragmatic description of early language development, *Journal of Psycholinguistic Research, 4,* 343–350.

Dukes, P. J. (1981). Developing social prerequisites. *Topics in Learning and Learning Disabilities, 1* (2), 47–58.

Dunn, L. M., and Dunn, L. M. (1981). *Peabody Picture Vocabulary Test (M)*. Circle Pines, MN: American Guidance Service.

Durkin, D. (1978–79). What classroom observations reveal about reading comprehension instruction. *Reading Research Quarterly, 14,* 482–531.

Durkin, D. (1981). Reading comprehension instruction in five basal reader series. *Reading Research Quarterly, 16,* 515–544.

Dweck, C. S., and Goetz, T. E. (1978). Attributions and learned helplessness, in J. H. Harvey, W. Ickes, and R. F. Kidd (Eds.), *New directions in attribution research (Vol. 2).* Hillsdale, NJ: Erlbaum.

Dweck, C. S., and Licht, B. G. (1980). Learned helplessness and intellectual achievement, in J. Garber and M. E. P. Seligman (Eds), *Human helplessness: Theory and application.* New York: Academic Press.

Flood, J., and Salus, M. W. (1982). Metalinguistic awareness: Its role in language development and assessment. *Topics in Language Disorders, 2* (4), 56–64.

Freeman, G. G. (1970). An educational-diagnostic approach to language problems. *Language, Speech and Hearing Services in Schools, 4,* 23–30.

Gordon, H. W. (1983). The learning disabled are cognitively right. *Topics in Learning and Learning Disabilities, 3* (1), 29–39.

Grice, H. P. (1975). Logic and conversation, in P. Cole and H. L Morgan (Eds.), *Syntax and semantics (Vol. 3). Speech acts.* New York: Academic Press.

Grieve, R., Tunmer, W. E., and Pratt, C. (1980). An introduction to the study of language awareness in children, in D. P. Leinster-Mackay (Ed.), *Language awareness in children.* Perth, Australia: University of Western Australia Press.

Gruenewald, L. J., and Pollak, S. A. (1973). The speech clinician's role in auditory learning and reading readiness. *Language, Speech and Hearing Services in the Schools, 4* (3), 120–126.

Gruenewald, J. P., and Pollak, S. A. (1984). *Language interaction in teaching and learning.* Baltimore: University Park Press.

Guilford, J. P. (1967). *The nature of human intelligence.* New York: McGraw-Hill.

Hagen, J. W., Barclay, C. R., and Newman, R. S. (1982). Metacognition, self-knowledge and learning disabilities: Some thoughts on knowing and doing. *Topics in Learning and Learning Disabilities, 2* (1), 19–26.

Hagerman, R. J. (1984). Attention deficit disorder: Diagnosis and treatment. From *The learning disabled child: Medical, psychological, and educational perspectives.* Paper presented at a conference (Symposia Medicus), San Diego.

Hakes, D. T. (1980). *The development of metalinguistic abilities in children.* Berlin: Springer-Verlag.

Hallahan, D. P., and Kauffman, J. M (1976). *Introduction to learning disabilities: A psycho-behavioral approach.* Englewood Cliffs, NJ: Prentice-Hall.

Halliday, M. A. K. (1973). *Explorations in the functions of language.* London: Edward Arnold Press.

Halliday, M. A. K. (1978). *Language as social semiotic.* Baltimore: University Park Press.

Hannah, E. P. (1977). *Applied linguistic analysis (II).* Pacific Palisades, CA: SemCom Associates.

Hasenstab, M. S., and Laughton J. (1982). *Reading, writing and the exceptional child.* Rockville, MD: Aspen Systems.

Haynes, W. O., and McCallion, M. D. (1981). Language comprehension testing: The influence of three modes of test administration and cognitive tempo on the performance of preschool children. *Language, Speech and Hearing Services in Schools, 12* (2), 74–81.

Hess, T. M., and Radtke, R. C. (1981). Processing and memory factors in children's reading comprehension skill. *Child Development, 52,* 479–488.

Hiscock, M. (1983). Do learning disabled children lack functional hemispheric lateralization? *Topics in Learning and Learning Disabilities, 3* (1), 14–28.

Hollinger, P. C. (1979). Violent deaths among the young: Recent trends in suicide. *American Journal of Psychiatry, 136,* 1144–1147.

Hollon, T. H. (1970). Poor school performance as a symptom of masked depression in children and adolescents. *American Journal of Psychotherapy, 25,* 258–263.

Hook, P. E., and Johnson, D. J. (1978). Metalinguistic awareness and reading strategies. *Bulletin of the Orton Society, 28,* 62–78.

Hunter, M. (1976). Right-brained kids in left-brained schools. *Today's Education,* November-December, 45–49.

Kagan, J. (1965). Impulsive and reflective children: Significance of cognitive tempo, in J. D. Krumboltz (Ed.), *Learning and the educational process.* Chicago: Rand-McNally.

Kinsbourne, M. (1983). Models of learning disability. *Topics in Learning and Learning Disabilities, 3* (1), 1–13.

Kirk, S. A., and Kirk, W. D. (1983). On defining learning disabilities. *Journal of Learning Disabilities, 16* (1), 20–21.

Knepflar, K. J., and Laguaite, J. K. (1985). Relaxation and hypotherapy: Applications for improving classroom skills, in C. S. Simon (Ed.), *Communication Skills and Classroom Success: Therapy methodologies for language-learning disabled students.* San Diego, CA: College-Hill Press.

Knight, N. F. (1974). Structuring remediation in a self-contained classroom. *Language, Speech and Hearing Services in Schools, 5* (4), 198–203.

Kotsonis, M. E., and Patterson, C. J. (1980). Comprehension-monitoring skills in learning disabled children. *Developmental Psychology, 16,* 541–542.

Kratoville, B. L. (1974). *Youth in trouble.* San Rafael, CA: Academic Therapy Publications.

Kronick, D. (Ed.) (1975). *What about me? The learning disabled adolescent.* Novato, CA: Academic Therapy Publications.

Lasky, E. Z., and Chapandy, A. M. (1976). Factors affecting language comprehension. *Language, Speech and Hearing Services in Schools, 7* (3), 159–168.

Lee, L. L. (1974). *Developmental sentence analysis.* Evanston, IL: Northwestern University Press.

Levine, M., Busch, B., and Aufseer, C. (1982). The dimension of inattention among children with school problems. *Pediatrics, 70* (3), 387–395.

Loban, W. (1976). *Language development: Kindergarten-grade 12.* Urbana, IL: National Council of Teachers of English.

Locke, J. L. (1969). Short-term memory, oral perception and experimental sound learning. *Journal of Speech and Hearing Research, 12,* 179–184.

Lupert, N. (1981). Auditory perceptual impairments in children with specific language disorders: A review of the literature. *Journal of Speech and Hearing Disorders, 46* (1), 3–9.

Luria, A. R. (1976). *Cognitive development—its cultural and social foundations.* Cambridge: Harvard University Press.

Maisto, A. A., and Sipe, S. (1980). An examination of encoding and retrieval processes in reading disabled children. *Journal of Experimental Child Psychology, 30,* 223–230.

Martin, B. (1975). Parent-child relations, in F. D. Horowitz (Ed.), *Review of child development research (4th Ed.)* Chicago: University of Chicago Press, pp. 463–540.

McCarthy, B. (1980). *The 4-Mat System.* Arlington Heights, IL: Excel, Inc.

Monroe, M. (1965). Necessary preschool experiences for comprehending reading, in *Reading and inquiry. International Reading Association Conference Proceedings* (Vol. 10). Newark, DE: International Reading Association.

Moore, D. R. (1971). Language research and preschool language training, in C. S. Lavetelli (Ed.), *Language training in early childhood education*. Urbana, IL: University of Illinois Press.

Nelson, N. W. (1983). Beyond information processing: The language of teachers, in G. Wallach and K. C. Butler (Eds.), *Language-learning disorders in children*. Baltimore: Williams & Wilkins.

Nippold, M. A., and Fey, S. H. (1983). Metaphoric understanding in pre-adolescents having a history of language acquisition difficulties. *Language, Speech and Hearing Services in Schools, 14* (3), 171–180.

O'Brien, C. A. (1983). *The language different child*. Tucson, AZ: Communication Skill Builders, Inc.

Ogbu, J. V. (1974). *The next generation*. New York: Academic Press.

Owings, R., Petersen, G., Bransford, J. D., Morris, C. D., and Stein, B. C. (1980). Spontaneous monitoring and regulation of learning: A comparison of successful and less successful fifth graders. *Journal of Educational Psychology, 72,* 250–256.

Phillips, I. (1979). Childhood depression: Interpersonal interactions and depressed phenomena. *American Journal of Psychiatry, 136,* 511–515.

Potter, R. E. (1973). Perhaps we have been in this business of specific learning disabilities longer than we know. *Language, Speech and Hearing Services in Schools, 4* (2), 84–86.

Pozanski, E., and Zrull, J. P. (1970). Clinical characteristics of overtly depressed children. *Archives of General Psychiatry, 23,* 619–623.

Prinz, P. M., and Ferrier, L. J. (1983). Can you give me that one? The comprehension, production and judgment of directives in language impaired children, *Journal of Speech and Hearing Disorders, 48,* 44–54.

Prutting, C. A. (1982). Pragmatics as social competence. *Journal of Speech and Hearing Disorders, 47,* 123–133.

Pullis, M., and Smith, C. D. (1981). Social-cognitive development of learning disabled children. *Topics in Learning and Learning Disabilities, 1,* 43–55.

Ramos, N. P. (1978). *Delinquent youth and learning disabilities*. San Rafael, CA: Academic Therapy Publications.

Rhodes, L. K., and Shannon, J. L. (1982). Psycholinguistic principles in operation in a primary learning disabilites classroom. *Topics in Learning and Learning Disabilities, 1* (4), 1–10.

Rosenthal, J. H. (1973). *Hazy? crazy? and/or lazy? the maligning of children with learning disabilities*. Novato, CA: Academic Therapy Publications.

Rosenthal, J. H. (1984). The natural history of learning disabilities. From *The learning disabled child: Medical psychological, and educational perspectives*. Paper presented at a conference (Symposia Medicus), San Diego.

Ryan, E. B., Ledger, G. W., Short, E. J., and Weed, K. A. (1982). Promoting the use of active comprehension strategies by poor readers. *Topics in Learning and Learning Disabilities, 2* (1), 53–60.

Sawyer, D. J. (1981). The relationship between selected auditory abilities and beginning reading achievement. *Language, Speech and Hearing Services in Schools, 12* (2), 95–99.

Sheridan, E. M. (1983). Reading disabilities: Can we blame the written language? *Journal of Learning Disabilities, 16* (2), 81–86.

Shulman, M. D., and Liles, B. Z. (1979). A sense of grammaticality: An ingredient of language remediation. *Language, Speech and Hearing Services in Schools, 10,* 59–63.

Siegelman, E. (1969). Reflective and impulsive observing behaviors. *Child Development, 40,* 1212–1222.

Simon, C. S. (1979). *Communicative competence: A functional-pragmatic approach to language therapy.* Tucson, AZ: Communication Skill Builders, Inc.

Simon, C. S. (1984a). Functional-pragmatic evaluation of communication skills in school-aged children. *Language, Speech and Hearing Services in Schools, 15* (2), 83–97.

Simon, C. S. (1984b). *Evaluating communicative competence: A functional-pragmatic procedure.* Tucson, AZ: Communication Skill Builders, Inc.

Slobin, D. I. (1978). A case study of early language awareness, in A. Sinclair, R. J. Jarvella, and W. J. M. Levett (Eds.), *The child's conception of language.* Berlin: Springer-Verlag.

Smyth, V. (1979). Speech reception in the presence of classroom noise. *Language, Speech and Hearing Services in Schools, 10* (4), 221–230.

Snyder, L. S. (1980). Have we prepared the language disordered child for school? *Topics in Language Disorders, 1* (1), 29–46.

Soenksen, P. A., Flagg, C. L., and Schmits, D. W. (1981). Social communication in learning disabled students: A pragmatic analysis. *Journal of Learning Disabilities, 14* (5), 283–286.

Sternberg, R. J., and Wagner, R. K. (1982). Automatization failure in learning disabilities. *Topics in Learning and Learning Disabilities, 2* (2), 1–11.

Swanson, H. L. (1982). In the beginning was it a strategy—or was it a constraint? *Topics in Learning and Learning Disabilities, 2* (2), x–xiv.

Tallal, P. (1983). *Central auditory dysfunction in language-impaired children* (short course). San Diego, CA: California Speech-Language-Hearing Association.

Torgesen, J. K. (1978). Performance of reading disabled children in serial memory tasks: A review. *Reading Research Quarterly, 19,* 57–87.

Torgesen, J. K. (1982). The learning disabled child as an inactive learner: Educational implications. *Topics in Learning and Learning Disabilities, 2* (1), 45–52.

Torgesen, J. K., and Greenstein, J. J. (1982). Why do some learning disabled children have problems remembering? Does it make a difference? *Topics in Learning and Learning Disabilities, 2* (2), 54–61.

Tough, J. (1977). *The development of meaning.* New York: John Wiley and Sons.

Tyack, D., and R. Gottsleben. (1974). *Language sampling, analysis and training.* Palo Alto, CA: Consulting Psychologists Press.

Van Etten, G. (1978). A look at reading comprehension. *Journal of Learning Disabilities, 11,* 42–51.

Vellutino, F. R. (1977). Alternative conceptualizations. *Harvard Educational Review, 47,* 334–354.

Vellutino, F. R. (1979). *Dyslexia: Theory and research.* Cambridge, MA: MIT Press.

Vetter, D. K. (1982). Language disorders and schooling. *Topics in Language Disorders, 2* (4), 13–19.

Vygotsky, L. S. (1978). *Mind in society: The development of higher psychological processes.* Cambridge, MA: Harvard University Press.

Weaver, P. A. (1978). Comprehension, recall and dyslexia: A proposal for the application of schema theory. *Bulletin of the Orton Society, 11,* 42–51.

Wells, G. (1973). *Coding manual for the description of child speech.* Bristol, England: University of Bristol School of Education.

Wertz, F. J. (1963). Adolescent underachievers: Evaluating psychodynamic and environmental stress. *New York State Medical Journal, 63,* 352–354.

Wiig, E. H., and Semel, E. M. (1976). *Language disabilities in children and adolescents.* Columbus, OH: Charles E. Merrill.

40   Simon

Wiig, E. H., and Semel, E. M. (1980). *Language assessment and intervention for the learning disabled*. Columbus, OH: Charles E. Merrill.

Wilgosh, L., and Paitich, D. (1982). Delinquency and learning disabilities: More evidence. *Journal of Learning Disabilities, 15* (5), 278–279.

Wong, B. Y. L. (1982). Understanding learning disabled students' reading problems: Contributions from cognitive psychology. *Topics in Learning and Learning Disabilities, 1* (4), 43–50.

Zinkins, P. W., and Gottlieb, M. I. (1983). Patterns of auditory processing and articulation deficits in academically deficient juvenile delinquents. *Journal of Speech and Hearing Disorders, 48,* 36–40.

TRANSITIONAL NOTE

Between each of the chapters in this volume, the editor will provide a "transitional bridge" by reviewing major points from the earlier chapter(s) and relating these to the content of the following chapter, as well as sometimes adding additional research findings. The purpose of these transitional sections is to provide cohesion within an edited volume. The various contributors have been chosen with purpose, and it is hoped that the transitional sections will demonstrate underlying compatible philosophies as well as fresh perspectives.

The first chapter in this book provides a description of the population about whom these two volumes have been written: the language-learning disabled student. In addition to this population description, a major philosophical tenet was stressed: Assessment of a student's classroom performance must include observations of all factors that affect performance. In the past, the emphasis has been on looking at what is wrong with student to the exclusion of analyzing how interacting variables, such as the content of the curriculum, instructional language and methodologies used by the teacher, and general classroom ambience have contributed to the student's learning difficulties.

In Chapter 2, Cantwell and Baker address the relationships among psychodynamic, educational, and communication variables in students who are referred for psychiatric or educational assessment. Their research, and that of others, suggests that a significant role is played by communication skill deficits in children who are referred for evaluation. Several of the following chapters provide specific communication evaluation suggestions.

CHAPTER 2

Interrelationship of Communication, Learning, and Psychiatric Disorders in Children

Dennis P. Cantwell
and
Lorian Baker

The content in this chapter was originally presented by Dr. Cantwell as two lectures that were part of a symposium, *The Learning Disabled Child: Medical, Psychological and Educational Perspectives,* San Diego, California (1984). The material has been transcribed by Charlann S. Simon and edited by Dr. Cantwell.

This chapter will address the following questions:

1. Are children with learning disorders "at risk" for psychiatric disorders? (Definitions of learning disorders and psychiatric disorders will be discussed and evidence will be presented from epidemiological studies that they are related).

2. What are the mechanisms of the association between learning and psychiatric disorders?

3. What is the interrelationship of communication, learning, and psychiatric disorders in children?

DEFINITIONS OF DISORDERS

Very often, whether or not a child is considered to have a learning disorder depends on how this term is defined. The definition of learning disorder I use is as follows: A child who has a significant deficit in performance in one or more of the academic subjects which is below the level that would be predicted on the basis of the child's age and IQ. (This differs from the PL 94-142 definition, which emphasizes the underlying processes.) In my conceptualization, there is a difference between learning disability and learning disorder. Disabilities are things that generally we do not see; we infer them from problems with performance. Problems in performance are defined as severe discrepancies between what could be expected for a child of a particular age and intelligence level and what he or she actually does.

There is little disagreement, regardless of the label used, that we are talking about a very heterogeneous group of children. There are likewise many reasons why they have problems in performance.

My definition of a psychiatrically disordered child is as follows: A child who shows a disorder of overt behavior, disorder of emotional state, disorder of social relationships, or disorder of cognitive functioning that is sufficiently severe and of sufficient duration to cause some distress or disability in adaptive functioning. A more specific description of the nature of each type of psychiatric disorder would be as follows:

1. Overt behaviors would include hyperactivity, aggressive behavior, truancy, and delinquency. Overt symptoms I refer to as "garlic symptoms," because they disturb the environment and people nearby.

2. Emotional symptoms would include anxiety or depressed mood. I call these "onion symptoms," because they make the child cry inside. Parents and teachers are much quicker to be upset by garlic symptoms than they are by onion symptoms. Very often they are not aware of the onion symptoms because the overt behavioral problems stand out so vividly.

3. Disorders of social relationships would include autism or related pervasive developmental disorders.

4. Disorders of cognitive functioning would include mental retardation.

If one or more of these disorders is present and is both severe enough and of sufficiently significant duration that it causes some degree of disability in adaptive functioning, it would be concluded that the child has a psychiatric disorder.

The five areas of adaptive functioning are (1) academic performance at school, (2) behavior at school, (3) peer relationships, (4) interpersonal relationships in the home, and (5) use of leisure time. Generally when I evaluate a child, I focus on how much impairment in these five areas of adaptive functioning the child is having as a result of whatever psychiatric disorder the child has. Psychiatric disorder in childhood, then, is defined relative to problems in adaptive functioning.

ARE LEARNING DISORDERED CHILDREN AT RISK FOR THE DEVELOPMENT OF PSYCHIATRIC DISORDERS?

This question cannot be answered from clinical samples. Observing that 75% of the children who present to the Neuro-Psychiatric Institute (at the University of California at Los Angeles) for psychiatric disorders also have learning disorders, that is not the same thing as estimating prevalence from the other way around. To come to any conclusions, children from nonreferred samples must be studied in order to evaluate what the interrelationship is between psychiatric problems in childhood and learning disorders in childhood. There are two epidemiological studies that demonstrate this type of research.

The classic report is the Isle of Wight study. Rutter and his colleagues went to the Isle of Wight, just off the south coast of England, and studied every child on the island in a certain age range (Rutter, Tizard, and Whitmore, 1970). They selected the Isle of Wight because the social class distribution is similar to England's as a whole and the population tends to be permanent. The population is, therefore, representative and stable. They studied the children in this location concurrently for mental (psychiatric) disorder (using the definition cited earlier), learning disorders (including intellectual performance), and physical or neurological disorders. They were able to look at the intercorrelations among these disorders. Their findings included the following:

1. Children who had overt behavior disorders (such as attention deficit disorder [ADD], hyperactivity, or oppositional disorders) had very high rates of learning problems, especially reading disorders.

2. Of the children who had reading disorders, 25% also had one of the overt psychiatric behavioral disorders.

3. About 5% of the children in general had overt psychiatric disorders, whereas 25% of those who had a significant reading disorder had overt behavior disorder; there was, then, a five times greater incidence than was found in the general population.

4. There was a *tendency* to have an increased rate of emotional disorders, such as generalized anxiety disorders, separation anxiety disorders, phobic disorders, or depressive disorders in children who had specific reading disorders, but it was not nearly as high as with the overt behavior disorders.

Findings from other epidemiological studies are essentially the same: they show very strong correlation between reading disorders and overt behavior disorders. Studies of juvenile delinquents show the opposite type of correlation: There are very high rates of reading disorders in children who become juvenile delinquents.

The second study, the Douglas National Child Development Study (Douglas, Ross, and Simpson, 1968), is a unique longitudinal study. Douglas identified all children born in one particular time frame in Great Britain and followed them through their entire lives. He has longitudinal data, therefore, in a number of developmental areas, one of which is in learning. Douglas found that the *average* academic attainment was low in all subjects who had overt behavior disorders. In other words, average academic achievement was low for *all* academic subjects (reading, spelling, and mathematics) in those children with overt behavior problems. Children who had emotional problems in this study did have low academic attainment, but they also tended to have lower IQ. It was, therefore, not necessarily as strong a correlation with *specific* learning disorders as it was with "learning backwardness," which they defined as behavior that was behind grade level but appropriate for IQ level.

WHAT ARE THE MECHANISMS AND WHAT IS THE ASSOCIATION BETWEEN LEARNING AND PSYCHIATRIC DISORDER?

Children who have learning disorders do have high rates of psychiatric disorder. That brings up the question of the mechanisms underlying that correlation. Three broad possibilities are suggested: (1) psychiatric disorder causes the learning disorder; (2) learning disorder directly or indirectly leads to psychiatric disorder; (3) both learning disorder and psychiatric disorder are related to each other because they are both related to some X factor that independently leads to both of them.

There is some evidence that all three of these possibilities may be valid, depending on the type of psychiatric disorder and whether or not the association with psychiatric disorder occurs in children who *fail to develop learning* or in those children who, after beginning to learn normally, have a drop in achievement.

Rutter has suggested seven possible mechanisms underlying the relationships between psychiatric and learning disorders. These are essentially breakdowns of the three broad possibilities listed previously:

1. Temperamental characteristics of the child.
2. The effect of anxiety on learning.
3. Psychosocial stresses of various types that occur at some critical period in the development of learning.

4. Lack of motivation to learn.

5. Avoidance of learning.

6. Impaired cognitive function that is secondary, resulting from various types of psychopathology.

7. Subtle underlying factors (genetic, familial, environment, communication disorder) that lead to both learning and psychiatric disorders.

Temperamental Characteristics

The New York Longitudinal Study (Thomas and Chess, 1977) provides some data on temperamental traits. This is a landmark study in child psychiatry in terms of the way it was done which resulted in a fresh view of child development. A pediatrician and a psychiatrist worked together in studying a group of infants whom they have continued to study; the study group is presently in its mid-thirties. What these researchers hypothesized and indeed demonstrated is that there are temperamental characteristics of children that are identifiable by the age of three months. It is not *content* but *process* that is involved. The important focus should be on *how* children do things rather than on *what* they do. There are some temperamental characteristics that are associated with learning problems and the development of psychiatric disorder in later life. These would include fidgety behavior, restless behavior, inability to stay with a task, and impulsivity. These temperamental characteristics may also be associated with later psychiatric disorder in some children. The association of psychiatric and learning disorders occurs because they are both related to the same temperamental characteristics.

The Effect of Anxiety on Learning

We have already seen that there is a tendency, in populations studied, for learning disordered children to have slightly elevated rates of emotional disorders, in which anxiety plays a characteristic role. It is thought that high anxiety inhibits performance of difficult, complex cognitive tasks, but it may be beneficial for simple tasks. Although there may be some common sense in this thinking, there is very little in the way of systematic research to support it. A lot seems to depend upon the child's attitude to the task, the setting in which the learning takes place, and the responses the child has previously encountered after success or failure. Thus, the relationship of various types of anxiety (phobic, generalized, separation) to learning disorders in childhood is unclear.

Stress at a Critical Period in the Development of Learning

We do know, from behaviors other than learning, that if a child experiences significant psychosocial stress during a critical developmental stage, effects of that stress are observable. For example, if a child experiences admission into a hospital during the time that bladder control is being developed, high rates of enuretic behavior are observed. This is particularly evident in boys. It is as if the learning of bladder control was inhibited by this significant psychosocial stress. For a child in the period when primary attachment formation is developing, a significant degree of psychosocial stress can interfere with the ability of the infant—up to about the age of two years—to develop a primary attachment. There may be some lasting impairment in the ability to form attachments and make enduring social relationships.

It is apparent, then, that in areas other than academic learning, some evidence exists that there are critical periods in which psychosocial stress can play a role. There does not, however, seem to be good evidence for only one critical period for the development of certain kinds of learning skills. I do not think there is good evidence that certain kinds of psychosocial stresses occurring at times when learning skills are being developed lead to permanent impairment. This, of couse, is based on the premise that there is an adequate substitution at a later period so that the development of learning skills will take place.

Lack of Motivation to Learn

Lack of motivation can develop *secondarily* in children who are learning disordered. They begin to feel that they are not making it and they say "The heck with it. I'll do something else." However, lack of motivation can be a *primary* factor leading to academic underachievement. Thus, anything interfering with motivation (depression, parental attitudes and expectations, poor relationships with teachers, obsessional and intrusive thoughts, and so forth) may have a negative impact on learning.

Learning Avoidance

There may be a subgroup of children and adolescents whose academic work falls off as a part of a rebellion against adult values or because learning in general comes to be associated in the child's mind with unpleasant feelings. Parents who spend an inordinate amount of time with their child's homework, giving a lot of negative feedback, can create a situation in which learning in general becomes a painful process and can lead to a learning avoidance phenomenon. Peer pressure can have a similar effect.

Impairment of Cognitive Function

There is good evidence, in the limited amount of work that has been done, that impairment of cognitive function due to psychiatric disorder (such as depression, attentional disorders, or schizophrenia) can negatively affect learning.

Individuals with such disorders often begin to learn normally and do not have a developmental learning disorder. They show regression in learning as the result of significant major depressive disorder or the serious thinking disorder of schizophrenia. These are two conditions in which a decrease in academic performance is often one of the first symptoms to develop.

Certain psychiatric disorders, by nature and definition, have behaviors that interfere with learning as their core set of symptoms; an example is attention deficit disorder (ADD). Children who have clear-cut ADD have a major problem in sustaining attention. They have somewhat less of a problem in selective attention. Sustained attention, however, is necessary for success in learning. In addition, ADD children also have impulsivity as one of their core systems. This is not only a behavioral impulsivity but also a *cognitive* impulsivity. They are nonreflective in their cognitive style. They tend to make decisions too fast and they make them on the basis of relatively inadequate logical processes. This is not a "thought disorder"; the children are just too impulsive.

All three of these examples of psychiatric disorder—depression, schizophrenia, and attention deficit disorder—are psychiatric disorders that by definition can be expected to interfere with the learning process.

Common Underlying Factors

The mechanisms involved in children who have developmental learning disorders and fail to learn properly are probably different from the mechanisms involved for the child who begins to learn normally and then begins to withdraw at some point. That is a very sensitive indicator of psychiatric disturbance. A case example is an eight year old boy whose grades suddenly went down. The mother also noted that he was crying every night and was socially withdrawn. He had recently asked her, "Mommy, what happens if we commit suicide? Do we go to heaven or do we go to hell?" It became quite clear that this boy had profound depression and suicidal ideas and needed to be hospitalized. The thing that the parents noticed first, however, was a dramatic drop-off in academic performance in a child who had had no signs of developmental learning disorder in the past.

One of the underlying disabilities common to both learning and psychiatric disorders is speech and language disorder. These disorders usually improve with time or with speech and language therapy but may lead independently to both learning disorder and psychiatric disorder. The nature of this relationship will be discussed in more detail in a later section of this chapter.

Implications for treatment depend upon the mechanisms involved. If there is an underlying disability, such as a speech and language disability, that leads independently to learning disorder and psychiatric disorder, the next questions to be asked are, "Is there a preventive aspect here? If the speech and language disorder is treated early and the child is functioning as well as possible in the speech and language area prior to school entry, do you avert the later secondary consequence of learning disorder? If a child has already developed some degree of learning or psychiatric disorder and also has an underlying speech and language disorder, if you treat the underlying problem and nothing else, will the other problems just disappear?"

When looking to the literature on psychiatric and learning problems, it is necessary to draw upon primarily one type of learning problem— reading disorder. For example, there is little information in other isolated academic areas, such as spelling or mathematics or learning inhibitions, which involve a failure to make further school progress. Most of the literature with regard to psychiatric disorder in children who show academic problems is related directly to those children who have reading disorder.

There is strong evidence against the view that specific reading disorder is due to some underlying neurotic problem. For example, studies of the general population indicate that the association is not, in general, with emotional-type disorders and learning disorders but rather with the overt behavior problems, which are not neurosis-based. Second, the sex ratio and prognosis for reading disorder are quite different from those for emotional disorders in children. Third, there is good evidence that reading disorder is probably multifactorial in origin.

There is psychoanalytic literature that has historical value but is of no pragmatic value. This literature suggests that reading disorder develops as the result of some neurotic conflict or some underlying neurotic conflict or underlying neurotic emotional disturbance. This view was based on clinic studies of children who came in with anxiety disorders and also had learning disorders. As stated previously, you cannot make comments on these associations when you have already started out with a population of children who were referred with one or more types of psychiatric disorder.

The available evidence, in my view, suggests that the emotional disorders are not the cause of significant reading disorder or, for that matter, any other kind of learning disorder. I do think that there is not only a possibility but a likelihood that some *secondary* emotional symptoms develop as a result of a learning handicap. Children who are not making it in school are not making it in their everyday work; school is the work of childhood. If a child goes six hours of the day to school and is told by teachers and by parents—either directly or indirectly—that he or she is not making it, then school becomes a negative experience that is strongly associated with failure and with the adverse responses to this failure.

What about the association between overt behavior problems and specific reading disorder? The best way to investigate this is to study three groups of children, such as was done in the Isle of Wight study (Rutter, et al., 1970).

1. A group with pure overt behavior disorders with no learning disorder.
2. A group with learning disorder with no overt behavior disorder.
3. A group with both disorders.

When you look at common background factors, you find that those who have overt behavior problems plus reading disorder are more like those with pure reading disorders than they are like those with pure behavior disorder. This suggests that there may be some indirect way that the reading disorder leads to the overt behavior disorders. Indeed, what seems to be the case is that those children who have both overt behavior disorders and reading disorders *and* those who have pure reading disorder are characterized by a set of symptoms, such as the following: short attention span, fidgety and restless behavior, and impulsivity—the cardinal characteristics of attention deficit disorder syndrome.

INTERRELATIONSHIPS AMONG COMMUNICATION, LEARNING DISORDERS, AND PSYCHIATRIC DISORDERS

Children who present with developmental speech and language disorders represent a fairly sizable proportion of the general population. In this chapter, the term "speech" refers to the production of speech sounds (and would be represented by behaviors such as articulation, voice, stuttering, and rate). The term "language" refers to the symbolic code, manifested in grammar, syntax, and processing of the symbolic code. At our clinic we use a relatively simple classification system with regard to the communication impaired population: (1) they have only speech problems, (2) they have only language problems, or (3) they have both speech and language problems.

About 6% of school children have delayed language acquisition, and about 1% have a very serious and very specific delay in language acquisition. Children with language acquisition problems are sometimes referred to as "aphasic," but this is not a good term because they do not lose their language; "dysphasic" is probably a better term because they are developmentally abnormal. Speech problems affect 16% of school-age children. About 5% of these children have speech deficits that are serious enough to be evident to even the casual observer. Approximately 5% of five year old children enter school with a degree of speech problem that makes them unintelligible to their teachers and peers. If this group *is* at risk for learning disorders or psychiatric disorders, we are talking about a relatively sizable group.

We do know that this is indeed a high-risk group. Early identification of communication impaired children and early referral are essential. Telling parents that "They'll outgrow it" is very poor advice. While children *can* recover without speech therapy, it is a relatively slow process, and normal language acquisition is a relatively rapid process. The language delayed child, although making some spontaneous progress, gets left farther and farther behind his or her peers. Correction of underlying difficulties (such as hearing loss or dental abnormalities) is insufficient. An inadequate foundation in early language development often makes it difficult for the child to develop language in normal patterns. During the untreated phase, secondary problems arise, which may make later management of the speech and language problem more difficult. It is these secondary problems (psychiatric disorders and learning disorders) on which I will concentrate.

Hearing loss is the most common cause of speech and language problems. The hearing loss is often difficult to determine and is variable over time. Although only high-frequency sounds are affected in some cases, recurrent bouts of otitis media can cause a general suppression of hearing level, which impairs access to language learning; the child is unable to profit from language modeling in his or her environment. With a high-frequency loss, the child hears sounds, but the sounds are distorted.

There is a wide range of normality in language acquistion. For example, the Newcastle (Fundudis, Kolvin, and Garside, 1979) study showed a vocabulary range for two year olds from 8 to 2000 words. As with all developmental aspects, boys are slower than girls and twins and later borns are slower than first borns.

Language disorders can range from blatant to subtle. Even for more severe cases, it may be difficult for a physician in an office setting to discern these problems because of a child's shyness or fear of doctors. Other children, who converse easily, are sometimes referred in school for "not listening," and subsequent assessment indicates subtle comprehension difficulties. Some children appear normal in structured speech and language testing, but in an unstructured setting, disorders of thought, language, and communication become evident. (A list of "high-risk" communication behaviors appears in Chapter 11 of this book.)

Some segments of the population have disproportionately high prevalence rates for language handicaps, such as those with mental retardation or hearing loss. Six of these high-risk groups are as follows:

Otitis media. Early history of recurrent otitis media seems to be associated with later language and learning problems.

Psychosocial deprivation. Severe psychosocial deprivation or understimulation in the home primarily affects vocabulary development; however, children from substandard dialectal backgrounds can sound very disordered, when in fact they are only mimicking what they hear at home.

Family history of communication problems. Children may have family histories of language and learning problems, particularly those that involve reading or spelling.

Speech mechanism abnormalities. Abnormalties of the speech mechanism (such as cleft palate and dysarthria) account for only 8% of speech problems, and the prognosis for completely normal speech is poor.

Neurological involvement. Neurological problems, which would include cerebral palsy, apraxia, and attention deficit disorder, produce conditions that range from quite obvious to quite subtle.

Learning disorders. These children evidence learning problems that are associated with auditory perceptual difficulties, speech sound discrimination, auditory memory, and dyslexia.

Children who belong to these categories are at high risk and should be carefully monitored by physicians and parents.

Why even hypothesize that a child with communication problems would be at high risk for psychiatric problems? First, we know that children with all types of handicaps are at risk for psychiatric disorders. Secondly, communication is what makes us human. Finally, language is intimately involved in many areas of child development: cognition, intelligence, play, and peer relationships.

Cantwell-Baker Study

Current observations on the relationships between communication problems and psychiatric disorders evolved from a study of children who presented at the Community Speech Clinic in Encino, California, located in the San Fernando Valley just outside Los Angeles. In a community of 1.1 million people, this is the only community speech and hearing clinic in the valley. We set up offices within the clinic for a three year period and saw every child who came in for a speech and language evaluation. This service was offered as a free, extra psychiatric evaluation, and the refusal rate was essentially zero. We did a detailed evaluation (psychological, speech-language and academic functioning) on each child, all components of which were done blind to one another. Details on this study methodology are presented by Cantwell, Baker, and Mattison (1979). Our findings were as follows:

1. Of the 600 children we saw, two thirds were male and 60% were less than six years old. About 30% were between ages six and 6.11, and in addition there was a small percentage of children over age 12 years who were appearing in a speech and language clinic for the first time. The study group, then, consisted primarily of a preschool population and secondarily of elementary school children. The mean age was 5.5 years.

2. About 50.3% of the 600 children had a diagnosable psychiatric disorder at the time they presented for evaluation. Of this population, 26% had an overt behavior disorder (ADD, oppositional disorder, or conduct disorder) and 20% had emotional disorders (anxiety, affective and adjustment disorders, and a few with elective mutism). The greatest number, then, had overt behavior disorders, with the anxiety behaviors being second. A very small percentage of children had severe psychiatric disorders, such as the 1% who were autistic. About 7% had unspecified problems or other illnesses.

As the data show, more than half of the children who presented at the speech and language clinic for communication problems were found to have psychiatric disorders at the time they presented for the communication problem. The 50.3% incidence among this communication impaired population needs to be compared with the incidence for the same age range in the general population in terms of psychiatric prevalence, which is about 10%. Psychiatric disorder, then, was five times more common in this communication impaired population. Second, the psychiatric problems seen in this population were also the most common seen in children who do not have speech and language problems (e.g., behavioral and emotional disorders).

When you compare those children who *did* have a psychiatric disorder with those who did *not* have a psychiatric disorder on a variety of variables,

**Table 2-1. Comparison of Learning Disabled Versus
Non-Learning Disabled Children—Developmental Variables**

	LD Group	Non-LD Group
Performance IQ (Mean)	108.1	104.9
Verbal IQ (Mean)	95.0	95.8
Developmental milestones (mean age in months)		
Crawling	7.8	8.2
Standing	11.4	11.7
Sitting	7.0	7.0
Walking alone	15.3	14.6
First word	19.5	18.0
First sentence	32.3	28.6

All results are nonsignificant.

the factors that most distinguish those who have psychiatric disorders are the speech and language factors: the presence of a *language* (as contrasted to a speech) disorder, the *severity* of the language or speech disorder, and the presence of auditory processing disorders.

Because of the age of the population, learning disorder was difficult to study. In fact, it was possible with about 200 of the 600 children in the study. Of these 200 children, when learning disorder was diagnosed—especially in reading—it was also observed that between 50% and 72% of the children had a history of developmental language disorder. Data indicate that at the time these 200 children presented for speech and language evaluation, about 21% had a history of learning problems.

Follow-up studies on children with speech and language disorders indicate that they are indeed at risk for learning disorders. A complete review of the literature is found in the report by Baker and Cantwell (1984), which discusses the educational outcome of children with speech and language disorders.

Are these two conditions (learning and psychiatric disorder) related to each other in this group of children with communication disorder? The findings from our study can be seen in Tables 2-1 to 2-6.

We paired children who had a definable learning disorder by age and performance IQ with a group of children with communication disorders, but who did not have a significant learning disorder. "Significant learning disorder" was defined by two criteria: (1) McLeod's formula (McLeod, 1978), and (2) the children had been rated by their teachers as failing at least one academic subject. What is evident in Table 2-1 with regard to

**Table 2-2. Matched Groups: Learning Disabled Versus
Non-Learning Disabled—Speech and Language Diagnoses**

	LD Group (Per Cent)	Matched Group (Per Cent)
Linguistic Group:		
Pure speech disorder	14	61*
Speech and language disorder	68	29
Pure language disorder	18	10
Expressive Language Disorder	71	39†
Receptive Language Disorder	46	25†
Auditory Processing Disorder	71	20*

*P = less than 0.001 (Fisher's exact test).
†P = less than 0.01.

**Table 2-3. Comparison of Learning Disabled Versus
Non-Learning Disabled Children—Factor Scores from Parent
Questionnaires**

Mean Total Factor Scores	LD Group	Non-LD Group
Conners Parent Questionnaire:		
Antisocial	0.1	0.1 factor
Anxiety factor	2.9	2.0*
Conduct factor	2.5	1.6
Hyperactivity factor	6.1	3.9†
Learning factor	3.0	0.8†
Perfectionism factor	1.0	0.9
Psychosomatic factor	1.5	1.6
Tension factor	1.3	0.7
Rutter Parent Questionnaire:		
Total factor score	17.9	14.3*
Antisocial factor score	2.5	2.0
Neurotic factor score	2.9	2.1

*P = less than 0.03.
†P = less than 0.01 (by t-test).

Table 2-4. Comparison of Learning Disabled Versus
Non-Learning Disabled Children—
Factor Scores from Teacher Questionnaires

Mean Total Factor Scores	LD Group	Non-LD Group
Conners Teacher Questionnaire:		
Conduct factor	2.9	2.6
Hyperactive factor	6.0	3.8*
Inattentive-passive factor	6.2	4.1†
Tension factor	3.2	2.7
Rutter Teacher Questionnaire:		
Total factor score	14.7	10.1*
Neurotic factor	2.2	1.3
Antisocial factor	2.6	1.7

*P = less than 0.03.
†P = less than 0.01 (*t*-test).

developmental variables is that the learning disorder and the nonlearning disordered groups (all of whom had communication disorders) did not differ in performance or verbal IQ, nor did they differ on nonlanguage milestones. The children were matched on age and performance IQ, but it turned out that on verbal IQ they were roughly the same as well. They do, however, differ in a variety of ways that are quite striking:

1. Table 2-2 indicates that the learning disordered group had a high rate of language disorder as opposed to pure speech disorder; 61% of our non-learning disordered group had a pure speech disorder, whereas 68% of the learning disordered group had a speech and language disorder and 18% had a pure language disorder, with no speech involvement. In any learning disorder subgroup of a communication disorder group, the subjects are more likely to have language involvement rather than just speech involvement. Expressive disorder, receptive disorder, and auditory processing disorder were all more common in the learning disordered group.

2. Table 2-3 shows results of the parent questionnaires. The learning disordered group was rated on the Conners questionnaire (Guy, 1976) as more anxious, more hyperactive, having more learning problems, and having poorer attention than the non-learning disordered group. On the Rutter parent questionnaire (Guy, 1976), they had a much higher total score of behavioral abnormality.

3. Table 2-4 shows the results of the teacher questionnaires. The teachers rated the learning disordered group on the Conners questionnaire

Table 2-5. Matched Groups: Learning Disabled Versus Non-Learning Disabled—DSM-III Diagnoses

	LD Group	Matched Group
Axis I:		
Psychiatrically Ill	86%	46%
Axis II:		
Developmentally Disordered		
(Excluding Learning Disorders)	14%	18%
Axis III:		
Medically Disordered	54%	64%
Axis IV:		
Psychosocially Stressed	74%	70%
Axis V:		
Level of Impairment:		
None	7%	39%*
Mild	32%	39%
Moderate/Severe	61%	22%
Level of Adaptive Function:		
GOOD, V. GOOD, SUPERIOR	25%	57%
FAIR	46%	32%
FAIR, V. POOR, GROSS	29%	11%

*P = 0.003.

Table 2-6. Matched Groups: Learning Disabled Versus Non-Learning Disabled—Types of Psychiatric Disorders

	LD Group	Matched Group
Oppositional disorder	3%	0
Attention deficit disorder	43%	18%*
Conduct disorders	3%	0
Affective disorders	14%	11%
Adjustment disorders	3%	14%
Other disorders	13%	6%

*P = less than 0.01.

as more hyperactive and more inattentive. On the Rutter questionnaire, the teachers gave the learning disordered group a significantly higher rating on total behavioral abnormality in the classroom.

Based on symptom ratings, then, both parents and teachers rate the learning disordered group as significantly more behaviorally deviant. Another notation is that teachers rated the children who had learning problems as being less shy; in fact, they were frequently considered to be leaders by students who did not have learning disorders.

4. Table 2-5 shows that 86% of the learning disordered children had some psychiatric diagnosis. They did not differ in medical disorders or on the amount of psychosocial stress in the family, but they had about twice the rate of psychiatric disorders, and their level of impairment in adaptive functioning was significantly greater. For example, in the non-learning disordered group about 78% have either no or mild impairment, as compared with only 39% in the group with a learning disorder. The learning disordered group, then, has more psychiatric disorders and more impaired levels of adaptive functioning. Lastly, when considering the *types* of psychiatric disorders this group evidenced, 43% (almost half) have ADD. The other disorders seen in Table 2-6 are not significantly greater than in the matched non-learning disordered group. One could conclude that the increase in psychiatric disorder, which is substantial, is caused by ADD with hyperactivity.

SUMMARY

As a group, children with communication disorders are at risk for the development of learning and psychiatric disorders. The strongest correlates of psychiatric disorders in the group of children who have communication disorder are speech and language factors. Within this communication disordered group, when you select out a group that has already demonstrated significant learning disorders, you selectively identify a group 86% of whom also have a psychiatric disorder.

It apppears to be that the communication disorder leads to the learning disorder, which then leads to the psychiatric disorder; alternatively, the communication disorder may lead independently to both, which is why there is a strong association.

We finished our three year study in 1978 and we now have followed up about 400 of the 600 children we originally saw. About 95% of them received speech and language therapy. Very few have had any other type of services. Our study was intended to evaluate this question: If you intervene in their underlying disability area (communication disorder), would you prevent later development of learning or psychiatric disorders, or both, in those who did not have these problems initially, or would you ameliorate the learning disorder or psychiatric disorder in most children who did have the disorder initially? The answer to both parts of the question is no. The prevalence rate of both psychiatric and learning disorders has actually gone up over the four to five year period despite the fact that 26% now show totally normal results on tests with regard to speech and language functioning. Of the other 74% who still have some degree of communication disorder, 90% have shown substantial improvement in their communication skills. The major observations from this follow-up study are as follows:

1. Communication disordered children are at risk for psychiatric and learning disorders.

2. It takes more than just speech-language therapy leading to remediation of the underlying speech and language disorder to prevent or treat learning and psychiatric disorders.

Results of this study would suggest certain assessment and intervention procedures. When a child presents for an evaluation of a suspected speech or language disorder, the following plan seems reasonable:

1. A comprehensive assessment of speech and language functioning, including hearing, should be done.

2. If physical or neurological disorder is suspected as a contributing cause of the communication disorder, the appropriate type of investigation should be done. If a physical or neurological disorder is found, appropriate therapy should be instituted.

3. Appropriate therapy for the communication disorder should be instituted.

4. If the child is suspected of having a psychiatric disorder (using the definition in this chapter), there should be a referral for a comprehensive psychiatric evaluation. The goals of this evaluation should be to answer the following questions:

a. Does this child have a psychiatric disorder (or disorders)?

b. Does the disorder(s) meet the criteria for one or more Diagnostic and Statistical Manual of Mental Disorders (DSM-III) (American Psychiatric Association, 1980) syndromes?

c. In this child, what are the likely etiological factors for the disorder(s) (e.g., family, genetic or biological factors, dynamics) and what are their relative strengths?

d. What are the factors that are maintaining the disorder(s)?

e. What are the factors that are maintaining normal development?

f. What are the strengths and competencies of the child and his or her family?

g. What is likely to be the natural history of this child's psychiatric disorder(s) if left untreated?

h. Is intervention necessary?

i. What intervention modalities are most likely to be effective for this child and his or her family?

The *tools* available to the clinician to use in the above diagnostic process include:

1. Interviews with parents about the child and the family.

2. Interviews with the child.

3. Parent and teacher behavior rating scales.

4. Laboratory studies (including psychological and educational testing).

Using these tools and going through this process will result in the type of information needed to plan a multimodality treatment program for psychiatric disorder.

REFERENCES

American Psychiatric Association (1980). *Diagnostic and statistical manual of mental disorders* (DSM-III) (3rd ed.). Washington, DC: Author.

Baker, L., and Cantwell, D. P. (1984). Primary prevention of the psychiatric consequences of childhood communication disorders. *Journal of Preventive Psychiatry, 2*(1), 75-97.

Cantwell, D. P., Baker, L., and Mattison, R. E. (1979). The prevalence of psychiatric disorder in children with speech and language disorder: An epidemiologic study. *Journal of the American Academy of Child Psychiatry, 18,* 450-461.

Fundudis, T., Kolvin, I., and Garside, R. F. (1979). *Speech retarded and deaf children: Their psychological development.* London: Academic Press.

Guy, W. (1976). *ECDEU assessment manual for psychopharmacology.* National Institute of Mental Health, Psychopharmacology Research Branch. Rockville, Maryland: U. S. Department of Health, Education, and Welfare.

McLeod, J. (1978, January). *Psychometric identification of children with learning disabilities.* Monograph of the Institute of Child Guidance and Development, University of Saskatchewan, Saskatoon, Canada.

Rutter, M., Tizard, J., and Whitmore, K. (Eds.) (1970). *Education, health, and behavior.* London: Longmans Green.

Thomas, A., and Chess, S. (1977). *Temperament and development.* New York: Brunner/Mazel.

TRANSITIONAL NOTE

Cantwell has shown how inadequate skill in communication can sometimes be associated with both learning and psychiatric problems. As he has said, "Being able to communicate is what makes us human." If there is a mismatch between what the environment expects of the human being and what the human being can provide, the result appears to be a performance deficit. If an individual is reminded of performance deficits with sufficient frequency, feelings of frustration, anxiety, lack of motivation, or anger surface. These, in turn, produce the "garlic symptoms" and "onion symptoms" that Cantwell describes.

Nelson, in Chapter 3, addresses four components of any communicative event—the sender, the receiver, the message, and the medium. By engaging in an analysis of the breakdown of a communicative event, a teacher might find that the problem does not consistently lie with the student's performance deficits. Since communication is a dynamic process, positive and negative factors are constantly changing. By trying to foster "a better match," Nelson encourages educators to assume nothing in terms of developmental behavior or "school knowledge" and, therefore, analyze or evaluate everything before making any snap decision about a student's "learning problem." From the observational information collected, teachers can modify the situation, the instructional content, or their own verbal delivery or teach students more productive learning strategies (or compensatory skills to cope with situations that cannot be altered). With a slightly different, but compatible, philosophy Gruenewald and Pollak (1984) address this issue. Their contributions, along with those of Nelson, provide the classroom teacher with valuable guidelines for a realistic appraisal of "the instructional situation." These evaluative guidelines heighten teacher awareness of variables that affect learning, but which frequently are not monitored. The consequence of no monitoring is that students with "learning disorders" or "different learning styles" are labeled "disabled" because they do not fit in. Nelson addresses implications for fostering a better match between teacher talk and child listening by providing specific monitoring and programming suggestions. When communication, learning, and psychological needs are approached with professional cooperation and a coordinated program, there is a greater possibility that the student with problems in any one of these areas will better understand the nature of difficulties and be better motivated to develop more productive coping skills.

Gruenewald, L. J., and Pollak, S. A. (1984). *Language interaction and teaching and learning.* Baltimore: University Park Press.

CHAPTER 3

Teacher Talk
and Child Listening—
Fostering a Better Match

Nickola Wolf Nelson

> Now before you start I want to check to see about my
> listeners.
> OK, Lisa was a good listener.
> Randy was fairly good.
> Eric / you were not good, you got almost all your work
> filled in / you weren't listening.

This sample of teacher talk from a first grade classroom teacher (Cuda and Nelson, 1976; Nelson, 1984) could be analyzed by computing length and syntactic complexity, by asking questions about the teacher's tone of voice and his or her speaking rate, or by determining the internalized meanings the teacher is conveying. We could also focus on the context or ask questions about the intended function of this teacher's comments. Last, we might contemplate the actual effects this segment of teacher talk might have had on the students involved.

If we were to ask questions only about teacher talking samples, however, we would have less than half the picture. Human communication is interactive. Conversational partners come to communicative interactions with needs, abilities, ideas, and expectations of their own. Some may facilitate the normal process of the interaction. Some may even improve it and make it richer. Others may interfere with either the accuracy or the effectiveness of the interchange.

Although the title of this chapter, "Teacher Talk and Child Listening," seems to imply a stream of conversation running in one direction only, that is clearly not what occurs in most classroom discourse. Those who are primarily acting as listeners influence the movement of the exchange in both verbal and nonverbal ways. They make comments, ask questions, provide correct or wrong responses, fidget, ignore, interrupt, and otherwise give overt or covert evidence of having their own ideas, understanding, and interest. Likewise, teachers are not only talkers. They also listen to their students and, in varying degrees, monitor the evidence, both verbal and nonverbal, that the classroom exchange is moving along as intended.

Nevertheless, Griffin and Hannah (1960) report that elementary school students spend over one half of their day listening to teachers talking, and estimates for high school students range as high as 90%. These conditions result in formalization of communicative interaction routines that are quite different from the usual back and forth turn-taking of dyadic (two-way) conversations. In doing most of the talking, teachers most often communicate simultaneously with 20 students or more. If each student were to attempt to take as many conversational turns as teachers the result would be chaotic.

It is the purpose of this chapter to consider the formalized communication events in the classroom, especially for children with language-learning impairments, who are so often overwhelmed by the demands of classroom communication. First, the question of what makes listening easy or difficult will be addressed. Potential points of mismatch will be identified. Then, a framework will be constructed for developing improved communicative processes in areas where mismatches occur, with suggestions being offered for improving classroom communication.

TEACHER TALK

A communicative event may be described as having four components: (1) a sender, (2) a receiver, (3) a message, and (4) a medium (Thompson, 1969). At first glance, it would seem to make sense to view complexity as an inherent feature of the message and to view difficulty as a feature of the receiver's speed and accuracy in comprehending the message. In practice, however, we often do not distinguish between the ways the terms "complexity," and "difficulty" are used. For example, we can say with equal appropriateness, "That is a complex subject," and "That is difficult material." However, as Slobin (1971) commented:

> The search for a reliable metric of syntactic complexity. . .has not been strikingly successful, and the reason for this failure is an important one. We soon discovered that understanding a sentence can depend as much upon the context in which it is used as upon its syntactic form. (p. 33)

Difficulty usually becomes operationally defined in terms of the relative success an individual experiences in processing stimuli. Operational definitions of *complexity* are more often based on word counts, transformational distance, and other structural features. However, such measurements are of little value unless they correspond at least partially to the difficulty listeners have in understanding messages encoded in a certain way. Much of this section called "teacher talk" focuses on how a message may become relatively more or less complex based on features beyond the linguistic message itself, making it relatively more "easy" or "difficult" for listeners to understand.

The perspective this chapter will take when discussing classroom discourse is to apply the categories of use, content, and form to analyze teachers' talking. These are the categories first suggested by Bloom and Lahey (1978) for addressing the topics of language development and language disorders. They have also been widely applied by researchers and clinicians.

Language Use in Teacher Talk

The classroom environment leads to a number of unique characteristics of language use that do not appear in less formal settings. Some of them have to do with the nature of the context in which the language is being used; some have to do with the functions it serves; and some relate to the conventions of turn-taking that are vastly different in the classroom than in usual two-way (dyadic) conversations. All are part of what language specialists call "pragmatics." In attempting to determine what makes listening easy or difficult, the multiple facets of classroom interaction need to be considered.

The context of the classroom and the teacher's purpose in talking motivate the initiation of the message and influence the selection of vocabulary and the content of the message. The relationship between the nonverbal context and the information inherent in the language itself is an important consideration for understanding how easy or difficult a message is to receive. Other unique features in the uses of teacher talk relate to opportunities for repair and functions of classroom language.

Contextual Support. Home talk and less formal conversation differ widely from school discourse in the demands they place on a listener's ability to understand language without contextual support. Parents and other familiar dyadic conversational partners can often make accurate assumptions about an individual child's world and word knowledge based on previous experiences, and they usually converse in familiar settings and routines that provide rich nonverbal contexts to aid the child's comprehension.

School discourse, on the other hand, makes additional demands on the listener's ability to understand language, which continues to become more context-free as age and grade level increase. Communication in the classroom relies more on the meaning being expressed within the teacher's spoken words or the written words of textual material. Cook-Gumperz (1977) called the first type of meaning—that typical of the home—"situated meaning," and the second type—that occurring in schools—"lexicalized meaning." For example, the mother of a small child might say, as she is gathering her purse, car keys, and jacket and pointing to her child's jacket, "Get your coat on and let's go," and he or she may comprehend what is expected without difficulty, partly as a result of receiving considerable support from situated meaning cues. The same child, however, may appear to be inattentive, of low intelligence, or obstinate if he or she fails to respond to the kindergarten teacher, who, using highly lexicalized meanings, might say something like, "OK now, when you have finished your work and cleaned up your work area, you may go to your lockers and get your wraps; then come back in here and line up to get ready to go to recess."

Opportunity for Repair. Differences between home and school discourse also exist in the degree to which circumstances lend themselves to making conversational repairs. If parents notice that a breakdown has occurred in the child's comprehension, revisions and repetitions may be made as needed, being tailored to fit the child and the situation. In the home situation described earlier, if the child fails to respond immediately, the mother may, depending on her own style and momentary store of patience, rephrase the directive several times, saying, for example, "It's over there on the chair; no; on the chair [then, moving toward it], right here!" Or she may simply grab the jacket and begin helping him put it on, saying, "Come on, let's get it on right now; we're late." In the classroom, however, teachers must try to accommodate the varying needs of all the listeners in their classrooms, and they often must do this with less prior knowledge of the individual student's experiences.

Functions of Classroom Language. Beyond the special characteristics of the classroom communicative context and its unique conversational repair strategies, the actual purposes of teachers' speech events are influential in determining how easy or difficult it is to comprehend teacher talk. Here, we are not so much considering "what language is as what language is for" (Hymes, 1972, p. xii).

A number of different categorical systems may be used for characterizing the functions of teacher talk. Much of the work that has been done to gain an understanding of the functions of language in classroom settings has come from British researchers. In particular, Sinclair and Coulthard (1975) devised an analytic system for categorizing the regularities of teaching events. In their system, lessons are made up of transactions, transactions are made up of exchanges, exchanges are made up of moves, and moves are made up of acts. Acts are the smallest units. Among the 22 different acts described by Sinclair and Coulthard are the following: nomination (labeling), reply (in response to student question or response), acceptance (acknowledging a student's comment), and evaluation (reflecting on the correctness or worth of a response). Some acts do not occur individually, but only as a part of larger moves in which the teacher shifts the direction of the the communication from one pupil to another. The following sequence is used by Burton (1981) to illustrate the relationship of moves and acts:

Teacher Moves:	Student Replies:
John, what's the capital of France?	
	Paris.
Paris, that's right.	
And Mary, what's the capital of Sweden?	
	Stockholm.
Stockholm, good girl.	

In this sequence, the first line of talk is considered to be an opening move, made up of nomination and elicitation acts. The student's answering move, "Paris," is a reply act. The teacher then produced a follow-up move (the second line of teacher talk) that consists of acceptance and evaluation acts, and then makes a new opening move (line three). This is followed by another reply and follow-up move. The repeated three-part structure of this example is typical of many teaching exchanges in that it comprises initiation, response, and feedback moves. Several exchanges may be part of the same transaction. The beginnings and endings of transactions are often framed with a small set of words and phrases that frequently appear in teacher talk, words like "right," "well," "OK," and "now." The teacher may also tell the students what the focus of the upcoming transaction will be.

Children who are able to use such focus and framing cues to detect the overall structure of classroom transactions and exchanges will find the task of understanding classroom expectations more manageable than those who are not. Conversely, teachers who make such topic shift cues more apparent may be facilitating the process for their students.

It can be enlightening to study how children actually view the functions and processes of classroom interaction sequences. Willes (1981) reports on a research technique in which she encouraged children beginning school to play teacher so that she could observe the expression of their concepts of what it is a teacher does in teaching. Based on the results of her observations, she was able to conclude for the normal children of her study that "children do not start formal schooling in simple ignorance of what to expect" (Willes, 1981, p. 80). Rather, they start school with some knowledge of the kinds of moves teachers make and develop further within the first seven to eight months of school. However, in Willes' study, the "playing teacher" game held little interest for the "least successful" children in the classroom. When one child did develop interest in the game, she adopted a style that showed her view of teachers as those who organize and control, and not as individuals who serve as sources of information or who check whether information has been assimilated. Among this child's comments as "teacher" were a high proportion of evaluative statements of the type, "They've been very naughty," "All of them have been very naughty. These children are doing very naughty," and then added, "The teacher's talking to thin air" (Willes, 1981, p. 83).

Cultural Mismatches. The preceding bit of discourse illustrates what Tough (1977) has viewed as hindrances to effective communication that spring from attitudes, assumptions, and expectations. Attitudes affect how individuals approach others and how they interpret what others say to them. This is true of both students and teachers. Tough continues by noting that, "in most talk the exchange of intended meaning is not fully realized; more than that, there is often so much of a mismatch between intended meaning and received meaning that what has been communicated is far from the intentions of the communicator" (p. 10).

If such a mismatch occurs among normal communicators of similar cultural backgrounds, consider the effects that language disorder or cultural difference might have on the accurate communication of meanings, particularly certain kinds of meaning. For example, Hymes (1972) was concerned not with meanings in the narrow sense of naming objects and stating relationships, but in the fuller sense of such acts as "conveying respect or disrespect, concern or indifference, intimacy or distance, seriousness or play, etc." (p. xiii). It may not be the words themselves, but rather nonverbal cues, such as tone of voice, body posture, facial expression, and proximity (or nearness) that communicate to a child at a level underlying the surface level of meaning how the teacher feels about the child. Such cues also suggest a model for how the child might feel about himself or herself.

The "self-fulfilling prophecy" aspects of teacher attitudes toward their students have received considerable attention since Rosenthal and Jacobson's book was published in 1968. Teachers have been found to communicate differential expectations for classroom performance that are not attributable to objective differences among children (Brophy and Good, 1970). Gerber (1981) views the probable results of this kind of emotional climate as interfering with the processing of information. She speculates that, as children fail to invest themselves in the active processing of the information, neither the information nor the strategy required to perform the language-related tasks is mastered.

Multilevel Discourse Aspects. In order to try to account for some of the multilevel aspects of discourse, Dore (1979) has developed a coding system, which includes the three major functions: (1) to convey content, (2) to regulate conversation, or (3) to express attitude.

In a study of teacher discourse that was analyzed using Dore's categories, Nelson (1984) found that many of the regulative functions performed by teachers were aimed at regulating not conversation but the behaviors of their students. Sinclair and Coulthard (1975) suggested that a distinction should be made between "elicitations," which they defined as requiring verbal responses (usually contentive in nature), and "directives," which they defined as requiring nonverbal responses (usually compliance with regulatory expectations). However, Hammersley (1981) has questioned the verbal-nonverbal breakdown and has offered the following two examples as evidence for the artificiality of such a distinction:

Example A

> T: Now, who can tell me where Israel is? Go on then, Jackson. (Pupil walks out to the front of the classroom and points to a place on the map drawn on the board.)

Example B

> T: Do you think that's clever?
> P: No.
> T: No what?
> P: No, sir.
>
> (Hammersley, 1981, p. 53)

Hammersley suggested that the teacher's utterance in Example A was elicitative even though it was framed as a directive, with an expected nonverbal response. The teacher's "No, what?" exchange in Example B might best be classified as directive, even though it required a verbal response.

McDermott (1977) described much of the process of teaching as a matter of getting organized, and commented that success in getting organized for learning depends on how well the participants communicate to each other the importance of the learning tasks. McDermott holds that "teaching is invariably a form of coercion" (p. 204). However, individual teachers handle the coercion differently. Some are direct and authoritarian; others are less direct. Neither approach is uniformly better or worse than the other. For example, a child may be no more likely to follow the gentle suggestion of question-commands, such as "Why don't you close the door?" than the more direct command, "Close the door." In fact, language disordered youngsters may be less inclined to follow the indirect commands, because they may not understand them. The child must understand that the question is not meant to be a question, but rather an imperative or directive (i.e., "Close the door"); it is not permissible to answer, "I am not closing the door because I don't feel like it."

Language Content in Teacher Talk

In addition to language use, the content of language events occuring in classrooms differs widely depending on grade level. Whereas in the earlier grades, greater emphasis is placed on learning to read and write and perform basic mathematical computations, in the later grades much of teacher talk centers on topics of substance in the content areas of science, geography, social studies, and literature.

Talking About Language (Metalinguistics). The process of using language to talk about language is called metalinguistics. If children are to be able to understand the metalinguistic talk of teachers even at kindergarten and first grade levels, they must first be able to view the abstract symbols of language (i.e., words, sounds, and letters) as objects in themselves. This requires a degree of both cognitive and linguistic sophistication that many language-learning impaired children lack. Consider, for example, the following segment of talk produced by a first grade teacher:

> What sound does /cat/ begin with?
> No / that's not what I asked.
> I asked what sound.
> Good / We have two letters that make a /k/
>   sound.
> "k" and "c" make the same / sound.
> How do you know / that cat / does not begin
>   with a "k"?
> Because I didn't put a "k" on the paper / so
>   you know it has to begin with a / "c."
> Use your sounds and figure out the other words.
>   (Nelson, 1984, p. 164)

In order for this sequence to have been communicative for a child, children must be able to process and understand language about language on a number of levels. They must be able to shift focus from words to sounds to letters to the teacher's strategy in setting up worksheets. Imagine the confusion of the child whose only strategy for comprehending speech is to listen for key content words and to assume that they are related in the usual way. Such a child might have heard the teacher's words "sound" and "cat" in the opening question and assume that the correct response must be "meow."

By the third grade, the content of teacher talk consists of a combination of focus on skills for learning and areas of knowledge. Teachers continue to use language to talk about language, but beyond the first grade, greater emphasis is placed on learning about language at the word level and in longer units than on the analysis of words into their component sounds. DeStefano (1978) has called such metalinguistic language the "language instruction register" (LIR), and views it as one of the registers (i.e., variety of language set apart from others by the circumstances of its use) that is important to literacy learning in America's schools.

Lexical items, such as "sound," "letter," "word," "sentence," "beginning sound," and "blend," are all part of the LIR for teaching reading. Such terms abound in kindergarten and first grade, and the development of a complex LIR continues into the upper grades as the relationship between written and spoken language becomes the topic of many exchanges within literacy lessons. For example, the following is a third grade teacher's explanation of the homonyms "mail" and "male:"

> OK, number two is mail.
> This is like / talking about a letter that you
>   received through the mail.
> We use this word to talk about a man or a boy
>   but it's not spelled like this.
>
> (Nelson, 1984, p. 167)

Talking About Content Areas (Metacomprehension). The shifts of content across grade levels represent shifts of degree more than of kind. Although learning skills predominate as topics in early grades, and knowledge areas predominate in later grades, teachers at all levels use language to introduce content areas and to lead discussions about areas of knowledge or material that the students have read, experienced, or viewed through audiovisual media presentations. Mishler (1972) provides examples from two different first grade teachers to illustrate how teachers can help their students organize information about the world.

Example 1

The teacher has just finished reading a story to the whole class about a detective, Big Max, who had been hired by a king to find a lost elephant.

> Teacher: Big Max (pause) used some words that go with detectives. Can you think of any? Right over here someone. (Several children speak at once; unclear response.)
> T: What does a detective have to look for when he's on his way to solving a case? Bill.
> Child: A clue.
> T: A clue. Can you think of any clues that Big Max found in this story, Eric?
> C: Hmmm. (pause) Tears.
> T: And who do those tears belong to?
> Class: Crocodile.

Example 2

The children have finished cleaning up after a free period of play, games, and art. The teacher has assembled them around her.

> Teacher: Can I see everybody over here? We're going to be seeing a very unusual movie this morning.
> Child: What's it about?
> T: I don't think I'm going to tell you, Stephen. I'm going to let you wait and find out.
> Class (chorus of complaints from several children): Aw!
> T: It's done with colors.
> Class (several children calling out; unclear): Colors. . .
> T: I don't think it's a story.

(Mishler, 1972, p. 271)

Mishler uses these two talk samples to exemplify a difference in teaching strategies. The first exchange is considered to be more directed and focused than the second. The teacher in the first episode focuses the attention of the class on certain specific features of the experience and provides a transition between past and present. She also underscores the importance of language. The children are being told that it is important to pay attention to particular words, since they may later be held accountable for having heard and understood them. The teacher provides a way to help the children conceptualize "a complex yet ordered world" and to understand that not only is it organized, but that language is one of the basic principles of its organization (Mishler, 1972, p. 272).

In Example 2, the world view constructed by the teacher is different. In the organizational system constructed by this teacher, the salient dimension is the relationship between the teacher and the children. She manages to attract their attention, and to elicit a question, but in response to the question, not only does not supply new information, but also denies the legitimacy of the question. In this classroom:

> The world of objects is vague and undifferentiated, and the children will be able to learn about it not by a directed search or inquiry but by behaving in an acceptable way to the teacher. There is no substantive or logical continuity between what one child says and what another says, and the connections between responses are mediated by the teacher.
>
> (Mishler, 1972, p. 274)

Differences in Discourse Style. The style of discourse and content of the interaction that the teacher selects can affect the quality of cognitive processing. Bruner (1965) has described two kinds of teaching: (1) the expository mode and (2) the hypothetical mode. In the expository mode, the speaker has a wide choice of alternatives and is planning and anticipating paragraph content; the listener is still focusing upon the words without being aware of the speaker's options. In the hypothetical mode, the teacher and student are in a more cooperative state. The student takes part in the formulation and at times may play the principal role in it. Rather than being "bench-bound listeners," students are aware of alternatives and may even have an evaluative attitude toward them. Research has shown that listeners vary in their abilities to take advantage of such cognitive opportunities.

Questions are more likely to be used in extended discourse between children and adults than they are in conversations among children. Questions provided in advance of verbal learning activities may facilitate the learning of the material, particularly short-term factual recall of material that can be used to answer memory questions (Ausubel, 1960). Allen (1970) explored the possibility that higher order questions (i.e., those that required some cognitive processing before answering) might enhance the facilitative effect of questions placed before lessons on social studies on learning and retaining the course content material. However, he found that students differed in their ability to make use of the advance organizers. The less able students were only able to use the more concrete, more specific, and less generalizable organizers. The students with higher ability were able to use the higher order questions for enhancement of learning as measured by a delayed retention test, although there was no advantage for memory for factual material as measured by a short-term retention test. Allen (1970) speculated that the differences may have had something to do with differences in the students' existing cognitive structures.

The size of content or comprehension units, whether they are words, sentences, or larger units of text, largely determines the demands the segment of teacher talk makes on a student's listening ability. Words and sentences that can be understood based on their literal meanings are more easily comprehended than those requiring inference or interpretation of figurative meanings. On a broader level, text that can be understood based on world knowledge of such life "scripts" as eating in a restaurant or going to the zoo, or on linguistic knowledge of "story grammars" (Stein and Glenn, 1979), which give narratives their structure (Westby, 1984) are more easily understood when one has had the opportunity to engage in and integrate such experiences.

Language Form in Teacher Talk

The form of the language used in teacher talk is the third major variable that may influence the ease or difficulty of processing it. Language form has both linguistic and supralinguistic aspects. Linguistic aspects include such elements as the phonology (speech sounds), morphology (smallest meaningful units), and syntax (sentence structure) of language. Supralinguistic elements include the teacher's speaking rate, intonation and stress patterns, fluency, and similar variables.

Complexity of Sentence Structure. Much has been written about the sentence structure of speech addressed to preschool children (Phillips, 1973; Snow, 1977; Wilkinson, Hiebert, and Rembold, 1981), but less information is available about the syntax of teacher talk to school-age youngsters. In one study (Cuda and Nelson, 1976), analysis of speech samples gathered from 27 teachers, with nine each at the first, third, and sixth grade levels, showed syntactical structures to be significantly more complex in speech addressed to sixth graders than speech addressed to either first or third graders.

First and third grade teachers used a high number of simple sentences (those with one subject and one verb). For example, a third grade teacher explained:

> Oh, would you get out your English books please? Yesterday we had words that sound alike. Today we have words that / look alike. But they are pronounced differently.
>
> (Nelson, 1984, p. 166)

Compare the structural complexity of that sequence with the following one spoken by a sixth grade teacher:

> Now in the first / uh / you know you have marginal lines that you must give attention to.
>
> You may need to use two sheets of paper, you may need to use one.

However, /uh/ amount you write depends upon the / what you are capable of doing, and some of you are capable of long paragraphs and /uh/ because you have more thoughts /uh/ on a particular matter.

(Nelson, 1984, p. 170)

Suprasegmental Variables. Suprasegmental variables, when used intentionally to augment the linguistic aspects of messages, are designed to be instrumental in making the intended meanings of messages clear to perceptive listeners. However, when suprasegmental factors are not planned to assist in imparting meaning but occur incidentally (e.g., in the form of hesitations, nonmeaningful pauses, midsentence reformulations, or rapid speaking rate), they can interfere with processing rather than aid it.

In comparing suprasegmental variables among first, third, and sixth grade teachers, first grade teachers have been found to speak both simply and slowly; third grade teachers speak as simply as first grade teachers but as rapidly as sixth grade teachers; and sixth grade teachers speak both complexly and rapidly. The speech of sixth grade teachers also includes significantly more hesitations than either first or third grade teachers. Often appearing to pause in the process of formulating their ideas into sentences, sixth grade teachers revise and restart sentences, repeat portions of sentences, and use such fillers as "um," "er," "OK," "alright," and "you know" more frequently than teachers of lower grades (Cuda and Nelson, 1976).

In most instances the use of intonation patterns to impart meaning facilitates the comprehension process. DeStefano (1978) found that students could comprehend more difficult material, such as "The Merchant of Venice" better when it was read aloud skillfully than by reading it themselves. DeStefano (1978) also pointed out that suprasegmental devices are sometimes essential for understanding sentence meanings within larger contexts. Contrastive stress is one of the strategies that is used for tying together aspects of spoken text at discourse levels. For example, the same four words, "You didn't say that," could have at least four different interpretations related to the surrounding context and communicated by the placement of primary stress:

You didn't say that. (Someone else must have.)
You *didn't* say that. (You couldn't have said that!)
You didn't *say* that. (Perhaps you wrote it instead.)
You didn't say *that*. (You said something else.)

(DeStefano, 1978, p.25)

Effects of Adverse Listening Conditions on Content, Form, and Use

Another set of variables that can influence the perceptual clarity of messages is associated with the environmental context in which speech is produced. High-quality teacher talk produced in a quiet classroom with minimal reverberation (i.e., one that results in little or no echoing) can facilitate comprehension. Conversely, comprehension may be made significantly more difficult when the room has hard floors and high ceilings, which are not conducive to good acoustics (Ross, 1978; Smyth, 1979). The difficulty a listener has in comprehending under poor conditions depends on the message, the context, and the listener.

The sophistication of the normal listener's linguistic system can compensate for environmental distortions by filling in message systems that have been distorted. Whether a task is an auditory or a visual one, if an individual is familiar with the vocabulary, sentence structure, and contextual meanings being communicated, the process of providing closure (i.e., supplying missing "perceptual" information) to distorted messages is made easier. This is because of the ability of normal listeners to make predictions based on what is known about the total language system, and then to test those predictions for goodness of fit, confirming that they make sense or not, and revising them if necessary, doing all of this at the same time they are receiving subsequent information (Goodman, 1973; Smith, 1975).

However, language-learning impaired students, being less firmly in control of the rules of language, are penalized to a much greater extent by adverse listening conditions. Because they know less about the language system, they must rely more on processing complete perceptual input and avoid taking short cuts. Anyone who is barely competent in a foreign language and has tried to converse in it can appreciate how fatiguing it is to have to listen for every surface level cue in order to follow the conversation and understand the meanings being conveyed. The demands of such a task may be a major factor in why so many language learning impaired students appear to have attention problems and look as if they do not listen.

CHILD LISTENING

Any number of factors can make it more or less difficult for a student to be able to comprehend teacher talk from one day to the next. Even normal children have what White (1980) calls "wobbly competencies," so that many factors affect them:

> A child is not a computer that either "knows" or "does not know." A child
> is a bumpy, blippy, excitable, fatigable, distractible, active, friendly, mulish, semi-
> cooperative bundle of biology. Some factors help a child pull together coherent
> address to a problem; others hinder that pulling together and make a child
> "not know."
>
> (White, 1980, p. 43)

In this section, the emphasis shifts from teacher talk to child listening. The two major issues to be addressed are (a) methods of measuring how well a child understands spoken language, and (b) factors within the child that make it relatively more easy or difficult for the child to be an effective listener.

Measuring Children's Comprehension

The size of units that children are expected to comprehend influence the style of processing in which they engage. Most formal tests of language comprehension are designed to measure comprehension of linguistic units no larger than words, phrases, or sentences, and they tend to require only understanding of literal meaning (Rees and Shulman, 1978). When sentences or words are taken out of context and are presented to the student with a set of pictures from which the "correct choice" is to be selected, there is no need or opportunity to consider the speaker's intention in producing the utterance or the broader context of the exchange. Some reading and language tests do include paragraph level comprehension items, but questions following these items tend to focus more on memory for factual material than on ability to draw inference beyond the material itself, a skill known to be important for comprehension in the larger sense (Wallach, 1984).

Another problem with the use of formal testing of language comprehension relates to the standardization process. The main purpose of administering standardized tests in a standardized manner is to draw conclusions about how the individuals being tested compare with a normative group along a certain dimension. However, if the subject of the evaluation differs culturally or experientially from the normative population on which the test was standardized, the results of the test for the individual become irretrievably interwoven with the cultural bias of the instrument, and it is inappropriate to draw conclusions about performance on the test (Vaughn-Cooke, 1983).

Whether or not one engages in formal test administration, it is important also to consider the evidence regarding a child's listening ability within naturalistic contexts. Conversational samples, transcribed with contextual notation where necessary, provide the richest information about a child's ability to handle the multiple demands of connected discourse. Such procedures are time consuming, however, and only provide information about regularities observed within the context of a particular exchange.

Careful observation of children by teachers within their own classrooms or by outside specialists can yield helpful diagnostic information about such things as attention, ability to retain a series of instructions, task orientation, repair strategies (such as asking a clarification question like, "What page did she say?"), or correctness of responses. For teachers, the most useful and practical strategies are those that are based on an ongoing sensitivity that allows them to tune in closely to the multiple verbal and nonverbal signs that individual children in their classrooms are comprehending or not.

Factors Affecting Children's Comprehension

Multiple factors within children affect their abilities to listen to and comprehend language input. Knowledge of the rule systems for language serves as the underlying "competence" that is essential before language can be understood. However, beyond competence variables are the "performance" variables that determine whether children will be able actually to use the knowledge they have of language at a particular time and place. Both types of variables will be reviewed in this section on child listening.

Beginning with *performance factors,* models for understanding the interaction of perceptual abilities and higher level processing are considered. The problems language-learning impaired children have in such areas as attention, memory for auditory input, auditory discrimination, and multiple levels of processing are interpreted within this framework. Next, *language competence factors* (i.e., knowledge of the rule systems of language use, content, and form) that can be expected to be particularly at risk in language-learning impaired children are reviewed.

Performance Factors

Language-learning disabled children seem to have particularly "wobbly" competencies. To the degree that they have not yet internalized the rules for understanding language intentions, language in context, language content, or language form, they experience difficulty understanding teacher talk. When such performance problems as attention and memory deficits, impaired discrimination, intermittent conductive hearing loss, or anxiety about self-worth are added to these potential areas of impairment, it is easy to see how a child might give up on following the communicative flow of the classroom and simply "not listen."

Skills such as auditory attention, retention, discrimination, and sequencing are frequently referred to as "auditory processing abilities." They are thought to interact with so-called "higher level comprehension abilities" to enable children to understand. Views of the nature of this interaction have shifted somewhat in recent years. Researchers like Rees (1973), Smith (1975), and Hedberg (1982) have increasingly begun to replace traditional unidirectional models of "bottom-up" information processing with "top-down" and bidirectional ones. In bottom-up models, sensory input is received, attended to, held in short-term memory, and perceived before it is comprehended or manipulated in any higher conceptual center of the brain. In bidirectional models, conceptual analysis affects perceptual processing as much as perceptual processing affects conceptual analysis. What an individual knows is viewed as being equally important as perceptual factors in determining what sensory information is "tuned into," perceived, and held in short-term memory.

The theoretical models of top-down and bottom-up processing correlate roughly with the competence and performance factors being discussed here. An individual's competence is the cognitive representation of knowledge that enables the use of top-down processing to assist in comprehending teacher talk or any other aspect of classroom communication. An individual's performance is influenced by bottom-up factors related to both internal and external variables that make it relatively more or less difficult to hear, discriminate, and understand what has been said. The more a person can rely on top-down abilities (or underlying competence), the less the acoustics of a room or teacher's speaking style can influence the degree of comprehension experienced. Conversely, the less underlying competence a child has for assisting in top-down processing, the more important it is to have perceptual clarity of messages.

The implications for planning special education opportunities for language-learning impaired children are that a two-pronged approach is necessary. Efforts should be made to provide activities that will strengthen underlying knowledge of the rules of language, while at the same time providing environmental adaptations to help children compensate for their language performance problems. Children who cannot remember more than one instruction at a time are unlikely to increase their auditory memory by practicing remembering strings of unconnected verbal information. However, environmental adaptations can be made in their classrooms to help them compensate for this performance deficit. Individualized evaluation and intervention can also be conducted to help them learn to use knowledge of the rules of language to "chunk" incoming information and relate it as efficiently as possibly to information stored in long-term memory.

Aspects of Language Competence

In order to assist students to develop the knowledge that will enable them to use top-down processing strategies, it is important to consider aspects of their language competence. Children with language-learning impairments are a heterogeneous group, and there is no one pattern of abilities and deficits that can be predicted for them. That is why individualized assessment by speech-language pathologists and other specialists is so important. However, it is useful to consider what kinds of competence within each of the rule systems (language use, language content, and language form) are most likely to be underdeveloped in language-learning impaired children so that they may be addressed during evaluation and intervention efforts.

Comprehension of Language Use. Children who have not learned to handle the specialized rules of classroom discourse will have difficulty with such acts as turn-taking or sorting out language that is used to regulate classroom activity from that used to convey content. They may not recognize that the functions of teacher talk vary, and that the illocutionary function (or intent) of teacher talk may be directly communicated at one time, but at another time the teacher may use only an indirect hint to communicate intent. For example, a teacher who requests her class to, "Think about the evidence in Chapter 3 regarding the economic and the social conditions that led to the Civil War," has combined functions of conveying content and regulating behavior, indirectly hinting that it is permissible for students to open their textbooks to Chapter 3 for a quick review. A teacher at a lower grade might say to students, "I would like to go to lunch, but this classroom is entirely too noisy and messy." In such an instance the indirect requests to be quiet and pick up are likely to be ignored, at least by some students, especially those with language-learning impairments. In either classroom, students with language impairments may be unable to process the language and may appear not to listen.

Language-learning impaired children may also be unable to detect the differences between teacher discourse that is designed to elicit verbal responses from that which is intended to direct nonverbal behavior. In the early grades, language-learning impaired children may be the only ones to respond to their teachers' requests for nonverbal responses (e.g., hand raising) to questions like, "Let's see; how many brought something for Show-and-Tell today," by blurting out verbal responses like, "I brought my truck." In the later grades, language-learning impaired children may appear to sullenly ignore all of the teacher's requests, because many have learned that it is better to be thought bored than dumb.

To compound their problems, when they have incompletely understood a classroom exchange, language-learning impaired children have difficulty identifying the problem, and they rarely seek clarification on their own. One fourth grader who could only remember three part instructions under optimal conditions, and who had difficulty understanding complex sentence forms, went to the pencil sharpener frequently during the schoolday and stood and stared rather than let his teacher know that he did not know what he was supposed to be doing. He also mastered the art of dropping his pencil and taking three minutes to pick it up. Another child might act out instead, but in either case, teachers and parents are likely to conclude that the children are not trying, and the children themselves are likely to conclude that they are somehow not as "good" as their classmates without understanding exactly why or how.

Comprehension of Language Content. In attempting to process language content, many language-learning impaired children have excessive difficulty making the rapid associations that allow listeners to (1) hear a new word, or hear an old word used in a new way, (2) conduct quick inventories of the word's semantic features that compare or contrast with features of other words in related categories, and (3) make fine adjustments in their internalized representations of meanings for aiding present and future comprehension. Related to these difficulties, semantic rigidity is often a major problem for language-learning impaired children. Words are more likely to be categorized in limited ways, with single concrete referents, and language-learning disordered children are often unable to make rapid associations or shifts of meaning relative to context.

A mother of a sixth grade language-learning impaired child described the effects that this type of literalness can have (Duncan, 1984). Her son, Wayne, had spent hours preparing his science fair project printing photographs to illustrate the effects of light on different grades of sensitized paper. The day he turned in the project he enthusiastically carried it to school, but returned in the afternoon, project in hand, threw it on the floor and gave it a kick. "It's no good," Wayne told his mother, "It's on two poster boards instead of three. The written stuff has to go under the pictures, not on the paper. And my name has to be on the back not the front. The other kids all had theirs right. They laughed at mine."

That evening, after he remounted the pictures, Wayne got a box of Christmas ornaments from the attic. "I'm going to string lights all around the edges," he told his mother, "The teacher says that a project's got to shine." When his mother told Wayne that she was sure his teacher did not mean "shine" literally, that it had to be good, not all lit up, Wayne insisted that his teacher said, "shine" (Duncan, 1984, p. 164). A few weeks earlier, Wayne had had a similar argument with his mother over the term "sandbank," because he could not understand that it did not mean a place to deposit money when you were at the beach.

In addition to their literalness, language-learning impaired children often have difficulty drawing inferences about meanings that are not directly encoded or those that are relatively context free. Skill in drawing conclusions based on information beyond what is directly given is expected even at the first grade level. An example is the following question in a workbook exercise:

Nan likes to look out.   Nan is _____.
It rains and rains.   (a) at the zoo
Nan can't go out.   (b) in the house
Nan can sit and read.

(Series R, Macmillan Reading, 1983)

In this exercise, the student must go beyond the meanings of the printed words to reach the appropriate conclusion, something that many language-learning impaired children cannot do. On another level, meanings that require metalinguistic levels of understanding also present particular difficulties to language-learning impaired children. Students cannot focus on language as an object when they still have limited understanding of the meanings of words and their primary uses (van Kleeck, 1984). In particular, the language of instruction for beginning or later stages of learning to read and write is likely to present difficulties to such children. For example, to talk about "threw" and "through" as being homonyms may make no sense to the language-learning impaired child. Such children need to learn such rules, not by being told them, but by being provided multiple examples that clearly demonstrate the regularities or contrasts being demonstrated.

Even if they are able to make the connections necessary to learn to read on a surface level, language-learning impaired children often have difficulty comprehending the broader meanings of the textual material they read or hear. It is this type of child who may pass through the early grades, perhaps repeating first or second grade, yet not be identified as being language-learning impaired until the third or fourth grade, when language becomes much more context free and larger units of discourse must be processed. Sounding out words in the first grade reader may be manageable, but reading and understanding the social studies text in fourth grade, and relating it to new information that was read two days ago, may be completely overwhelming.

It is often observed that children who have difficulty comprehending connected discourse or text also have difficulty expressing their own thoughts in a connected fashion. One 9 year 10 month old boy, who was repeating the third grade and receiving services at a university reading clinic, but who had not been identified as learning disabled or language impaired, responded to the question, "What makes your principal a really good principal?" with the following bit of discourse:

> If you get at a fight at school and somebody called you a name and you slugged
> 'em in the mouth, um, you know and they have to write about 50 sentences,
> the other has to write about 100, is, we don't allow swearing. That's good 'cause
> I don't like to swear.

This sample demonstrates a lack of topic cohesiveness and also shows the difficulty language-learning impaired children have in using language to talk about general categories rather than specific cases. Such children often tend to interpret all events egocentrically as younger children would, even though they are not mentally retarded.

Comprehension of Language Form. Many language-learning disordered children experience excessive difficulties using grammatical rules to understand sentences produced by their teachers. They may try to rely on strategies that consist of identifying key content words and using the literal meaning of those words to attempt to understand the teacher's intent. Or, as the following segment of discourse from a third grade teacher illustrates, children may make premature decisions about what is intended, responding only to a portion of their teacher's instructions, and end up as an example of what not to do:

> One word in each paragraph does not make sense. This is your paragraph right
>   here / and there's one word in there that does not make sense / and
>   that's where you put your X / on the word that doesn't make sense.
> Well, she has these X'd and circled and everything else.
> That wouldn't be right, would it?
> Then you should circle the word here / that should go in there.
> (Nelson, 1984, p. 167)

This segment of teacher talk also illustrates sentences formed with "logicogrammatical" rules that are used frequently in teachers' instruction-oriented discourse. Language-learning impaired children who demonstrate problems with syntax in their own language formulation, who rarely use complex sentences, and who get caught up in excessive "mazes" and "tangles" when they attempt to do so (Loban, 1963; Simon, 1981) often have particular difficulty understanding sentences formed with logicogrammatical rules.

Logicogrammatical rules generate syntax that is used for directions that must be followed in sequence or in which syntax must be decoded to understand the logical relationships being presented. An example of such a sentence would be the directive (with an expected nonverbal response), "After you get out your math books, turn to the first section in Chapter Five and do the first 10 problems." Sentences that use a phrase sequence ordering that is different from usual, or that require a different order of compliance, present particular difficulties. Language-learning impaired children often decode sentences in terms of rigid subject-verb-object patterns, and they misunderstand sentences that violate that order. For example, sentences like, "John was hit by Susan," may be understood as "John hit Susan." In another example, language-learning disordered children may interpret, "Before you go outside, finish your work," as giving them permission to go outside and then come back to finish. This is because they are processing each component ("go outside" and "finish your work") in the order in which it was heard rather than in relation to the way these phrases were syntactically encoded.

Language-learning impaired children also have difficulty making use of such grammatical morphemes as plurals, verb agreement markers, and "function words," such as *is, are, of, the, for,* and so forth, to predict words in workbook, textbook, or listening tasks. This reduces the efficiency of their listening and reading and can lead to errors. For example, in matching workbook sentences—(a) He calls the dog, (b) The dogs jump, or (c) The girl calls the dog—to a picture of a boy calling a dog (with the dog pictured jumping over a low bush and running toward the boy), the child who does not use the verb agreement and plural marker information available in the choices, could select (b) ("The dogs jump") and not understand why the teacher marks this an error.

Phonological problems that some language-learning impaired children exhibit can also affect their ability to understand a number of academic tasks. In particular, phonological problems may result in (1) difficulty in making sound-symbol associations, (2) problems in sequencing sounds and syllables in efforts to "sound out" words, (3) encoding sound and syllable patterns in order to spell words, or (4) decoding sound and syllable patterns in order to read or understand unfamiliar words. Comprehension abilities of children who have excessive problems with the phonological elements in particular, and language form in general, are often more susceptible to any distortion of speech as well. Rapid speaking rate, dysfluency of teacher talk, and the presence of background noise may all lead language-learning impaired children to be excessively penalized.

FOSTERING A BETTER MATCH

Alleviating the problem of mismatches in teacher talk and child listening can be approached from several perspectives. It is important to identify which aspects of children's language competence are involved in their unique language-learning impairments and which performance factors might be interfering with comprehension within classroom contexts. It is also useful to examine the classroom contexts and identify which factors within a particular classroom setting might be adjusted to increase the likelihood that language-learning impaired children might become successful students. In this section, suggestions are outlined for (a) teacher contributions, (b) teacher or context related variables, and (c) child contributions to the process of fostering a better match between teacher talk and child listening. The categories of language use, content, and form are used to outline the suggestions within each section.

Teacher Contributions

In order to study the problems a language-learning impaired child is having in a particular classroom, teachers and special educators are urged to use videotaped or audiotaped samples of classroom interactions. Such samples can yield insights about points of completed communication events, points of failure of communication, and points where communication occurred, but where the meanings apparently received by one or more of the students were not the same as those intended by the teacher.

When reviewing a tape or its transcription, it is useful to go over it several times: the first time listening or looking for examples of language use, next considering content, and finally analyzing aspects of language form that appear to act as obstacles or facilitators of communication. Taping one hour of classroom interaction on a monthly or bimonthly basis gives teachers a chance to observe changes in their own communication skills as well as those of their students. The transcripts yield a variety of types of information. Although it would be overwhelming to try to do an exhaustive analysis, examples of areas that may be selected based on particular questions of interest posed by the teacher and other educational personnel are summarized here.

Analyzing Language Use

1. Count the number of conversational turns taken by the teacher and the students and compute the proportions for various types of events. There are no "right" or "wrong" proportions, but the teacher could take a look at what is occurring and question whether what is occurring is optimal for the purpose of the moment or whether improvements could be made. Focus could also be directed at determining whether particular students take too many or too few turns.

2. Study the kinds of intentional communicative acts performed by the teacher and the students (particularly those involving the child who is having difficulty) using either Dore's (1979) categories of (conveying

content, regulating conversation, or expressing attitude) or Sinclair and Coulthard's (1975) categories (labeling, responding, acknowledging, and evaluating). A new set of categories could also be created to fit the sample itself.

3. Examine aspects of the teacher's verbal and nonverbal style that may unintentionally be conveying negative evaluative judgments.

4. Analyze the degree to which requests are directly or indirectly expressed, such as, "Please be quiet so I can hear Susan's question" (stated directly), as opposed to, "I didn't hear Susan's question because some people were talking" (stated indirectly), remembering that "polite-indirect" requests are often more difficult for language-learning impaired children to comprehend (Vetter, 1982).

Analyzing Language Content

1. Focus on identifying meanings that are relatively more "situated" (i.e., context bound) versus those that are relatively more "lexicalized" (i.e., context free) and therefore likely to be more difficult for children who are language impaired. For example, two third grade teachers presented two different types of activities with different styles of language, one teacher using language that was highly context-bound to introduce a math lesson, saying:

"The blue line's on top / Put your finger on 7 / on the blue line / on top."

Another teacher used highly lexicalized and metalinguistic meanings in a language lesson:

"Sometimes it's easier if we pick / one noun / and we put an adjective with it / Because we can think of lots of adjectives that can describe one noun / where it might be difficult to think of an adjective to describe another noun"
(Nelson, 1984, p. 168).

Neither of these methods is inherently "better" than the other. The point is that either lesson may present difficulties to the language-learning impaired child, and for different reasons.

2. Consider how much of the curriculum requires students to use metalinguistic levels of processing. An example would be the second sample of teacher talk quoted above.

3. Look at teacher-student interactions in which new information is introduced and analyze how comprehension is probed. For example, are questions asked at a variety of levels that require varying cognitive organizational strategies, and does the teacher match the cognitive demands of questions with the cognitive skills of students? To be specific, does the teacher ask some "product-oriented" (who, what, where, when) questions that elicit key factual information and direct these to students who appear to have less well developed cognitive strategies and also ask some "process-

oriented" (how, why) questions that allow other students to draw inferences and perform logical operations on the material?

4. Analyze teacher methods for checking that students have understood the content presented. In classroom settings it is tempting to use the positive acknowledgments of just a few students to confirm that all students have understood a particular explanation or assignment. What strategies of verbal and nonverbal checking has the teacher developed to ensure that the least capable child or language-learning impaired student has understood the topic or directions in addition to the academically achieving child?

Analyzing Language Form

1. Perform an informal analysis of linguistic complexity used by the teacher. Determine the relative use of simple sentences (those with only one subject and one verb), compound sentences (those with two main clauses that are combined with a conjunction like "and," "but," or "or"), and complex sentences (those with one sentence embedded in another, conjoined with conjunctions like "before," "while," "except," or relative pronouns like "who," "which," or "that").

2. Determine if the teacher offers students an array of verbal and nonverbal stimuli (skillful teachers often do this at an empathic level). For example, are explanations clearly marked with discourse devices like, "Now listen everyone, . . . ," and produced with clear pauses (called "phrase junctures") that surround the essential information? One might also consider whether important content is presented at slower speaking rates, with key ideas encoded using less complex sentence structures and major points spoken with contrastive stress.

3. Note whether or not students are gradually introduced to more complex sentence structures and more lexicalized meanings. For example, a teacher who uses a complex sentence structure to present some new information may then rephrase the information using more simple structure. For example, she might start by saying, "Except for whales, elephants are the largest mammals," and then continue, saying, "You see, elephants are very big, but whales are even bigger. There are no animals bigger than whales."

4. Consider the degree to which the teacher varies form of messages to introduce more abstract concepts that may not be the central focus of the lesson, but may be at the "developing edge of competence" and within the reach of some of the students. For example, in the sequence about elephants and whales, the category of "mammal" could be explored further, asking students to name some other mammals. This was the type

of focusing strategy Mishler (1972) suggested that one of the teachers he observed used effectively (see the section on language content in teacher talk, earlier in this chapter). Are specialized devices of language form used to mark the difference between essential information, such as "Now this is the most important thing. . .," and optional information, such as, "You might also want to think about. . ."? Although language-learning impaired children usually do not automatically take advantage of such markers when they occur, special intervention may enable them to benefit from such focusing strategies if they are a part of the teacher's usual discourse style.

A Review of Teacher and Context Related Variables

By combining consideration of such linguistic variables as sentence length and complexity with consideration of such supralinguistic variables as speaking rate, pause placement, and hesitation phenomena, decisions can be made about which strategies the teacher is already using well and which might be altered to benefit the student. Although individualization within the group context is the ideal, with different strategies being adapted to the needs of different students, this may be difficult to achieve. Most students benefit from the meaningful placement of pauses and the use of contrastive stress and varied speaking rate to signal new or especially important information. Such techniques can be used in classrooms without penalizing either the language proficient or language impaired students in those rooms.

Room acoustics are also an important area of consideration (Ross, 1978; Smyth, 1979) when analyzing the interacting effects of teacher and environmental variables on the performance abilities of language-learning impaired children. High rates of reverberation, which result in an echoing effect, adversely affect signal-to-noise ratios and may make it particularly difficult for some children to attend and to comprehend lesson content. To measure classroom acoustics objectively, audiologists may be sought to assist teachers. Objective ratings are obtained using sound level meters. In rooms that are particularly "bouncy" with respect to sound, absorptive material may be applied to the walls to reduce the amount of extraneous noise that could interfere with reception and perception of the teacher's instructional language. For example, carpet squares applied to portable room dividers or to classroom walls are effective. Other creative options may also be explored. As another example, it was possible to reduce the noise characteristics in one classroom by about 10 decibels (dB) merely by thumbtacking plastic apple packing dividers (which look like oversized egg cartons) to the bulletin board strip around the top of the chalkboard that encircled the room. School board members may also be more willing to pay for carpeting the floor of a classroom in a noisy old building if it is presented as a need for "sound treatment," as opposed to "looking good."

Another way of creating a more favorable signal-to-noise ratio is to use a standard public address system within a classroom. One school district in southern Illinois (Wabash and Ohio Valley Special Education District, 1980) found dramatically positive results for all students, not just the learning disabled ones, by amplifying the speech of a classroom teacher who presented the standard curriculum. While amplification could also be accomplished by providing FM transmitter units to teachers and fitting individual students with receivers, as is done with some hearing impaired students, this is far more expensive than the loudspeaker system found effective in Illinois. The loudspeaker system is also consistent with the federal requirements that all handicapped children be educated in the "least restrictive environment," since children using such a system are educated almost entirely within regular classroom settings.

Child Contributions

A language-learning impaired student's Individualized Education Plan (IEP) specifies the services that are considered most appropriate in serving that student's particular educational needs. Various combinations of placements in regular and special education classrooms and speech-language pathology services may be designed. The "least restrictive" educational environment provides an opportunity for the child to be educated with peers to the maximum extent possible. The child's IEP also specifies what special education programming is to be provided in individual or small group contexts to develop abilities that are deficient or otherwise interfering with the child's functioning. Attempts are made to identify factors in the areas of both language competence and language performance.

All children who are having comprehension difficulties in the classroom should have thorough audiologic examinations as part of their original assessments and should have follow-up monitoring if they exhibit even "mild" (15 to 20 dB) hearing losses. Children who are not hearing well, even if their losses are mild, have an extra disadvantage on top of "wobbly" language competencies that make it especially difficult for them to process the language of the classroom. It is generally necessary for language-learning impaired children to have clearer speech signals in order to understand spoken language. The fuzzy or muffled signals that accompany conductive hearing loss accentuate the listening problems these children have, and it is important to try to prevent them from occurring.

The special education programming for a language-learning impaired child is based on a comprehensive view of the child's abilities and areas of difficulty that will assist in planning activities to develop the child's ability to process aspects of language use, content, or form so that they will be more compatible with teacher talk. Activities might be planned in any of the following areas:

Developing Language Use

1. A dialogue approach, such as that described by Blank (1973), may provide the most effective format for intervention. In this approach, adults use carefully structured experiences and requests in a conversational format to help students acquire uses of language, particularly for manipulating abstract content.

2. Conversation between adult and child can be structured to elicit improved pragmatic communicative behaviors, such as turn-taking, topic-maintenance (Miller, 1978), or understanding indirect requests. Occasions may be constructed that require the use and interpretation of such rules, first in more direct forms, and gradually in more indirect ones.

3. Particular communicative functions may be identified that are difficult for the students to use, such as requesting clarification when they do not know what to do, or providing clarification to listeners as necessary.

Developing Language Content

1. A need for traditional "vocabulary" training may be indicated by formal evaluation procedures. Examples would be problems with (a) prepositional or relational terms like "many-few" and "largest-smallest," (b) words that are used to convey abstract attributes, such as "shy" or "elusive," (c) words that may have multiple meanings, like "broke" and "state," (d) words that may have figurative meanings in addition to their concrete meanings, such as "to eye something one wants to buy," or to make a school project "shine," (e) words that have more concrete referents but are unfamiliar to the student, like "auditorium" or "wigwam," and (f) morphologic units that must be bound to other words but affect word meaning, such as "un-," "dis-," "-tion," and "-ly."

2. Beyond the word level, activities may be designed to help the child develop competence with conversational units that are increasingly complex and context free. For example, on a relatively concrete level, the child might be given practice in completing workbook-like activities using the instructional language of classrooms (Rush, 1977), such as, "Draw a circle around the largest number."

3. For developing higher order semantic organizational abilities, the Boning (1976) Specific Skills Series provides individual exercises for developing written language comprehension and may also be adapted for oral language interaction. A variety of skills is covered, including "Getting the Main Idea" and "Mastering Multiple Meanings."

4. Westby (1984 and Chapter 7 in the companion volume, *Communication Skills and Classroom Success: Therapy Methodologies for Language-Learning Disabled Students*) has suggested ways in which children's own narrative skills may be developed for facilitating their comprehension of textual material.

5. Older children and elementary, junior high, and secondary school students need to be given assistance to develop outlining and notetaking skills.

Developing Language Form

1. Activities can be designed to develop those articulatory, morphological, and syntactical abilities that have been identified as deficient in individualized assessment.

2. In the areas of language form, it is often appropriate to design more structured activities (Nelson, 1979). Multiple opportunities are provided to practice producing syllables, words, phrases, and sentences that exemplify regularities of target phonemes, morphemes, or structures.

3. Opportunities for using new language forms also need to be woven into more naturalistic settings to become automatic, and classrooms are important contexts for doing this (Nelson, 1981).

4. Developing language expression skills has also been found to be a facilitator of language comprehension, even when the problems of comprehension are subtle. For example, Tyack (1981) worked with a 10 year old child whose problems in comprehending classroom instruction and written textual material were related to failure to acquire the rules for forming complex sentences. The intervention program Tyack described included practice in formulating complex sentences of a variety of types as well as practice in comprehending them, and the results were positive in both areas.

SUMMARY AND CONCLUSIONS

In this chapter, a variety of variables in both teacher talk and child listening have been reviewed that affect the relative difficulties language-learning impaired children experience in classroom settings. Suggestions have been presented for adjusting (1) aspects of teacher discourse and (2) environmental characteristics to assist children to compensate for problems of language performance. Suggestions have also been made for providing intervention that will strengthen (3) the child's basic language competence in the areas of use, content, and form. The rationale for this approach is that more firmly established competence for the rules of language provides an active component of processing systems to make them more resistant to outside interference.

The above suggestions are far from exhaustive. They are provided primarily as examples. This chapter concludes with a restatement of the earlier caution to view any suggestions not as general prescriptions, but as areas to consider in analyzing the individual characteristics of teacher talk, child listening, and learning contexts to foster a better match.

REFERENCES

Allen, D. I. (1970). Some effects of advance organizers and level of question on the learning and retention of written social studies material. *Journal of Educational Psychology, 61*, 333–339.

Ausubel, D. P. (1960). The use of advance organizers in the learning and retention of meaningful verbal material. *Journal of Educational Psychology, 51*, 267–272.

Blank, M. (1973). *Teaching learning in the preschool: A dialogue approach.* Columbus, OH: Charles E. Merrill.

Bloom, L., and Lahey, M. (1978). *Language development and language disorders.* New York: John Wiley & Sons.

Boning, R. A. (1976). *Specific skill series* (2nd ed.). New York: Barnell Loft, Ltd.

Brophy, J. E., and Good, T. L. (1970). Teachers' communication of differential expectations for children's classroom performance. *Journal of Educational Psychology, 61*, 365–374.

Bruner, J. S. The act of discovery (1965). *On knowing: Essays for the left hand.* Cambridge, MA: Harvard University Press.

Burton, D. (1981). The sociolinguistic analysis of spoken discourse. In P. French and M. MacLure (Eds.), *Adult-child conversation.* New York: St. Martin's Press.

Cook-Gumperz, J. (1977). Situated instructions: Language socialization of school age children. In S. Ervin-Tripp and C. Mitchell-Kernan (Eds.), *Child discourse.* New York: Academic Press.

Cuda, R. A. (1976). Analysis of speaking rate, syntactic complexity and speaking style of public school teachers (unpublished master's thesis). Wichita, KS: Wichita State University.

Cuda, R. A., and Nelson, N. W. (1976). Analysis of teacher speaking rate, syntactic complexity and hesitation phenomena as a function of grade level. Paper presented at the annual meeting of the American Speech-Language-Hearing Association, Houston, TX.

DeStefano, J. S. (1978). *Language, the learner and the school.* New York: John Wiley & Sons.

Dore, J. (1979). Conversation and preschool language development. In P. Fletcher and M. Garman (Eds.), *Language acquisition.* Cambridge, MA: Cambridge University Press.

Duncan, L. (1984). When smart kids can't learn: A mother's painful search for answers. *Ladies' Home Journal, 101* (2), 64, 163–164.

Gerber, A. (1981). Problems in the processing and use of language in education. In A. Gerber and D. N. Bryer (Eds.), *Language and learning disabilities.* Baltimore: University Park Press.

Goodman, K. S. (1973). Psycholinguistic universals in the reading process. In F. Smith (Ed.). *Psycholinguistics and reading.* New York: Holt, Rinehart and Winston.

Griffin, K., and Hannah, L. (1960). A study of the results of an extremely short instructional unit in listening. *Journal of Communication, 10,* 135–139.

Hammersley, M. (1981). Putting competence into action: Some sociological notes on a model of classroom interaction. In P. French and M. MacLure (Eds.), *Adult-child conversation.* New York: St. Martin's Press.

Hedberg, N. L. (1982). Language learning disabilities appraisal: Bottom-up and top-down processing. *Communicative Disorders, 7*(4), 45–59.

Hymes, D. (1972). Introduction. In C. B. Cazden, V. P. John, and D. Hymes (Eds.), *Functions of language in the classroom.* New York: Teachers College Press.

Loban, W. (1963). The Language of Elementary School Children. National Council of Teachers of English Research, No. 1. Champaign, IL: National Council of Teachers of English.

Macmillan Reading. Series R workbook. (1983). *You can, I can too, we can read.* New York: Macmillan.

McDermott, R. P. (1977). Social relations as contexts for learning in school. *Harvard Educational Review, 47,* 198–213.

Miller, L. (1978). Pragmatics and early childhood language disorders. *Journal of Speech and Hearing Disorders, 43,* 419–436.

Mishler, E. G. (1972). Implications of teacher strategies for language and cognition: Observations in first-grade classrooms. In C. Cazden, V. P. John, and D. Hymes (Eds.), *Functions of language in the classroom.* New York: Teachers College Press.

Mishler, E. G. (1975). Studies in dialogue and discourse. II. Types of discourse initiated and sustained through questioning. *Journal of Psycholinguistic Research, 4,* 99–121.

Nelson, N. W. (1979). *Planning individualized speech and language intervention programs.* Tucson, AZ: Communication Skill Builders.

Nelson, N. W. (1981). An eclectic model of language intervention for disorders of listening, speaking, reading and writing. *Topics in Language Disorders, 1,* 1–24.

Nelson, N. W. (1984). Beyond information processing: The language of teachers and textbooks. In G. Wallach and K. G. Butler (Eds.), *Language learning disabilities in school-aged children.* Baltimore: Williams & Wilkins.

Phillips, J. (1973). Syntax and vocabulary of mothers' speech to young children: Age and sex comparisons. *Child Development, 44,* 182–185.

Rees, N. (1973). Auditory processing factors in language disorders: The view from Procrustes' bed. *Journal of Speech and Hearing Disorders, 38,* 304–315.

Rees, N., and Shulman, M. (1978). I don't understand what you mean by comprehension. *Journal of Speech and Hearing Disorders, 48,* 208–219.

Ross, M. (1978). Classroom acoustics and speech intelligibility. In J. Katz (Ed.), *Handbook of clinical audiology* (2nd ed.). Baltimore: Williams & Wilkins Company.

Rosenthal, R., and Jacobson, L. (1968). *Pygmalion in the classroom: Teacher expectations and pupils' intellectual development.* New York: Holt, Rinehart and Winston.

Rush, M. L. (1977). *The language of directions.* Washington, DC: Alexander Graham Bell Association for the Deaf.

Simon, C. S. (1981). *Communicative competence: A functional-pragmatic approach to language therapy.* Tucson, AZ: Communication Skill Builders.

Sinclair, J. McH., and Coulthard, R. M. (1975). *Towards an analysis of discourse.* London: Oxford University Press.

Slobin, D. I. (1971). *Psycholinguistics.* Danville, IL: Scott, Foresman and Company.

Smith, F. (1975). *Comprehension and learning.* New York: Holt, Rinehart and Winston.

Smyth, V. (1979). Speech reception in the presence of classroom noise. *Language, Speech, and Hearing Services in Schools, 10,* 221–230.

Snow, C. (1977). The development of conversation between mothers and babies. *Journal of Child Language, 4,* 1–22.

Stein, N. L., and Glenn, C. G. (1979). An analysis of story comprehension in elementary school children. In R. O. Freedle (Ed.), *New directions in discourse processing* (Vol. II). Norwood, NJ: Ablex.

Thompson, J. J. (1969). *Instructional communication.* New York: Van Nostrand Reinhold Company.

Tough, J. (1977). *Talking and learning.* London: Drake Education Associates.

Tyack, D. L. (1981). Teaching complex sentences. *Language, Speech, and Hearing Services in Schools, 12,* 44–48.

van Kleeck, A. (1984). Metalinguistics and language disorders in children: Does meta- matter? In G. P. Wallach and K. G. Butler (Eds.), *Language learning disabilities in school-age children.* Baltimore: Williams & Wilkins.

Vaughn-Cooke, F. B. (1983). Improving language assessment in minority children. *ASHA, 25,* 29–34.

Vetter, D. K. (1982). Language disorders and schooling. *Topics in Language Disorders, 2*(4), 13–19.

Wabash and Ohio Valley Special Education District (1980). (F. E. Glassford, Director, Norris City, IL.) *Mainstream amplification resource room study (MARRS).* Paper presented at the annual meeting of the American Speech-Language-Hearing Association, Detroit, MI.

Wallach, G. P., (1984). Later language learning: Syntactic structures and strategies. In G. P. Wallach and K. G. Butler (Eds.), *Language learning disabilities in school-age children.* Baltimore: Williams & Wilkins.

Westby, C. E. (1984). Development of narrative language abilities. In G. P. Wallach and K. G. Butler (Eds.), *Language, learning disabilities in school age children.* Baltimore: Williams & Wilkins.

White, S. H. (1980). Cognitive competence and performance in everyday environments. *Bulletin of the Orton Society, 30,* 29–45.

Wilkinson, L. C., Hiebert, E., and Rembold, K. (1981). Parents' and peers communication to toddlers. *Journal of Speech and Hearing Research, 24,* 383–388.

Willes, M. (1981). Learning to take part in classroom interaction. In P. French and M. MacLure (Eds.), *Adult-child conversation.* New York: St. Martins' Press.

APPENDIX 3-1

ANALYSIS CHECKLIST
FOR CLASSROOM INTERACTIONS

This informal assessment protocol is designed for use by teachers and communication consultants who wish to foster better matches between teacher talk and child listening by analyzing current situations so that they may adjust the environment and provide individualized intervention when indicated.

1. How complex are the teacher's messages?
   a. How often is information embedded in complex sentences that violate expected subject-verb-object word order or have other complexities?
   b. How concrete or abstract is the vocabulary used, and what contextual cues are provided to make new word meanings clear?
   c. How many meaning segments are provided when the teacher gives directions?
2. How much background or contextual support is available?
   a. Is there any experience base for the content being covered?
   b. Does the child know the classroom routine so that certain directions can be predicted?
   c. Are pictures or demonstrations included as comprehension aids?
3. How much repetition or revision of a message is built into teacher talk, and how much does the child seem to benefit from such verbal input?
   a. Does the child act only after observing what others are doing?
   b. Does the child ask clarification questions?
   c. Does the child seem to act on an intuitive sense about what is expected, and if so, how effective does this strategy appear to be?
   d. Does the child appear to give up when the listening demands become too great?
4. Are the regularities of classroom interactions and expectations understood by the child?
   a. Has direct teaching taken place to acquaint the child with classroom routines?
   b. Is the child expected to grasp intuitively and then remember what is appropriate and expected?
   c. Is the student prepared for transition from one expectation to another?

d. Does the teacher always assume the leader or control role, or does he or she sometimes shift to being a resource of information and check to see whether the information has been assimilated?

5. What is the child's general attitude toward school, the classroom, the teacher, pursuing a curriculum and interacting or competing on a substantive level with peers?
   a. What are the child's attitudes in these areas compared with nonacademic attitudes?
   b. What do the child's assumptions appear to be?
   c. What are the child's expectations?

6. Does the teacher assume the students comprehend the nature of the task or are discussion probes developed so that student or teacher expectations can be clarified?
   a. Is the topic for the discussion introduced?
   b. Do the students know why they are doing the task?
   c. Do they have requisite skills to perform the task?
   d. Are they allowed a "question or clarification" period rather than being expected to show complete comprehension immediately or being penalized for asking clarification questions?

7. Are both teacher and students aware of nonverbal communication that relays attitudes and expectations?
   a. Does the teacher monitor vocal tone, body stance, and proximity to students during instruction?
   b. Is the student aware of how nonverbal behaviors communicate attitudes and expectations to the teacher?

8. On a continuum between "direct authoritarian" and "guidance-oriented" styles, where could the teacher's style be rated?
   a. When a child does not follow a "guidance-oriented" approach, is the ability to comprehend indirect regulatory requests considered?
   b. Does the child realize that commands can be stated as imperatives, suggestions, or questions?
   c. Does the teacher use the same style consistently or vary the style?
   d. Are variations in style designed to facilitate students' comprehension or are they merely reflections of the teacher's mood that day?

9. In reviewing evidence of a child's performance, does there seem to be a pattern of successes and failures?
   a. Can a relationship be established with a particular teacher personality type, linguistic accent, or class size?
   b. Do difficulties relate to newness of task demands?
   c. Does success vary depending on whether or not the material being covered relates directly to the student's experiences or interests?

d. Does success relate to the intrinsic cognitive demands of the subject being studied?

10. Does the teacher prepare the students for switching from thinking about language as a mode of communication to viewing it as an object of discussion (e.g., thinking about the beginning sounds of words)?
    a. Does the teacher engage in task analysis to determine the types of knowledge and abilities each lesson demands?
    b. Are students given transitional statements as the teacher switches from talking about words, to sounds, to letters representing sounds?
    c. Do the students understand the underlying definitions and concepts for such exercises as "sound blending" and "homonym" identification?

11. Does the teacher provide some cognitive organization of a topic domain before launching into specific content related to the topic?
    a. Have students had an opportunity to share their conceptualization of certain words or story passages?
    b. Has the teacher provided an overview of the topic and included comparisons of how content is similar to experiences the students have had?
    c. Is an overall "schema" developed that is the result of combining past experiences, conceptions, inferences, and expectations?
    d. Are students directed toward the most important features and vocabulary of the learning experience, or are they expected to distinguish essential from supportive or irrelevant material on their own (this might be a skill that could be addressed directly in intervention, if lacking)?
    e. Is teaching style didactic, or does it encourage listener participation in testing hypotheses and alternative views or solutions?
    f. Is the student able to participate in and profit from an active involvement in learning, or does the student exhibit difficulty in engaging in this type of give-and-take educational interaction?

12. Does the teacher modulate speaking rate and inflection during instruction?
    a. Is the rate slowed as new information is presented?
    b. Are there pauses between major segments of information?
    c. Is the rate comfortable enough that the teacher does not have to revise content midphrase or use vocal fillers during delivery?
    d. Is vocal inflection varied to provide emphasis or communicate mood?

13. What is the quality of the listening environment?
    a. What is the amount of competing noise from outside sources?

  b. How much reverberation of sounds that are generated by classroom activity occurs?

  c. Are there variations in teacher volume depending on the size of the group?

  d. Can the child attend to directions when nearby conversations are in progress?

14. What factors are considered in observing a child's comprehension?

  a. Is the size of the unit to be comprehended considered?

  b. Is listening measured in naturalistic contexts or in unusually quiet contexts?

  c. Does the child have verbal and nonverbal means of letting others know he or she does not understand something?

15. Is it possible to isolate and describe a student's language processing problems related to contextual and complexity variables?

  a. Is auditory attention observed in a variety of contexts for a variety of tasks?

  b. How good is the student's memory for auditory input of a variety of types?

  c. What evidence is there that the student is able to perform auditory sequencing in such tasks as (1) saying multisyllabic words, (2) spelling, and (3) formulating expression in speaking and writing?

  d. What evidence exists regarding the child's auditory discrimination abilities in quiet and in noise, for longer utterances as well as individual words, and for detecting first, last, and middle sounds in workbook type activities (recognizing the metalinguistic nature of such tasks)?

16. Is there some adaptability in teacher style to accommodate students' problems?

  a. What checking and facilitating strategies are used for students who have difficulty remembering multilevel directives (possibilities include writing assignments on the chalkboard, tape recording instructions, and checking over notes)?

  b. When multiple bits of pertinent factual information are embedded in a series of complex sentences, does the teacher provide enough processing time, review, and checking to ensure that students do not feel lost?

  c. Is there an awareness that some students may understand simple sentences stated in active voice, but not those stated in passive voice or sentences with such clausal connectors as "although," "except," and "however" that affect the relational meanings expressed within the sentence?

  d. Are there strategies for assisting students to relate new information with information they have stored in long-term memory?

17. In analyzing a student's knowledge of the rules of language *use,* are rules for how language is used to communicate for various purposes and in various contexts considered?
    a. Does the child observe conventions for turn-taking during class discussions?
    b. Is the child capable of distinguishing (and complying with) teacher talk intended to regulate behavior from that for conveying subject matter?
    c. Does the student comprehend both direct and indirect ways a teacher can tell students to do something?
    d. Does the child seem to be aware of circumstances in which responses should be verbal (e.g., when a choral response is expected or in one-to-one dialogue) and those in which they should be nonverbal (e.g., when raising one's hand to be called on or during seatwork)?
    e. Does the child ask clarification questions to fill in details missed, and does the teacher have a method for allowing these in a minimally disruptive way (perhaps assigning a "buddy" to be available to answer the student's questions of a limited number)?
18. In analyzing a student's knowledge of language *content,* are meaning units of a variety of size and types considered?
    a. Are there multiple-meaning words in the textual material and, if so, does the student understand the meaning per context?
    b. Can the student categorize concepts efficiently and do so in a systematic way?
    c. Does the student comprehend figurative language?
    d. Can the student go beyond what is directly stated in content and make inferences?
    e. Can the student demonstrate his or her knowledge of such metalinguistic concepts as homonyms and antonyms by giving examples of each and describing the characteristics of each?
    f. Does the student relate new information with content studied a few days (or hours) earlier?
19. In analyzing the student's knowledge of the rules of language *form,* are syntactic, morphological, and phonological rules considered for both oral and written language?
    a. Does the student comprehend multilevel directions stated in complex syntax?
    b. Can the student make sound-symbol associations?
    c. Can the student use sequences of sounds and syllables based on phonics rules to "sound out" new words?
    d. Do the student's reading, speaking, writing, and spelling errors provide useful information about his or her linguistic processing abilities?

20. Is a team approach to intervention a real possibility?
    a. Do regular and special education administration systems support this kind of ecological approach to improving communication in classrooms, and are positive attempts being made to enlist their help and keep them informed?
    b. Are parents and children enlisted as active partners in identifying points of communicative mismatch and fostering improvements?

TRANSITIONAL NOTE

Anytime we can break a phenomenon into its component parts, we can analyze not only the dynamic interrelationships among components but also the integrity of any one component. Analysis heightens awareness. Increased awareness leads to better monitoring or modification of teaching style and provides guidelines for helping students prepare for the educational setting. When educators monitor and modify behavioral and situation components, they can share the reasons for doing so with the student. At the same time, students need to become more aware of what the educational context expects of them. A rationale, then, for developmental programming or the development of compensatory strategies, or both, can be based on a sensitive analysis of interacting factors in the educational context. Nelson, in Chapter 3, has made a comprehensive analysis of these factors and has provided educators with a list of questions to pose regarding the student's behavior, the curriculum content, the context, and instructional practices.

Creaghead and Tattershall, in Chapter 4, also consider possible mismatches between the teacher, the curriculum, and the textbook expectations, as well as the child's perception and awareness of the "student role." There are certain aspects of the student role that are quite different from the "child role." An example would be raising your hand if you want to say something. This signal is expected by the teacher; it allows the teacher to maintain control over a group of 30 to 40 individuals. In other types of conversation, however, such a large number of people do not participate, so the signal is not needed. The student must learn that raising one's hand is an expected behavior preliminary to expressing one's thoughts in the classroom setting. This action signals the teacher that the child wants to participate, and it also permits the teacher to control *when* the child will participate.

This example is only one of many rules that are part of the "school game." Learning to play the school game is an important factor in classroom success and in acquiring a positive self-image as a student. The more familiar we are with situational expectations or social rules of a context, the more likely we are to appear competent and successful. Creaghead and Tattershall outline features of classroom interactions and behavioral expectations based upon "scenarios." Scenarios are useful to people because they allow us to predict what will happen and what is expected. We have an "airport scenario," for example that allows us to predict how much time we need to complete the check-in procedure, go through security, get a boarding pass, and prepare for departure. If a child knows the "classroom scenario" in contrast to the "baseball game scenario" or the "going to the movies scenario," it will be possible to enter the classroom with an implicit understanding of what is expected. In addition, with increased exposure to a particular contextual scenario, students learn to refine the "school scenario" to accommodate differences in teaching style or subject content.

In the following chapter, the reader will be able to look at the nature of classroom pragmatics through a fresh pair of spectacles; it will be possible to rethink some basic expectations and assumptions on which adults act. Doing so raises an individual's level of sensitivity so that he or she begins to look at students from *their* side of the teacher's desk. This fresh view can have a direct impact on the types of systematic observations made about the level of sophistication of a student's classroom scenario. Once analyzed, behaviors and concepts that are necessary but not yet developed can be incorporated into the student's educational programming objectives.

CHAPTER 4

Observation and Assessment of Classroom Pragmatic Skills

Nancy A. Creaghead
and
Sandra S. Tattershall

A sixth grade teacher was asked the following question in early September, "What is the hardest thing about starting school?" Her answer was, "Teaching the children my routine."

When children enter school, they must learn how to be students, how to operate in a new situation. Many children function well in school, but there are those who never seem to know "When to say or do what, to whom and how much," to paraphrase Hymes (1971). In order to identify and help these children, we need to specify the pragmatic requirements of classrooms.

Teachers frequently complain about students' inability to follow directions, to understand abstract language, to learn the classroom routine, or to complete tasks independently. Mehan (1979) observed that classroom lessons have overall organizational schemes and specific interactional sequences that require certain behaviors and communication skills from children—i.e., learning the routine. In light of the apparent school requirements, what are the skills that children need in order to function effectively? These skills include the ability to make appropriate presuppositions about school and what is required to succeed there; to predict content in oral and written communication based on available clues; to sample effectively from the school environment; and to correctly confirm or deny their predictions.

We have chosen to discuss three underlying competencies in order to illustrate the interaction between these communication skills and effective learning in school:

1. Understanding of classroom routine and other specific formats for school conversations and written material.
2. Ability to follow and give oral and written directions.
3. Ability to comprehend and use nonliteral language.

UNDERSTANDING FORMATS FOR CLASSROOM COMMUNICATION

One thing that we need to know about children who are having difficulty in school is whether or not they appreciate and can make predictions based on the overall schemas of various communication situations. It is important for children to be familiar with these formats and to know the classroom routine and expectations. This will make them more comfortable in school, and they will be evaluated more positively by teachers. Some oral communication formats include (1) parties, (2) meetings, (3) interviews, (4) classrooms, (5) home, (6) talking to close friends, and (7) talking to strangers. Written communication formats include (1) stories, (2) poems, (3) textbooks, (4) formal letters, (5) friendly letters, and (6) memos.

Classroom Routines

Schultz (1979) states that "the task faced by children entering school for the first time is . . . to figure out what the appropriate contexts are for interaction and to figure out what behavior is considered appropriate in each of the different contexts" (p. 272). He suggests that teachers may expect children to know these rules early in the school year. He gives the example of a kindergarten child who was evaluated by the teacher as being naive and immature because she was unable to follow certain classroom procedures by the fourth day of school.

A brief case study may help to illustrate the importance of knowing and attending to the school routine. Walter is an example of a preschool child with normal intelligence who is already exhibiting difficulty in this area. In his very structured nursery school, the teacher's daily routine for recess is to announce to the children that as she calls their names, they should put on their coats and get in line for recess. Then she calls the children's names one by one; they go to their lockers, put on their coats, and get in line. Except for Walter. When his name is called, he is not attending; even when the teacher gets his attention, Walter does nothing. When she tells him to go to his locker, he does that, but does not put on his coat. At each step, the teacher must provide the next direction in the original sequence. This preschooler is very likely to have difficulty in school. Compare his responses to those of a four year old girl who learned an important part of the nursery school routine on the very first day of school. When her mother asked, "What did you do at school today?", she replied, "We learned to sit in rows." In other words, there are some children who seem to intuitively abstract school rules from the very beginning. In contrast there are children with maturation, attention, or memory problems who do not.

Mehan (1979) suggests that classroom lessons have an overall structure that requires specific types of interactional skills on the part of the student. The rules for classroom interaction may be different from the rules for conversations outside of school. Mehan suggests two differences. First, turn taking in school is different from turn taking in conversations. In conversation, it is possible that the current speaker may select the next speaker, but more frequently, the next speaker is self-nominated. In classroom interaction, however, the next speaker is almost always selected by the teacher, which allows him or her to keep control over the lesson. Second, conversations generally include a two part interaction sequence. One participant may ask a question and the other responds. In school, we see a three part sequence wherein the teacher asks a question, the child responds, and the teacher evaluates the response.

In order to function well in school, children must be able to follow these and other classroom interaction rules. Mehan notes further that children must integrate rules about appropriate classroom form with appropriate content. Consider the child who knows the correct interactional rules, but who does not know the answers. He may raise his hand every time the teacher asks a question, but when called upon say, "I forget." On the other hand, there are also children who know the answer but fail to raise their hands before giving it. Both responses may be evaluated negatively by the teacher, but for different reasons.

The child faces additional problems in figuring out the rules for interaction at school. For example, Green and Wallat (1979) state that the context that determines appropriate interaction coincides with the overall structure of lessons only on a gross level. In other words, the overall structure of a reading lesson may be as follows: The children read a story in their readers. When finished, the teacher asks each child a question which he or she answers orally. The rules for appropriate behavior may change depending on whether the child has had his or her turn, whether he or she knows the answer, or whether or not the answer he or she provides is correct. In this case following the rules requires on-the-spot analysis and adjustment. The context is always changing because it is being created by the participants as they interact.

Other classroom rules are tacit and therefore never communicated directly to the students. In one author's grade school, the superintendent came around to each class every year before Halloween to spell out the rules about vandalizing school property, and again on the day of the first snow to give the rules about throwing snowballs. He was never seen the rest of the year, which means that no such edicts were given for a multitude of other rules governing day to day conduct. Students are unlikely to be given explicit directions on such things as how to address the principal, when a question may be asked, or when and how often it is possible to tease the teacher.

Finally, in addition to the above problems, rules may be not only tacit but also ambiguous to the student (Mehan, 1979). Mehan gives the example that the child must determine when the teacher's "you" means that a certain child should respond and when it means that the invitation is open to all. For example, if the teacher says, "You may go to the library now," the child must be attentive to cues in the overall context in order to determine whether the teacher means the whole class, another child, or the individual himself.

In a research project, the authors of this chapter asked third grade children questions about the rules in their classroom and the behaviors which they thought were pleasing or irritating to their teacher. We found that the children agreed that not talking was the most important rule and that the teacher was most pleased with nontalkers and most irritated with talkers. The children were also able to agree on the teacher's behavior when irritated and on her strategies for keeping order. It is clear that most children learn both the stated and the unstated rules of school easily. Other children may not be able to attend to rules given to the class as a whole, may be unable to generalize stated rules to new situations, or may not use nonverbal and verbal cues for learning unstated rules.

Other Formats

Knowledge of classroom formats is of utmost importance for school-age children, but this information is not sufficient for children's successful participation in all aspects of school life. For example, children must also have routines or scenarios for social interaction with peers on the playground and in the cafeteria, for talking to the principal, and for interacting with their teachers.

These different types of communication interactions have unique frameworks, which Lund and Duchan (1983) call speech event frames. The frame will determine the specific roles of the participants and the appropriate behaviors for opening and closing the event as well as the appropriate interaction throughout. Schank and Abelson (1977) use the term "script" for the general organization of speech events, such as going to a restaurant. Children must acquire various new scripts for school. They construct these scripts on the basis of their experiences, and, in turn, the scripts guide their expectations in future situations of the same type.

It has been demonstrated that children do develop these scripts. For example, three and four year old children have an overall structure for discourse in conversations (Keenan, 1974; Lindfors, 1980). Children as young as two years of age have begun to modify their patterns of speech depending on the age of the listener, and by four and five years, they have a variety of formats for speaking to listeners of different ages (Ervin-Tripp, 1977). Lindfors (1980) notes that during the elementary school years, children continue to refine rules for conversations and learn the structure for more formal types of interactions, such as group discussion, meetings, and debate.

Written Language Formats

Understanding the relationship of format to content is also important as students try to comprehend written language. Goodman and Burke (1980), Holdaway (1979), and Smith (1978) observe that effective reading involves a process of making reasonable predictions about the expected content and sampling the text to confirm or deny the prediction. Predictions may be based on syntactic, semantic, and even phonological information. However, recent researchers have become interested in the effect of the larger context—the discourse. There is evidence that connected discourse aids comprehension (Goetz and Armbruster, 1980), as does prior knowledge about the nature of the discourse provided by such elements as a title or picture (Bransford and Johnson, 1972; Dooling and Lachman, 1971). One factor, then, which may shape the good reader's initial prediction regarding content is the overall format of the material—i.e., whether it looks like a story, a cartoon, or a letter. Feeley (1982) examined the ability of second, third, fourth, and fifth grade children to identify the subject area of textbooks based on their viewing of sample textbook pages with the words made unreadable. The subject areas were language arts, science, social studies, mathematics, and reading. She found that as a group the children were approximately 60% correct in their identification. The second grade children were significantly less able to make correct identifications than the third, fourth, or fifth graders. The most easily identified texts were reading (78.2% correct) and mathematics (75.5%); the least was language arts (42.7%).

DIAGNOSTIC QUESTIONS

In order to identify and to help those children whose communication and learning problems may be related to difficulty in making use of formats, we need to answer the following kinds of questions.

1. What does the child know about
   — the school and classroom rules.
   — the general routine followed in the classroom.
   — the rules for various types of communicative interactions.
   — written formats.

2. What are the child's formats or routines for various activities and communicative contexts? Are these routines conventional or idiosyncratic?

3. Can the child use the information about existing formats in order to make predictions about the content and to control his or her own performance?

4. Is the child so bound to the format or routine that he or she does not see alternatives?

WHAT TO DO: DIAGNOSIS AND REMEDIATION

Classroom Routines

What can the classroom teacher or the speech-language pathologist do to find answers to the questions outlined above? This section will provide activities for specifying the child's information about formats and suggestions for using formats in learning and communication.

Table 4–1 shows a sample questionnaire that a teacher might administer to the entire class to find out how most children perceive the rules and routines of the school and classroom. The information can be used to identify those children who (1) do not know the rules, (2) perceive the routine differently, or (3) are not able to recognize subtle clues to identify the wishes and feelings of others.

Table 4-1. Questionnaire Regarding Classroom Routine and Rules

1. What does your teacher do or say when he or she is angry with the class?
2. What really makes your teacher mad or angry?
3. What is the most important thing that you should always do in class?
4. What is the most important thing that you should never do in class?
5. How do you know when it is time to go inside after recess?
6. What is the first thing that you should do when class begins?
7. What does your teacher do or say when she is going to say something really important?
8. What is the last thing you should do before you go home at the end of the day?
9. When is it OK to talk out without raising your hand at school?
10. How do you know when your teacher is joking or teasing?
11. What does your teacher do when it is time for a lesson to begin?
12. When is it all right to ask a question in class?

A first step in remediation may be to specify those classroom rules that are generally understood but not taught. For example, teacher's signals for quiet in the classroom vary from turning the light off, flicking the light, raising his or her voice, and speaking quietly to more idiosyncratic systems. One of the authors recalls an elementary teacher who stood for a very long time in front of the class with her arms outstretched in front of her saying nothing until all of the students were quiet. Some children may need to be taught these signals in a formal manner through role playing or open ended stories. Role playing can be a valuable way to highlight, then rehearse, appropriate classroom routines. There will always be certain children who are very adept at imitating the idiosyncratic behavior of the teacher. The teacher whose ego is strong may be able to employ those young actors to make such behaviors clearer to students who do not pick them up automatically. Open ended role play situations as well as open ended stories can be used to investigate or remedy children's ability to make predictions based on an overall format. Open ended stories have been used as a strategy for evaluating pragmatic knowledge. Ramsey (1979) used 22 stories to evaluate five, six, and seven year old children's ability to specify appropriate communicative intents and listener-appropriate forms for expressing them. The following is an example of the test items. The same situations could also be used for role playing.

> You are at your friend's house where you are getting all dressed up for a Halloween party. You can't reach your buttons in the back. What would you do? How would you say that?

You are alone in your classroom with your teacher and you are getting ready for the big school play, but you can't reach your zipper on the back of your costume. What would you do? How would you say that?

(Ramsey, 1979)

Wiig (1982a, b) used similar tasks to assess and enhance children's knowledge of appropriate speech acts in given contexts.

Written Language Formats

It has been demonstrated that school-age children are able to identify the general nature of written materials based on only the overall format (Feeley, 1982). Figure 4–1 shows written language formats that the reader will recognize as a business letter, a friendly letter, a newspaper, and a story with dialogue. Presentation of these and similar materials can demonstrate children's knowledge of familiar visual formats. A more important consideration, however, is whether the child can predict potential content on the basis of the format. For example, preschool children can learn the outline of a simple story structure that enables them to predict the following sequence: a setting statement, a problem or goal, a series of episodes, and a resolution. Older elementary school children should be familiar with a variety of written language formats. They should know, for example, which of the following words are appropriate for the friendly letter and which for the business letter, and they should be able to match the words with the format.

committee	party
manufacturers	friends
consistent	happy
correspondence	note
sincerely yours	love
Mrs. Smith	Aunt Jane

The first three pairs of words differ in content and signal topics expected in a business versus a friendly letter. The second three pairs differ in style although meaning is similar.

Effective use of ormats is also important for the child's own ability to write. One author has observed a nine year old learning disabled child who was unable to start the task of writing a business letter. When shown the overall format like that in Figure 4–1, the child was able to begin the task, but he wanted to keep the picture as a guide while writing. Children can be given practice in writing specific types of material when provided with appropriate formats. They can also be asked to create a format after exposure to a number of specific examples.

Figure 4–1. Four written language formats.

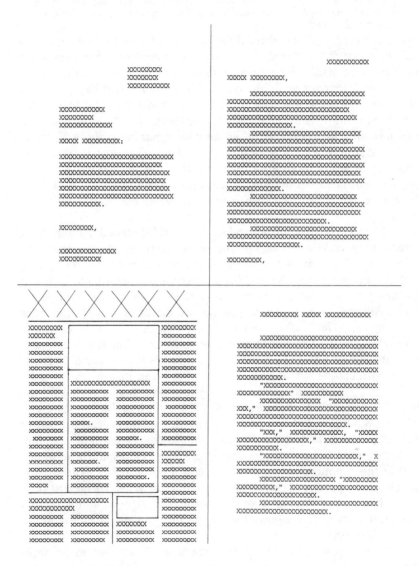

GIVING AND FOLLOWING ORAL DIRECTIONS

Understanding directions and their purpose, form, and place in classroom routines is critical to effective school performance. Suppose a third grade teacher gives the following directions to her class:

"All right, class. Put away your arithmetic workbooks. Take out your reading workbooks, and turn to page 37. Do all the problems and, when you are finished, close your books, put down your pencil and raise your hand so that I can come around to check your work."

Can third graders follow these directions? If we consider only attention and memory factors, even adults cannot remember more than seven unrelated commands. How then could an eight year old function in this third grade? Perhaps he or she could if it is not the first day of school. If we agree that some third graders would know what to do and some would not, what is the difference? What does the successful child know in order to follow these directions? The child must recognize in the above directions what is old information (that reading always follows arithmetic in this class) and what is new ("page 37"). Some parts of the teacher's remarks are well-known classroom routines. The successful child ignores those parts, focuses on the critical new information, and does not overtax his or her memory.

Mehan (1979) and Sinclair and Coulthard (1975) found that directives, informatives, and elicitations were the major constituents in school lessons. Directives and informatives specified procedure and occurred in the opening and closing phases of a lesson. For example, a teacher set up the lesson by saying, "These four people over to Martin . . . . Now these four people . . . . Alberto, turn around so you can see the blackboard" and ended it by saying, "That's all for this morning." Elicitations, both verbal and nonverbal, involved exchange of academic information and occurred in the instructional phase of lessons. For example, the teacher elicited a choice ("Now, which one is that one?"), a product ("and then it says to point to _____"), an opinion or interpretation ("Jeannie, what do you think?"), and a metaprocess comment ("Carolyn, how did you remember where it was?"). In order to participate in the content or learning part of the lesson, then, children must know what procedures to follow—i.e., how to do their part. Given the importance of directions in Mehan's observations and in the comments of teachers in general, it behooves us to explore children's competence or performance vis-à-vis directions. We need to know what children presuppose, what they focus on or ignore, and what they understand about directions. One way to find this out is by examining children's directions to others.

Current information tells us that preschoolers' directives are primarily direct imperatives until the age of four years; when indirect requests such as hints appear. Five year olds use twice as many indirect requests as four year olds, and they sometimes give directions without stating the goal, as in "Pretend this is my car" (Ervin-Tripp, 1977; Garvey, 1975).

In an attempt to explore oral directions of school-aged children, the authors have designed and used a barrier task. A child is asked to give (or follow) oral directions using a three-dimensional scene, which must be reproduced by a listener seated beside the speaker. A barrier separates the speaker's prearranged three-dimensional scene from the listener's empty cardboard base with "loose" objects to be placed in accordance with oral directions. The speaker must direct the listener to reproduce the original scene. The speaker may observe the listener's board and revise directions when necessary, but the listener may not look at the speaker's board. We have used adults as listeners and children as speakers; however, any combination is possible using this instrument.

> The following directions are given to the speaker: "You have a picture. Your picture is finished. I have the same toys but my picture is not finished. You be the teacher. I can't see your picture so tell me how to make my picture exactly like yours. I might do something wrong. You can look at my picture and tell me how to make it right. Tell me in words; don't use your hands."

In a recent study directed by the authors at the University of Cincinnati, the barrier task was used to study the oral directions given by first graders, third graders, fifth graders, and college students. The results showed that first graders identified objects with nouns but that they sufficiently differentiated only 42% of referents from similar nonreferents. They chose objects to be placed on the board randomly without an apparent plan. Their directions were more successful in placing objects in the intended general area (69% of objects) and in achieving correct orientation (31%) than in directing placement to the exact location (4%). Few revisions occurred. Brown (1983) noted that these first graders did reformulate messages not understood by the listener, but they failed to provide adequate new information. Messages tended to be ambiguous rather than distinctive ("Put the cat in the corner—no, the other corner"). Whitehurst and Sonnenschein (1981) reported similar results with five year olds in a series of referential communication studies and concluded that young children can compare referents and nonreferents but do not know that this is relevant (and necessary) in communication. "The young child does not know that to communicate referentially is to describe differences" (Whitehurst and Sonnenschein, 1981, p. 139).

The third graders in the Cincinnati study (Miller, 1983) were more successful in discriminating similar referents and nonreferents (86% correct) and were more orderly in giving directions. They typically directed placement of all objects in one general area, then moved to another general area. They directed 95% of objects to the correct general area, 49% to the correct orientation, and 20% to the exact location. Although they did not give many more directions than first graders (third grade = 43; first grade = 40), third graders' directions apparently were more effective.

Fifth graders showed a predictable developmental improvement on most measures (Buerkle, 1983). They were successful in placing 85% of objects in the exact location and 36% in the correct orientation. They gave more directions (56 versus 43) but revised less than third graders. They took half the amount of time to complete the task (6.2 minutes versus 11.1 minutes for third graders). By fifth grade, children were more specific on their first attempts at directions and more effective in achieving their goals through oral directives.

College students were predictably quite able to give directions, but often were redundant in details given. In their apparent attempts to leave nothing to chance, they provided more than the distinctive characteristics required for appropriate communication (Nelcamp, 1983).

DIAGNOSTIC QUESTIONS

When using this barrier task as an assessment instrument, a child's performance can be judged using the following diagnostic questions.

For speakers:

1. Did the child attend to the listener and notice if the directions were effective?
2. Did he or she revise when necessary? What kinds of revisions?
3. Did he or she take responsibility for communication failure or blame the listener?
4. Did he or she give efficient directions, i.e., complete one general area rather than selecting objects randomly?
5. Did he or she identify objects by distinctive characteristics?
6. Did he or she depend on oral language or were gestures used?
7. What did the child focus on in her or his directions?
8. Did he or she give irrelevant information?

For listeners:

9. Did he or she attend to directions?
10. Did he or she presume too much or follow explicitly?
11. Did he or she request clarification?
12. Did he or she take responsibility for his or her part in communication failure?

Additional diagnostic questions need to be asked regarding the child's comprehension and use of written directions.

1. Does the child read the directions at all or simply note the format?
2. Does the child read all of the directions or just the first one?
3. Does the child add something not required by the written directions?
4. Do the child's written directions include a topic sentence? Does he or she explain the task in the correct sequence?
5. Do the child's written directions reflect awareness of multiple or predictable directions?

WHAT TO DO: DIAGNOSIS AND REMEDIATION

Oral Directions

The diagnostic questions (Nos. 1 to 12) regarding oral directions and responses address Hymes' definition of pragmatics: *when* (2, 4) to say *what* (5, 7, 11) to *whom* (1, 3, 12) and *how much* (5, 8) and help define the appropriateness of the child's skills in using directives. We can thus identify the child's knowledge of the critical components in informative messages (Glucksberg, Krauss, and Higgins, 1975):

1. A comparison component in which the speaker determines which attributes distinguish a referent from nonreferents.
2. A listener component in which the speaker acknowledges the listener's communication needs.
3. An evaluative component in which the speaker recognizes, rejects, and revises uninformative messages.

We can also observe the child's spatial perspective-taking ability, which reportedly relates to age and overall task performance (Coie, Costanzo, and Farnill, 1973).

After observing the child in this oral direction activity and answering the diagnostic questions, specific remediation measures can be instituted using the same barrier task.

From our experience with the barrier activity, it appears that ambiguity is a major issue in directions. Younger children do not recognize ambiguity and older children can't correct it in their revisions until fifth grade. In giving oral directions to children, then, we should focus on and model referent versus nonreferent distinctions. Children could profit from observing, identifying, giving, and responding to ambiguous versus discriminating directions. Particular attention could be given to pertinent adjectives and relative clauses appropriate to referents in a barrier task.

The following remediation activities using the barrier activity are suggested:

1. Have the child hand each object to the listener while giving directions for placement to focus his or her attention on the listener.

2. Have the listener repeat each direction as it is given to allow the speaker to appreciate how his or her directions sound.

3. Have the listener give communication and perceptual feedback stressing the critical information needed ("Tell me which cat—the one standing, the one with the ball, or the big cat?").

4. Have the listener request clarification ("I'm confused") to draw attention to his or her communication needs.

5. Let the speaker change places with the listener to appreciate a different perspective.

6. Let speakers observe others in the same role and see what works and what does not.

7. Remove the barrier after the activity and have the listener and speaker discuss difficulties encountered.

8. Model ambiguous versus distinctive directions.

9. Set a time limit for a second trial to encourage more efficient directions (and perhaps more complex sentences).

10. Have speaker and listener teams write directions. Have another child construct the three-dimensional scene using the written directions, then let speaker and listener teams compare it with the original preset scene and revise directions as necessary.

The barrier game has shown broad application for illustrating effective and ineffective communication skills in clinical practice. Children who are good communicators use complex sentences in order to specify particular objects on the board. They demonstrate their ability to depend on oral language rather than gestures, while some children need their gestures. Others find it difficult to take the speaker's perspective even in a side-to-side arrangement. Some children continue beyond the critical age of seven years (Robinson, 1981) to blame the listener for communication failure. This barrier activity lends itself to investigation and remediation of these and other direction-giving skills.

Written Directions

A study by one of the authors of this chapter examined responses from fourth and sixth graders to written directions; results suggest that children attend primarily to visual format in completing worksheets and may need help in also focusing on written directions. This is especially true for younger children or poor readers. Teachers could give children practice in predicting the directions and then confirming through comparison with uncovered printed directions. Unpredictable "tricky" directions could be used more often to wean children from overdependence on visual format. Children could also profit from writing directions for others to follow. Students could rewrite confusing directions in textbooks or identify the poor directions for a multiple choice test. Teachers and speech-language pathologists could use the child's pattern for written directions: topic sentence, followed by single propositions in sequence.

COMPREHENDING AND USING NONLITERAL MEANINGS

It has been suggested that ambiguity may make it difficult for some children to learn school routines and to understand directions. Ambiguity also may interfere with some children's comprehension.

The language of adults is filled with nonliteral meaning, including similes, metaphors, proverbs, idioms, and jokes. The language itself includes extensive examples of words that can have two or more different meanings (run, can, crab) and potentially ambiguous sentences ("Flying airplanes can be dangerous").

Classroom teachers observe and the literature indicates that language and learning disabled children may have difficulty with comprehension and use of nonliteral language (Nippold and Fey, 1983; Wiig and Semel, 1980). Chukovsky (1963) and Gardner, Kircher, Winner, and Perkins (1975) observe that preschool children use language in novel ways that may indicate purposive metaphorical usage or may reflect lack of specific word meanings or strategies to deal with vocabulary deficits. Examples like the following illustrate young children's novel use of language:

"Would you higher the swing?"

"He's in the Mark unfan club." (Lindfors, 1980)

"I'm a whyer; you're a becauser." (Chukovsky, 1963)

Children with language or learning problems may persist in using novel forms because of the same factors that cause preschoolers to use them—lack of sufficient proficiency with language. Unlike their normal peers, who may use such forms on purpose, they may not recognize the incongruency or humor in their utterances and be hurt or confused when others laugh.

Lund and Duchan (1983) report studies suggesting that normal elementary school–age children may reject nonliteral language usages and may even argue that metaphors do not make sense or cannot be true. Nippold and Fey (1983) conclude that there is a marked increase in competence with figurative language during the ages nine through twelve.

The development of the comprehension and use of figurative language has been studied in a variety of ways. Asch and Nerlove (1960) asked children from three to twelve years old to describe double-function terms such as "hard." They found that the youngest children used the terms only in relationship to objects. As they got older, they saw the figurative meaning as a separate vocabulary item. Most children under twelve years were not able to explain the relationship between the two meanings. Pollio and Pollio (1974) used three tasks to observe the development of figurative forms in the written language of third, fourth, and fifth grade children. When asked to write an imaginary story, all of the children used more "frozen" or commonly used figurative forms than novel forms, but the use of all figurative forms decreased across grade levels! When asked to write as many sentences as possible in response to double-function terms (run), the number of frozen forms was still higher but both novel and frozen forms increased across grades. Finally when children were asked to describe similarities between pairs of words (box, can), they used more novel forms, and both types increased across grades. It appeared that the children's ability to use figurative language when needed increased across grade levels, but their spontaneous production in creative writing decreased. The authors suggested that children may view the latter task as one requiring accuracy rather than creativity.

Winner, Rosenstiel, and Gardner (1976) asked children to select the best of four choices to explain metaphors such as "After many years of working at the jail, the prison guard was a hard rock that could not be moved." They found that six and seven year olds' interpretation of the metaphors tended to be magical or metanymic (both parts of the metaphor interpreted literally, but not related as identical). An example of a magical response might be, "The king had a magic rock, and he turned the guard into another rock," while a metanymic interpretation might be, "The guard worked in a prison that had hard rock walls." Although eight year olds continued to give magical and metanymic responses, eight to ten year olds also used primitive metaphors, such as, "The guard had hard tough muscles." Ten to fourteen year olds chose more genuine metaphorical answers, such as, "The guard was mean and did not care about the feelings of the prisoners" (p. 29); however, ten year olds were not yet able to explain them. Unlike the ten year olds, fourteen year olds were able to describe more than one similarity between the two terms in a metaphor. The authors concluded that children first achieve spontaneous production of metaphors, then comprehension, and finally the ability to explain them. This suggests that school materials designed to teach comprehension and use of figurative language should not require metalinguistic explanations of metaphors until adolescence.

Westerbeck (1983) presented multiple choice verbal and pictoral answers for 25 common idioms used in sentences to children in grades 1 through 8. Some of those included were, "I'd like to go out and play, but it's raining cats and dogs," and "That movie we saw yesterday was for the birds." She found that six year olds were 60% correct in choosing the idiomatic meaning; seven year olds were 80% correct; and after eight years, all ages were nearly 100% correct.

John-Steiner, Irvine, and Osterreich (1979) found that when five to fourteen year old children were asked to give images in response to nouns, their responses included more visual images ("There's snow on the top of the mountain") than those of adults, which tended to include more abstractions ("The mountains give a sense of the majesty of nature"). The children gave more close-up descriptions ("There's a bird in the tree"), while the adults provided an overall view ("It's a pretty woods"). Chukovsky (1963) confirmed that school-age children's poems tend to contain clear visual images and few adjectives.

Some of the research involving use of nonliteral language by children has been directed toward their comprehension and telling of jokes. It appears that it is not until adolescence that children understand the full range of requirements for telling jokes (Lund and Duchan, 1983). Before six years, children do not tell ready-made or previously heard jokes. At four and five, their humor tends to be original, made-up silly stories. Five year olds find riddles to be meaningless. Wolfenstein (1954) reported a five year old who, when told a riddle, said, "My [older] brother knows those; I don't" (p. 139). McGhee (1972) suggests that external clues are important to young children's recognition of humor. Five year olds will be more likely to laugh when the speaker says, "Here's a joke." During the ages six to ten children tell riddles. They repeat jokes with an exact verbal formula. It appears that the form of the joke is all-important (Lund and Duchan, 1983). Wolfenstein (1954) suggests that during this stage, telling jokes is more of a science than an art. It is important to use the exact words of the joke. It appears that during the early elementary years riddles that require an answer are most frequent:

"Why did the moron throw the clock out the window?"

"Because he wanted to see time fly."

During prepuberty and early adolescence, riddles with no answer become popular:

Did you ever see a horsefly?

In both cases, linguistic ambiguity is the basis for the humor. It appears that children learn to appreciate ambiguous meanings in jokes during elementary school years (Schultz and Horibe, 1974).

Wolfenstein (1954) suggests that as they enter adolescence children begin to see that often jokes should be relevant to the situation. They begin to tell jokes that depend on "artistic" skill in telling. Adolescents understand the requirements for jokes, are able to discriminate between humor and nonhumor, can explain why something is funny, and can create alternate answers for riddles.

Language arts books and workbooks begin to include lessons on nonliteral meanings at about the third and fourth grades. A survey of some commonly used workbooks at these grade levels (Barnes, Burgdorf, and Wenck, 1974; Harris, 1976) showed lessons on similes ("The orchestra sounded like a barnyard chorus"), metaphors ("The lake was a mirror"), imagery ("The leaves whispered to the trees"), idioms ("Let's bury the hatchet"), slang expressions ("I'm broke"), humor ("A bike can't stand up by itself because it is two tired"), exaggeration ("It was so hot that we started to melt"), reality versus fantasy ("The chocolate dog jumped off the table"), slanted arguments ("The saints in heaven would approve"), homonyms ("rose," "bark").

The research suggests that elementary school children are not adept at explaining nonliteral language or at understanding all of the specific meanings involved in metaphors or jokes. What is it then that allows them to function adequately in a world that is filled with such usages? What is it that sets learning disabled children apart from their peers in this area of language or that prevents them from comprehending information that contains such language? This question is partially answered by determining those factors that are necessary for comprehension and use of figurative language.

DIAGNOSTIC QUESTIONS

Questions that need to be answered include:

1. Is the child able to deal with the abstract or is he or she bound to concrete interpretations?

2. Is the child able to see two possible alternatives or does the first learned, the concrete, or the most obvious alternative stick in his or her mind so that he or she cannot see another possibility?

3. Is the child able to use the context to interpret ambiguous meaning?

4. Is the child able to read and interpret the subtle contextual clues that tell when it is appropriate to use various nonliteral forms?

WHAT TO DO: DIAGNOSIS AND REMEDIATION

In asking questions three and four, we are hypothesizing that at least one deficit involved here is related to our overall premise that comprehension and use of old and new information is an underlying factor in the language differences of learning disabled children. Making use of context, subtle clues, and the overall situation is a common theme that may tie deficits in those areas to deficits in other areas of language use.

Knowing the answers to the above questions, however, may not suffice for selecting remediation procedures for use of nonliteral language. It was suggested earlier that normally developing school-age children may not be proficient in this area. Our next task is to identify as accurately as possible what normal children know about and how they use nonliteral language.

As stated earlier, beginning at about the third grade, language arts texts and workbooks include materials that give practice in dealing with nonliteral language. Many of these materials can be adapted for working with the children we have discussed. Several children's books include humorous pictures of the literal meaning of figurative forms which can be used as a starting point for identifying the nonliteral (Gwynne, 1970, 1976).

For some children, experience with figurative language may be the primary goal. Hearing impaired children, for example, may fail to comprehend or use figurative language because of their inability to hear all of the information required to understand, i.e., the total verbal context in which it occurs, the specific wording required for the full impact, or the novel intonation patterns used. It has been suggested that teachers and clinicians may inadvertently add to the problems of hearing impaired children by failing to use nonliteral language with them (Iran-Nejad, Ortony, and Rittenhouse, 1981). The desire to make information clear and comprehensible to the child may cause us to be very concrete and thus further reduce the child's opportunity to experience nonliteral language. One job of the speech-language pathologist may be to provide increased exposure to such language. One clinician, for example, instituted a "Joke of the Day" and made sure that she told certain of her clients a new joke every day.

Other children, however, may require more specific intervention regarding the ability to deal with the abstract and to see alternatives. It may be helpful to ask language impaired children to draw pictures depicting sentences containing idiomatic or metaphorical expressions. Explicit explanation or discussion may be required. Asking the child to paraphrase expressions or to draw or describe both literal and nonliteral interpretations can provide experience in flexibility. It is important that at least sentence level, if not paragraph material, be used in teaching nonliteral language, because it is the context that often provides clues to meaning and that determines appropriate use. For some children, the restrictions on use may be the primary problem. These children may have the ability to decipher the meaning of abstract language, or they may be able to learn how to deal with it when specifically taught. However, they may fail to use nonliteral language because they cannot determine when it is appropriate, or they may use expressions inappropriately, which will make them seem odd and socially inept to their peers and to adults. With these children the presentation of figurative language in appropriate contexts is of utmost importance and may well be combined with explicit discussion of some of the restrictions on use. Role playing and monitored experience in a variety of settings are strategies for enhancing appropriate use. One clinician reported that she worked and worked on teaching a repertoire of jokes, idioms, and slang expressions to a teenage boy. She often wondered if he really used them outside of therapy. She was gratified when the boy's sister reported that at the bus stop he had exclaimed from under his umbrella, "It's raining cats and dogs!"

A note of caution: in teaching jokes and idioms the clinician needs to be aware of the generation gap. Using expressions that are frequent in adult conversation or were popular when "we" were children can be disastrous. Listening to the child's peers or using other children as teachers is an important strategy for assuring age-appropriate language use.

Inappropriate intonation frequently signals difficulty in the use of figurative language. Faulty intonation patterns may either interfere with intended meaning or make language sound stilted instead of helping the child seem more "with it." Teaching appropriate intonation is a difficult task, but it is important that the clinician be aware of its integral role in use of figurative language. Exaggeration of such patterns may be helpful for some children.

CONCLUSION

This chapter has discussed some specific skills needed in classrooms: knowledge of classroom routine and specific communication sequences in schools; recognition of formats for written materials and the implications for predicting meaning; facility with oral and written directions; comprehension and use of nonliteral language. We have stressed the importance of appropriate presuppositions that determine students' attention to old and new information when predicting, sampling, and confirming information in school. In order to pay attention, children seem to need a balance of old information for context and a new twist worthy of note. Therefore, as we see it, a basic pragmatic skill required in classrooms is the ability to properly balance old and new information in comprehending or expressing ideas in both oral and written language. Diagnostic and remedial procedures were described for pertinent school language skills.

A checklist of communicative skills required in school appears in Appendix 4-1.

REFERENCES

Asch, S., and Nerlove, H. (1960). The development of double function terms in children, in B. Kaplan and S. Wagner (Eds.). *Perspectives in psychological theory.* New York: International Universities Press.

Barnes, D., Burgdorf, A., and Wenck, S. (1974). *Reading, thinking and reasoning skills program.* Austin, TX: Steck-Vaughn Company.

Bloom, L., Hood, L., and Lightbown, P. (1974). Imitation in language development: If, when and why. *Cognitive Psychology, 6,* 380–420.

Bransford, J., and Johnson, M. (1972). Contextual prerequisites for understanding: Some investigations of comprehension and recall. *Journal of Verbal Learning and Verbal Behavior, 11,* 717–726.

Brown, J. (1983). Communication skills of normal first grade children involved in a direction giving task using a barrier game. Unpublished masters thesis, University of Cincinnati.

Buerkle, J. (1983). A study of communication and revision strategies used by fifth graders involved in a direction giving task within the context of a communication barrier game. Unpublished masters thesis, University of Cincinnati.

Chukovsky, K. (1963). *From two to five.* Berkeley, CA: University of California Press.

Coie, J., Costanzo, P., and Farnill, D. (1973). Specific transitions in the development of spatial perspective-taking ability. *Developmental Psychology, 7,* 21–23.

Dooling, D., and Lachman, R. (1971). Effects of comprehension on retention of prose. *Journal of Experimental Psychology, 88,* 216–222.

Ervin-Tripp, S. (1977). Wait for me roller-skate, in S. Ervin-Tripp and E. Mitchell-Kernan (Eds.), *Child discourse.* New York: Academic Press.

Feeley, R. (1982). The identification of the physical format of school textbooks by normal learning second, third and fourth/fifth grade students and a group of learning disabled students. Unpublished masters thesis, University of Cincinnati.

Gardner, H., Kircher, M., Winner, E., and Perkins, D. (1975). Children's metaphoric productions and preferences. *Journal of Child Language, 2,* 125-141.

Garvey, C. (1975). Requests and responses in children's speech. *Journal of Child Language, 2,* 41-63.

Glucksberg, S., Krauss, R., and Higgins, E. (1975). The development of referential communication skills, in F. Horowitz (Ed.), *Review of child development research* (Vol. 4). Chicago: The University of Chicago Press.

Goetz, E. and Armbruster, B. (1980). Psychological correlates of text structure, in R. Sprio, B. Bruce, and W. Brewer (Eds.), *Theoretical issues in reading comprehension.* Hillsdale, NY: Lawrence Erlbaum Associates.

Goodman, Y., and Burke, C. (1980). Reading Strategies: Focus on Comprehension. New York: Holt, Rinehart and Winston.

Green, J., and Wallat, C. (1979). What is an instructional context: An exploratory analysis of conversational shifts across time, in O. Garnica and M. King (Eds.), *Language, children and society.* Oxford: Pergamon Press.

Gwynne, F. (1976). *Chocolate moose for dinner.* New York: Messner.

Gwynne, F. (1970). *The king who rained.* New York: Messner.

Harris, P. (1976). *Moccasins and marvels workbook.* New York: Harper and Row.

Holdaway, D. (1979). *Foundations of literacy.* New York: Ashton Scholastic.

Hymes, D. (1971). Competence and performance in linguistic theory, in R. Huxley and E. Ingram (Eds.), *Language acquisition: Models and methods.* New York: Academic Press, pp. 3-28.

Iran-Nejad, A., Ortony, A., and Rittenhouse, R. (1981). The comprehension of metaphorical uses of English by deaf children. *Journal of Speech and Hearing Research, 24,* 551-556.

John-Steiner, V., Irvine, P., and Osterreich, H. (1979). A cross-cultural investigation of children's imagery, in O. Garnica and M. King (Eds.), *Language, children and society.* New York: Pergamon Press.

Keenan, E. (1974). Conversational competence in children. *Journal of Child Language, 1,* 163-183.

Lindfors, J. (1980). *Children's language and learning.* Englewood Cliffs, NJ: Prentice Hall.

Lund, N., and Duchan, J. (1983). *Assessing children's language in naturalistic contexts.* Englewood Cliffs, NJ: Prentice-Hall.

McGhee, P. (1972). On the cognitive origins of incongruity in humor: fantasy assimilation versus reality assimilation, in J. Goldstein and P. McGhee (Eds.), *The psychology of humor: Theoretical perspectives and empirical issues.* New York: Academic Press.

Mehan, H. (1979). Learning lessons: Social organization in the classroom. Cambridge, MA: Harvard University Press.

Miller, M. (1983). Revision strategies employed by normal third grade children: An analysis of communication competence within the context of a communication barrier game. Unpublished masters thesis, University of Cincinnati.

Nelcamp, V. (1983). Referential specification and revision behavior of college age adults in a direction giving task. Unpublished masters thesis, University of Cincinnati.

Nippold, M., and Fey, S. (1983). Metaphoric understanding in preadolescents having a history of language acquisition difficulties. *Language, Speech and Hearing Services in Schools, 14,* 171-180.

Pollio, M., and Pollio, H. (1974). The development of figurative language in children. *Journal of Psycholinguistic Research, 3,* 185-201.

Ramsey, B. (1979). "What would you do?"—a study of children's knowledge of selected communicative intentions and illocutionary speech acts. Unpublished masters thesis, University of Cincinnati.

Robinson, E. (1981). The child's understanding of inadequate messages and communication failure: A problem of ignorance or egocentrism? in W. Dickson (Ed.), *Children's oral communication skills.* New York: Academic Press.

Schank, R., and Abelson, R. (1977). Scripts, Plans, Goals and Understanding. Hillsdale, NJ: Lawrence Erlbaum Associates.

Schultz, J. (1979). It's not whether you win or lose, it's how you play the game, in O. Garnica and M. King (Eds.), *Language, children and society.* Oxford: Pergamon Press.

Schultz, T., and Horibe, F. (1974). Development of the appreciation of verbal jokes. *Developmental Psychology, 10,* 13–20.

Sinclair, J., and Coulthard, R. (1975). Towards an analysis of discourse: The english used by teachers and pupils. Oxford, England: Oxford University Press.

Smith, F. (1978). *Reading without nonsense.* New York: Columbia University Teachers College Press.

Westerbeck, S. (1983). Comprehension of idioms by first through eighth grade children. Unpublished masters thesis, University of Cincinnati.

Whitehurst, G., and Sonnenschein, S. (1981). The development of informative messages in referential communication: Knowing when versus knowing how, in W. Dickson (Ed.), *Children's oral communication skills.* New York: Academic Press.

Wiig, E. (1982a). *"Let's talk"—developing pro-social communication skills.* Columbus, OH: Charles Merrill.

Wiig, E. (1982b). *The "Let's talk" inventory for adolescents.* Columbus OH: Charles Merrill.

Wiig, E., and Semel, E. (1980). *Language assessment and intervention for the learning disabled.* Columbus, OH: Charles Merrill.

Winner, E., Rosenstiel, A., and Gardner, H. (1976). The development of metaphoric understanding. *Developmental Psychology, 12,* 189–297.

Wolfenstein, M. (1954). *Children's humor.* Glencoe, IL: Free Press.

APPENDIX 4-1

COMMUNICATIVE SKILLS REQUIRED IN SCHOOL

KNOWLEDGE ABOUT THE SCHOOL ROUTINE

In the classroom and school, the child

_____ knows routine for activities like starting the day, going to lunch, ending the day.

_____ knows routine for participating in lessons, i.e., preparing necessary materials, knowing when to ask and answer questions, changing from one lesson to another.

_____ is able to deviate from the routine when appropriate.

_____ is able to read the teacher's strategies for cuing a given routine.

_____ participates effectively in peer routines such as games, sports, verbal exchanges.

KNOWLEDGE ABOUT COMMUNICATIVE ROUTINES

In communicative interactions with adults and peers, the child

_____ knows when to talk.

_____ takes turns appropriately in conversation.

_____ initiates conversation.

_____ has more than one style of interaction, i.e., can change style depending on the listener, situation, etc.

_____ exhibits appropriate greetings and closings for different listeners and situations.

ABILITY TO USE FORMATS AS AN AID TO COMPREHENDING WRITTEN LANGUAGE

When presented with written material, the child

_____ is able to recognize various types of written material on the basis of the format, i.e., textbook versus leisure reading, type of textbook, etc.

_____ is able to predict workbook directions on the basis of the page format.

_____ is able to predict content on the basis of the title, subheadings, or pictures.

_____ is able to confirm or deny predictions after reading the content.

GIVING AND FOLLOWING ORAL DIRECTIONS

In a barrier task, the child as speaker

_____ clearly identifies pertinent objects.

_____ specifies location adequately.

_____ watches listener to check communication.

_____ revises directions when necessary.

_____ takes responsibility (does not blame listener) when directions do not work.

In a barrier task, the child as listener

_____ follows directions exactly.

_____ follows general direction, but proceeds further on presumed information.

_____ requests clarification when direction is unclear.

GIVING AND FOLLOWING WRITTEN DIRECTIONS

In a written directions task, the child as writer of directions

_____   states the overall objective in a topic sentence.
_____   uses single proposition sentences.
_____   sequences directions appropriately.
_____   gives enough but not too much information.

In a written directions task, the child as reader of directions

_____   follows multiple directions.
_____   notes unpredictable procedures in an otherwise predictable set of directions.
_____   notes unpredictable directions.

COMPREHENSION AND USE OF FIGURATIVE LANGUAGE

When confronted with oral and written communication, the child

_____   can restate figurative meaning of simple similes, metaphors, and idioms.
_____   can draw pictures to illustrate figurative meanings.
_____   uses idiomatic expressions that are used by peers.
_____   uses idiomatic expressions appropriately for context and listener.
_____   is able to comprehend material that is loaded with figurative language.
_____   is able to figure out the meaning of an unknown figurative expression when given an appropriate context.

TRANSITIONAL NOTE

Creaghead and Tattershall have presented information regarding the observation of how well a student has "learned the routine" of the classroom and functions in the role of a student. Although some children seem to abstract rules from experiencing or just observing a situation, others may need direct teaching on those operational or procedural rules. In particular, Creaghead and Tattershall have focused on rules such as the following:

1. Turn-taking in class and how it differs from turn-taking in conversation.

2. Developing strategies for holding pertinent information in short-term memory until called on by the teacher.

3. Learning that although some rules are stated explicitly (or phrased as direct commands), others are implicit and communicated through body language or intonational patterns or given as indirect suggestions.

4. Becoming aware of necessary shifts in communication behavior depending upon the context and the person with whom you are interacting.

What needs to be encouraged is a combination of educator awareness to observe the degree of sophistication of a student's classroom pragmatic rules and the development of productive scenarios for students who have not acquired them spontaneously.

Vetter (1982) has presented a series of excellent questions for teachers to ask that serve as guidelines for systematic observation of classroom skills in the following areas:

I. Language
   A. Phonological system (articulation, auditory discrimination)
   B. Semantic system (level of vocabulary, degree of word-finding problems)
   C. Syntactic system (grammatical accuracy, understanding of subject/object relationships, sensitivity to ambiguity or anomaly)
   D. Pragmatics (rules of discourse, politeness, eye contact, classroom rules such as raising hand to gain recognition, requesting clarification, interpret direct and indirect requests)

II. Thinking
   A. Information processing (attention span, figure-ground distractions, short-term memory, rehearsal strategies, solid experiential background, long-term memory, associative skills, evaluation)
   B. Conceptual information (conceptual notions, supportive language)
   C. Integration and association of information (integration of new with old information, ability to make use of analogies, level of language formation in attempting to demonstrate that integration of information has taken place)

Calfee and Sutter (1982) have presented guidelines for the analysis of a student's communication skills during a classroom discussion. In particular, they recommend observing the following:

1. Range of discussion methods (comparing, explaining, enumerating, and so forth)
2. Turn-taking that was natural (as contrasted to holding up a hand)
3. Ability to elaborate, refer to, or amend previously stated information
4. Support for assertions by providing evidence (from experience, empirical proof, authority, or logic)
5. Variety of types of questioning tactics used by the leader and participants
6. Ability to evaluate the quality of the discussion
7. Social relations between the "target student" and the other group members
8. Characteristics of the setting (such as ambient noise or where the person was seated) and how they affected people

In Chapter 5, Calvert and Murray describe the Environmental Communication Profile. Their system of observation, from which the profile is derived, aids the educator, clinician, and student in better understanding behaviors and situations that foster or inhibit proficient communicative interactions in various contexts, including the classroom. The authors emphasize the dynamic relationship among communication-related variables. They do not focus solely on what the child is doing or not doing effectively, but they also analyze how the child's environment is affecting functional communication. Once analyzed, it is possible to capitalize on the environment in which the child is expected to communicate and use this environment to stimulate communication skills. As they state, this evaluation procedure places "equal emphasis on the analysis of environmental events and the communicative act itself." The rationale of evaluation procedures such as this is that communication is dynamic and must consider the interaction of four variables: the speaker, the listener, the content, and the context.

Calfee, R., and Sutter, L. (1982). Use of discussion to observe thinking, speaking, and listening skills. *Topics in Language Disorders, 2*(4), 45–55.
Vetter, D. K. (1982). Language disorders and schooling. *Topics in Language Disorders, 2*(4), 13–19.

CHAPTER 5

Environmental Communication Profile: An Assessment Procedure

Mary B. Calvert
and
Sharon L. Murray

The pragmatic revolution is here (Lund and Duchan, 1983). We as speech-language pathologists and teachers have climbed on the bandwagon—because it makes sense. It focuses our efforts on the development of functional language, which has direct application to a child's social and emotional growth. As a result of the "revolution," methods for analyzing functional language and communication interactions are flooding the literature on child language and communicative disorders. (For a comparison over a short two year period refer to Miller, 1981, Chapter 4, and Lund and Duchan, 1983, Chapter 3.) There is less information on methods for treatment, but the pace in this endeavor is accelerating as well (Creaghead and Margulies, 1982; Kunze, Lockhart, Didow, and Caterson, 1983; Lucas, 1980; Musselwhite, St. Louis, and Penich, 1980; Newhoff and Wilcox, 1981; Simon, 1979; Wiig and Bray, 1983).

A brief look at recently described observational systems shows that we are gaining an awareness of the role significant others (and varying contexts) play in stimulating functional communication (Frankel, 1982; Newhoff, Silverman, and Millet, 1980; Schwartz, 1983). In the systems developed to date, however, the predominant focus is on children's communicative intents (Coggins and Carpenter, 1981; Dore, 1978; Halliday, 1977; Prutting and Kirchner, 1983; Tough, 1976; Wollner and Geller, 1982) and their discourse abilities (Creaghead and Margulies, 1982; Gallagher and Darnton, 1978; Lund and Duchan, 1983). Generally the observational method recommended is to videotape children in a natural interaction so that multilevels of analysis are possible. This implies that staff time and resources should be made available, which is not always possible.

One of the challenging tasks we have as clinicians and teachers is to select the method, or methods, that suit our needs, the needs of communicatively handicapped children, and the resources of our facility.

We need to analyze not just what the child is doing, or not doing, but also what the environment is doing, or not doing, to increase functional communication. For those of us in school settings, the classroom is the ideal environment for analyzing and developing language use because we should be capitalizing on classroom events to stimulate functional communication. In order to do this we must

1. Analyze the child's functional language.

2. Find out what events stimulate language use.

3. Develop intervention goals and objectives to increase language use in the classroom.

4. Coordinate activities between the individual therapy sessions and activities in the classroom.

5. Provide feedback to teachers and parents regarding the effectiveness of their efforts.

The purpose of this chapter is to share a method for analyzing the communicative interactions of children with language impairments in their school setting. We developed a system that placed equal emphasis on the analysis of environmental events and the communicative act itself. For example, if a child answers a teacher's question with a head nod, we record both the teacher's cue (a question) and the child's communicative act (nonverbal gesture). In addition, we would record the function of the child's head nod as "acknowledgment." We hypothesized that after we recognized the events that seemed to foster functional language, we could arrange the class environment to increase these events and thereby increase a child's language use. We also needed a system that could be accomplished without extensive videotape analysis; very few of us have the luxury of time or the budget to permit multiple videotape viewings.

The result of our endeavor was the Environmental Communication Profile (ECP), which we use to analyze a communicative interaction on three levels:

1. Function of the child's communicative interactions (e.g., giving information, getting information).

2. Communicative act (i.e., verbal or nonverbal) and type (e.g., declarative, question).

3. Environmental events that precede the communicative act (e.g., teacher question, peer eye contact, environmental noise).

The charting system is easy to learn and is intended as a live observation tool that is not dependent on numerous videotaped samples at a later time. The observer tallies ongoing behavior within a time limit and at set intervals. For example, observations could be made of a daily teacher-directed activity for 5 to 10 minutes each, or of playground activity once per week for 10 to 15 minutes. The observer may wish to monitor play and classroom activity for comparison. We have used 10 minute samples taken once a week during a teacher-directed activity. In this way a baseline is established and then a method is available to monitor the effects of pragmatic language intervention. Preferably three observations are made for each setting to establish an adequate baseline. From the information gathered by these observations, decisions can be made regarding intervention. This method is intended to be a quick, easy, multilevel analysis, without dependency on videotapes, that has direct implications for milieu intervention. We found that an observer could learn the tallying system within two observation sessions; in fact, our inter-rater reliability quotient within two sessions was 0.92, which means the system is easy enough to allow for agreement between raters viewing rapidly occurring events.

BRIEF DESCRIPTION OF THE CHART AND PROCEDURE

Setting the Stage

Before we begin our analysis, decisions need to be made regarding the following questions:

1. Who is the best person to make the observations? Since the impact of the ECP information will be on classroom interaction and on the speech-language sessions, it is designed so that clinician, teacher, volunteer, or aide would be able to do the observations.

2. When would be the best times to make the observations? Our goal is classroom interaction; therefore, a loosely framed activity that allows for group exchange would be one of the observation periods. (See Lund and Duchan, 1983, for a discussion of "frames.")

3. How should the child be observed? Our experience has been that an observer's presence in the classroom is soon forgotten by the children. There must be close coordination with the teacher so that class disruption is kept to a minimum.

4. How long should the observation take place? Once again we suggest the amount of time per observation be kept within reason. We use 10 minute periods.

5. How often should observations be made? This decision is more dependent upon staff availability than anything else. We use weekly intervals. The critical aspect of this decision is that the intervals must be

regular, i.e., same day, same time, same class activity. This consistency is the only way to document changes in behavior during therapeutic intervention.

6. Which children should be observed? This should be determined by a consensus from the professionals working with the children, including the teacher, speech-language clinician, learning disabilities specialist, and so forth.

Procedure for Charting

The observer charts three aspects of the communicative interaction simultaneously: (1) the function of the child's communicative act, (2) the kind or type of act, e.g., verbal or nonverbal, declarative or question, and (3) the environmental event that "cues" the child's communicative act. The observer marks the type of act and type of cue simultaneously and assigns a code to the communicative act, which corresponds with a function or communicative intent.

Charting the Child's Communicative Act

The observer charts the child's communicative act according to the following categories: *verbal* acts are declarative/command, question, echolalia, perseveration, other (jargon, loud vocal behavior); *nonverbal* acts are tactile, action gesture, facial expression, eye contact, no response (see Appendix 5-1 for an example of the recording form. This may be reproduced). The observer puts an X in the square corresponding to the type of communicative act. For example, the utterance "I want that!" would be charted as a verbal, declarative/command (Table 5-1).

Charting the Environmental Event

The environmental event that is judged by the observer to have cued the child's communicative act is charted according to whether it was verbal or nonverbal, who or what provided the event (teacher, peer, self), and the categories of events (Table 5-2). If the example "I want that!" was preceded by a peer's taking something from the child under observation, the event would be marked with an X under *Nonverbal,* peer, action/gesture (Table 5-2).

Charting the Child's Functional Rating (Communicative Intent)

Any of the available systems that focus on communicative intent can be selected. We selected and modified a system developed by Yoder and

Table 5-1.

X₅ declarative/command	V
question	E R
echolalia	B
perseverative	A
other	L

Table 5-2. Example of charting the environmental event for "I want that!" when cued by the action of a peer.

ENVIRONMENTAL EVENTS																
VERBAL								NON-VERBAL								
TEACHER			PEER			SELF			TEACHER				PEER			
QUESTION	DECLARATIVE/COMMAND	DECLARATIVE/COMMAND TO OTHER CHILD	QUESTION	DECLARATIVE/COMMAND	DECLARATIVE COMMAND TO OTHER CHILD	SELF-DIRECTED	CHILD INITIATED TO TEACHER	CHILD INITIATED TO PEER	EYE CONTACT	ACTION/GESTURE	FACIAL EXPRESSION	NO RESPONSE	EYE CONTACT	ACTION/GESTURE	FACIAL EXPRESSION	NO RESPONSE	NOISE/ENVIRONMENT
												X					

Reichle (1977). Using a selected system, the observer determines the child's intent and assigns the corresponding number to the communicative act. In our example "I want that!", the rating is a 5, representing "Expressing one's own intentions." The number is placed with the X beside the communicative act (Table 5-1).

The list of functional ratings is as follows:

0 *Other*   Communicative act that does not seem to fit any other category, including inappropriate

		acts that seem to have no communicative function (e.g., echolalia, perseveration).
1	*Giving Information*	A self-initiated verbal or nonverbal communicative act or one in response to a question or statement that provides information (e.g., "That's a Bingo game").
2	*Getting Information*	Requesting information verbally (question form or declarative with appropriate intonation) or nonverbally (facial expressions or gestures) (e.g., "What's that?").
3	*Describing Events*	Providing more information about an event (e.g., "The score was 5 to 7. We won!").
4	*Getting Another Person(s) to:*	
	Do Something	Initiating a verbal or nonverbal command with the intent that the person will perform (e.g., "Tie my shoelace").
	Believe Something	Attempts to convince a person of a personal belief (e.g., "I didn't take the cookies!").
	Feel Something	Attempts to convince a person to feel a certain way (e.g., "You have been a bad boy!").
5	*Expressing One's Own:*	
	Intentions	Relating one's own intentions to a person through verbal or nonverbal communicative acts (e.g., "I'm gonna hit you!").
	Belief	Expressing one's own belief or opinion (e.g., "I think you're mean!").
	Feelings	Reflecting one's own feelings or emotions (e.g., "I don't like spinach!").
6	*Indicating Desire for Further Communication*	
		A verbal or nonverbal cue that signals another to continue to communicate (e.g., "Oh, really?").
7	*Entertainment*	Intended for another person's enjoyment (e.g., making a funny face).
8	*Learning New Behavior*	
	Rehearsal	Repetition of an instructional task.
	Reinforcement	Strengthening the new schema.
	Feedback	Auditory or visual feedback (e.g., Adult: "It's on the table behind the pencil sharpener." Child: "... table ... behind sharpener").
9	*Social Rituals*	Socially accepted ways of exchanging greetings (e.g., "Bye, nice talking with you").

10   *Personal Gratification*

Intended for one's own satisfaction (e.g., singing the alphabet).

11   *Compliance*

Complying with a request through verbal or nonverbal communicative acts (e.g., Adult: "Say Hello to Susan." Child: "Hello").

Below are examples of completed forms from 10 minute observational sessions to demonstrate how we can interpret the information directly from the profile.

Example A₁

The observational setting is a writing task in the classroom. The environmental cues are teacher questions and statements, with one statement directed to Sherry by a peer. Sherry's communicative acts are all statements in response to the teacher. Her utterances had the function of giving information and therefore were given a "1" as the code for function. She did not respond to the peer, so the "no response" column was marked. (See chart on page 142.)

Example A₂

In another observational setting, lunchtime, the ECP showed questions and a statement from the teacher, and Sherry's communicative acts were either statements to give information or actions. One action was given the function code of "1" for giving information. Another action, in response to eye contact from a peer, was coded as "5" because Sherry gave a gesture that signaled her own intent (e.g., motion such as shoving). There was one instance of eye contact in response to a teacher action (nonverbal cue) that was coded as "6" because Sherry's eye contact signaled a desire for further communication. (See chart on page 143.)

We can see at a glance that Sherry's communicative acts are primarily verbal, and although she is responding to others, she is not initiating communication interaction. In addition, the functions of her verbal acts seem quite restricted to giving information that is asked for.

Example B₁

The observational setting for Roger is seatwork activity in the classroom. The environmental cues that predominate Roger's communicative acts are his statements to the teacher. The functions of his

Example A₁

CHILDREN'S HEARING AND SPEECH CENTER
ENVIRONMENTAL COMMUNICATION PROFILE
Mary Balfour Calvert/Sharon L. Murray

EXAMPLE A1

CHILD'S NAME: Sherry
DATE: 10-3-80   CA: 12-1
ACTIVITY: reading   TIME: 2:10-2:20
RECORDER: MC

(note: whining, stary)

ENVIRONMENTAL EVENTS

NON-VERBAL

PEER:
- NOISE/ENVIRONMENT
- NO RESPONSE
- FACIAL EXPRESSION
- ACTION/GESTURE
- EYE CONTACT

TEACHER:
- NO RESPONSE
- FACIAL EXPRESSION
- ACTION/GESTURE
- EYE CONTACT

SELF:
- CHILD INITIATED TO PEER
- CHILD INITIATED TO TEACHER
- SELF-DIRECTED

VERBAL

PEER:
- DECLARATIVE/COMMAND TO OTHER CHILD
- DECLARATIVE/COMMAND
- QUESTION

TEACHER:
- DECLARATIVE/COMMAND TO OTHER CHILD
- DECLARATIVE/COMMAND
- QUESTION

CHILD'S COMMUNICATIVE INTERACTIONS

NON-VERBAL:
- NO RESPONSE
- EYE CONTACT
- FACIAL EXPRESSION
- ACTION/GESTURE
- TACTILE

VERBAL:
- OTHER (jargon, loud vocal behavior)
- PERSEVERATIVE
- ECHOLALIA
- QUESTION
- DECLARATIVE/COMMAND

Example A₂

CHILDREN'S HEARING AND SPEECH CENTER
ENVIRONMENTAL COMMUNICATION PROFILE
Mary Balfour Calvert/Sharon L. Murray

CHILD'S NAME: Shawn

DATE: 11-25-80 CA: 13-2

ACTIVITY: Lunch TIME: 12:05-12:15 Eating

RECORDER: MC

Shawn
Showldana

ENVIRONMENTAL EVENTS

NON-VERBAL

PEER:
- NOISE/ENVIRONMENT
- NO RESPONSE
- FACIAL EXPRESSION
- ACTION/GESTURE
- EYE CONTACT — X X

TEACHER:
- NO RESPONSE
- FACIAL EXPRESSION
- ACTION/GESTURE — X
- EYE CONTACT

VERBAL

SELF:
- CHILD INITIATED TO PEER
- CHILD INITIATED TO TEACHER
- SELF-DIRECTED

PEER:
- DECLARATIVE/COMMAND TO OTHER CHILD
- DECLARATIVE/COMMAND
- QUESTION

TEACHER:
- DECLARATIVE/COMMAND TO OTHER CHILD
- DECLARATIVE/COMMAND — X
- QUESTION — X X X X

CHILD'S COMMUNICATIVE INTERACTIONS

NON-VERBAL:
- NO RESPONSE — o/X o/X
- EYE CONTACT — X
- FACIAL EXPRESSION
- ACTION/GESTURE — X s/X
- TACTILE

VERBAL:
- OTHER (jargon, loud vocal behavior)
- PERSEVERATIVE
- ECHOLALIA
- QUESTION
- DECLARATIVE/COMMAND — X X X

Example B₁

CHILDREN'S HEARING AND SPEECH CENTER
ENVIRONMENTAL COMMUNICATION PROFILE
Mary Balfour Calvert/Sharon L. Murray

CHILD'S NAME: ROGER

DATE: 10-16-80 CA: 10-11

ACTIVITY: work TIME: 9:00-9:10 SEAT

RECORDER: MC

ENVIRONMENTAL EVENTS

NON-VERBAL

PEER
- NOISE/ENVIRONMENT
- NO RESPONSE
- FACIAL EXPRESSION
- ACTION/GESTURE
- EYE CONTACT

TEACHER
- NO RESPONSE
- FACIAL EXPRESSION
- ACTION/GESTURE
- EYE CONTACT

VERBAL

SELF
- CHILD INITIATED TO PEER
- CHILD INITIATED TO TEACHER
- SELF-DIRECTED

PEER
- DECLARATIVE/COMMAND TO OTHER CHILD
- DECLARATIVE/COMMAND
- QUESTION

TEACHER
- DECLARATIVE/COMMAND TO OTHER CHILD
- DECLARATIVE/COMMAND
- QUESTION

CHILD'S COMMUNICATIVE INTERACTIONS

NON-VERBAL
- NO RESPONSE
- EYE CONTACT
- FACIAL EXPRESSION
- ACTION/GESTURE
- TACTILE

VERBAL
- OTHER (jargon, loud vocal behavior)
- PERSEVERATIVE
- ECHOLALIA
- QUESTION
- DECLARATIVE/COMMAND

communicative acts are to give information and use a social ritual. In three cases of 13 (approximately 23%), Roger's communicative acts serve no communicative function and are perseverative in nature. (See chart on page 144.)

Example B2

A few weeks later Roger was again observed during seatwork. This time the environmental cues were predominantly questions by a peer. Roger responded in 7 of 13 cases with a function rating for giving information. He also initiated questions to the teacher in order to get information. He gave no response to three of his peer's questions. The function ratings that predominate this observation period are giving information and asking for information, and there are no communicative acts judged as nonfunctional. (See chart on page 146.)

We now can take the baseline information (such as that provided above) and form an impression regarding the following:

1. The amount of functional communicative acts and variety of functions.

2. Ways in which the environment is facilitating or failing to facilitate communicative interactions.

3. The type of communicative acts being relied upon by the child.

(A reproducible ECP form appears in Appendix 5-1.)

THERAPEUTIC PROGRAMMING—OR WHAT DO WE DO NOW?

Let's look further at these two children to see how we use the information in order to generate therapeutic goals.

Case Study: Sherry

Sherry was 12 years old. She had been in a program for children with specific language learning disabilities for three years. Her management of language structure and vocabulary were equivalent to the four to five year level. When we analyzed the ECP baseline data, we found that 80% of Sherry's utterances related to a single function: giving information in response to a direct statement or question from a peer or teacher (Fig. 5-1). She was not asking questions specifically. When we analyzed the environmental cues, we learned that she was doing very little self-initiating.

Example B₂

CHILDREN'S HEARING AND SPEECH CENTER
ENVIRONMENTAL COMMUNICATION PROFILE
Mary Balfour Calvert/Sharon L. Murray

CHILD'S NAME: ROGER

DATE: 12-6-8?   CA: 11-1

ACTIVITY: work   TIME: 8:05-?05   SEAT-

RECORDER: MC

(Handwritten notes: "asking new questions" / "Roger")

ENVIRONMENTAL EVENTS

NON-VERBAL

PEER
- NOISE/ENVIRONMENT
- NO RESPONSE
- FACIAL EXPRESSION
- ACTION/GESTURE
- EYE CONTACT

TEACHER
- NO RESPONSE
- FACIAL EXPRESSION
- ACTION/GESTURE
- EYE CONTACT

VERBAL

SELF
- CHILD INITIATED TO PEER
- CHILD INITIATED TO TEACHER   X X X ... X
- SELF-DIRECTED

PEER
- DECLARATIVE COMMAND TO OTHER CHILD
- DECLARATIVE/COMMAND
- QUESTION   X X X X X X X X X

TEACHER
- DECLARATIVE/COMMAND TO OTHER CHILD
- DECLARATIVE/COMMAND
- QUESTION

CHILD'S COMMUNICATIVE INTERACTIONS

NON-VERBAL
- NO RESPONSE   X X X
- EYE CONTACT
- FACIAL EXPRESSION
- ACTION/GESTURE
- TACTILE

VERBAL
- OTHER (jargon, loud vocal behavior)
- PERSEVERATIVE
- ECHOLALIA
- QUESTION   X X X
- DECLARATIVE/COMMAND   x x x x x x ... x

Figure 5–1. Sherry: Communicative acts.

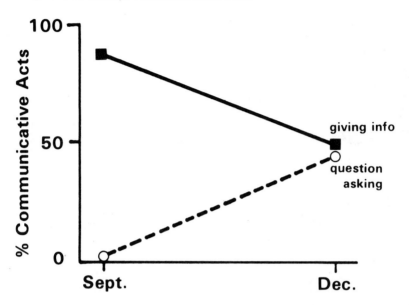

In addition, and quite importantly, the predominant cues were directions and questions from others (Fig. 5–2). Opportunities that encouraged Sherry's questions were not occurring in the classroom. With this information we were able to write an appropriate long-term goal and the following objectives for intervention.

Goal. Increase Sherry's use of questions.

Objective for Individual Sessions. Sherry will increase her use of "Can I?" in a category game to 100% criterion level in 12 sessions.

In therapy, the "Can I?" question form was introduced through games in which Sherry had to ask for specific items. The therapy session was structured, for example, so that Sherry would need to ask for specific items during a game, such as "Can I have (*the monkey*)?" Writing for Sherry was a strength; therefore, she wrote the question each time she used one. In this way she was not only able to enjoy the functional properties of the utterance, but was also able to analyze its syntactical components. The structure was provided (*Can I*), and Sherry completed the question: "*Can I have the monkey?*" (see Fig. 5–3).

Objective for the Classroom. Sherry will demonstrate carryover of "Can I?" in the classroom to 100% in appropriate context by the end of 12 weeks.

In the classroom there had to be a need for Sherry to ask questions so that she could be more actively involved in the learning process; therefore, the classroom environment was restructured so that the teacher set up

Figure 5–2. Sherry: Environmental cues.

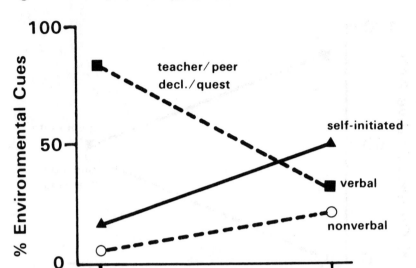

situations to encourage questions. For example, the teacher would instruct Sherry to go to the easel and paint without giving her a paint brush. The teacher and Sherry charted Sherry's "Can I?" questions for reinforcement and documentation of progress. In this way, Sherry was engaging in auditory evaluation of a teacher's directive and then asserting herself appropriately so that she could complete the directive.

Objective for Individual Sessions. Sherry will use wh-question forms when shown pictures to 100% correct criterion level in 12 sessions.

Objective for the Classroom. Sherry will demonstrate carryover of wh-questions into spontaneous situations in the classroom as measured by the ECP at the end of 12 weeks.

In therapy, Sherry was required to ask the clinician wh-questions about various pictures presented to her. She was given the Question Bug (Fig. 5–4) as a visual cue. She was initially required to write the questions she used to inquire about pictured content (see Fig. 5–5 for sample questions). Gradually the written language was removed and Sherry was required to ask questions on a conversational level with the clinician. For example, "*What* did you do this weekend?" "*Who* did you go with?" The Question Bug was again provided as a stimulus and then faded. Gradually other students visited the therapy session to have conversations with Sherry. Following each session, a probe sheet was completed *by Sherry,* critiquing

Figure 5-3. "Can I" questions.

Can I _____

Can I _____

Can I _____

Can I _____

Can I _____

Can I _____

Can I _____

Can I _____

her conversation. For example, she checked yes or no to statements such as, "I asked a Why question," "I looked at Mrs. Calvert," and "I asked 3 questions" (Fig. 5-6).

Sherry's progress was documented by the ECP at the end of 12 weeks for a total of 11 individual sessions (Fig. 5-1). Sherry demonstrated an increase in question-asking from 0 to 50% of her communicative acts and a corresponding increase in self-initiating, reflecting the increase in question-asking (Fig. 5-2).

Case Study: Roger

Roger was 11 years old. He had been in a program for children with specific language learning disabilities for four years. His verbal language was fragmented and perseverative in terms of both structure and content.

Figure 5-4. Wh- questions.

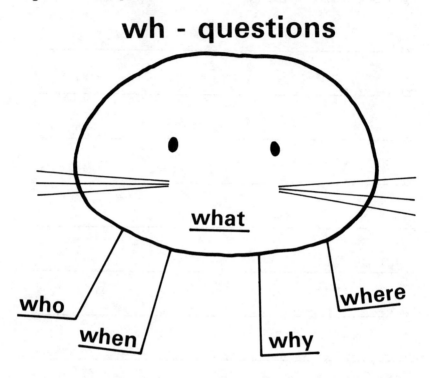

wh - questions

what

who

when

why

where

He used long strings of loosely connected words which served limited function in communicative interactions. Baseline information from the ECP indicated Roger responded to very few environmental cues. His communicative interactions were primarily self-directed (Fig. 5-7). For example, Roger would commonly go about his activities with self-directed comments, such as "Roger go play, now," "Roger eat 12 o'clock," "Daddy go work," "Roger go school." As a result of his self-directed behavior, 50% of Roger's communicative acts (or use of language to interact with others) were nonfunctional in context (Fig. 5-8). Probably the most critical piece of information the data gave us was that when Roger *did* interact, his functional communicative acts were directed toward the teacher and one particular child. As a direct result of this information, we provided opportunities for the two children to be together as much as possible, e.g., lunchtime, errands, seating assignments. In addition, we wrote the following goals and objectives for intervention:

   Goal. Roger will decrease verbally self-directed and nonfunctional utterances in spontaneous speech.

Figure 5-5. Question asking: pictures.

What are the children doing?

They are having a party.

Whose birthday is it?

It is Bobbi's Birthday.

Where are the presents?

There on the floor by the couch.

When will he open the presents?

After they eat the cake.

Why are they having a party?

They are having a party because

It is Bobbi's Birthday.

Objective. Within 12 therapy sessions Roger will generate three utterances to describe a picture for a conversational partner who does not have access to the picture without digressing from the subject.

In the individual therapy sessions, Roger was asked to generate three utterances about a picture. He was presented the Boston Cookie Theft Picture (Goodglass, 1972) and instructed to "tell me everything you see happening in the picture." A communicative efficiency rating was established using the method developed by Yorkston and Beukelman (1980). Initially Roger used two utterances that referred to the picture and 11 that

Figure 5-6. Conversational analysis.

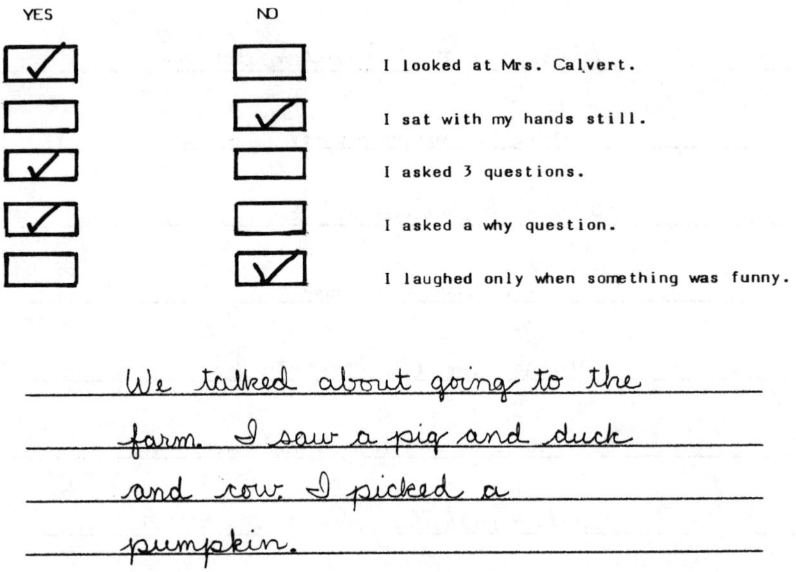

YES   NO

☑   ☐   I looked at Mrs. Calvert.

☐   ☑   I sat with my hands still.

☑   ☐   I asked 3 questions.

☑   ☐   I asked a why question.

☐   ☑   I laughed only when something was funny.

We talked about going to the farm. I saw a pig and duck and cow. I picked a pumpkin.

digressed (Fig 5-9). The clinician gave verbal feedback to maintain Roger's attention to the task. After 12 sessions, Roger used ten different utterances to describe the picture and digressed only five times.

Objective. Roger will describe a scene he is observing without digressing from the topic by the end of the 12 sessions.

In the individual therapy sessions Roger was asked to describe a scene he was observing. This helped focus his attention to specific events in his environment. The clinician questioned him as he was observing a scene to increase his awareness and attention to detail that could be shared (Fig. 5-10). Gradually the sample questions were faded.

In the classroom the teacher reinforced this strategy by asking Roger to describe both routine and special events in which the class was involved as they occurred. For example, he would be asked to describe the class visit to the circus, or the class routine involved in an art experience.

Objective. Roger will sequence a three-part picture story in which he participates in the supportive art work and then describe the activity to 100% criterion level by the end of 12 sessions.

Figure 5-7. Roger: Environmental cues.

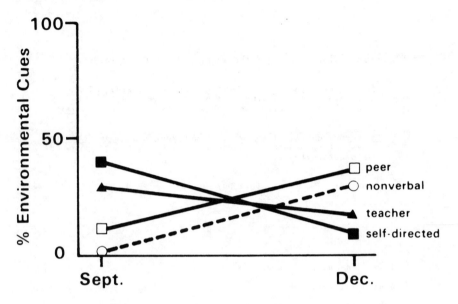

Figure 5-8. Roger: Communicative acts.

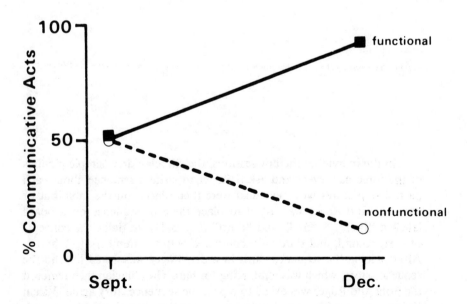

Figure 5-9. Description of Cookie Theft Picture by Roger.

```
"This picture kid get the washing, to get the washer.

He's gettin the cookie. He's gettin the cookie. (To
clinician: "Can I take this out?"). He's gettin the
cookie. He's gettin the cookie. He's going up the chair.

Got you cookie. I got you. I got you, kid. Open the door.
Does not open nother two door. Does not getting the washer.
He's gettin the cookie.

No tuff. No tuff. This boy, gum.
```

```
Time: 1 minute, 10 seconds

# of syllables: 108

# of content words/units: 6
```

(18) Communicative efficiency - the lower the number, more efficient.

In the individual therapy sessions, the clinician drew simple pictures of the three-part event and asked Roger to write a sentence about each part. The pictures with sentences were then placed on the table out of sequence and Roger was asked to place them in sequence on a board labelled "first," "second," and "third" (Fig. 5-11). Initially, the concepts of first, second, and third were *combined* with the numbers 1, 2, and 3. After placing the sequence cards in order, Roger was asked to read the sequence story, which was reinforcing for him. The clinician then removed the print and Roger was asked to repeat the sequence story again. Visual finger cuing, such as showing one finger for first, two fingers for second, and three fingers for third was used when necessary.

Figure 5-10. Observation of a scene.

What is Damone doing?

Where is Mr. Miller?

What game is Michael playing?

What is Tanya doing?

Who is doing math?

Where is Joe?

Who is doing speech?

Who is working alone?

Who is working with Miss Zara?

What is on Joe's desk?

Figure 5–11. Sequencing events.

Sequencing Events

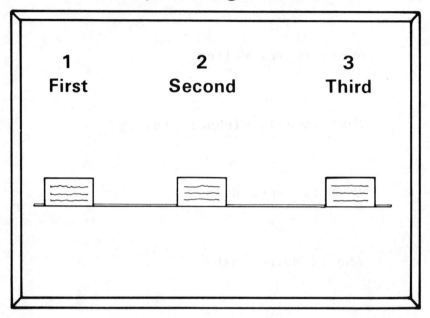

In the classroom, the teacher asked Roger what he had done in therapy. Roger used the sequence cards he and the therapist had drawn and then described the sequence of events (Fig. 5–12). This was the culmination of an interpersonal act (i.e., drawing a sequential story with the supportive aid of the clinician) and also provided an introduction to verbally relating a sequence of events.

Objective. Roger's classroom environment will be restructured to increase his functional communicative interactions by 50% at the end of 12 weeks.

In the classroom, Roger had one peer who was able to get and maintain his attention and stimulate functional communicative acts. Therefore, this peer was incorporated into Roger's daily classroom and play activity goals and objectives. In the individual therapy sessions, this same child was included as the listener in barrier game activities. In this type of activity, the visual fields of the speaker and listener are separated, which necessitates that they communicate with the same degree of clarity that would be needed if two conversational partners were in separate rooms. For example, "Pick up this one" would not be effective because the listener could not read

Figure 5-12. Three part sequence cards.

3 Part Sequence Cards

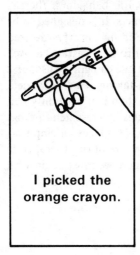

I picked the
orange crayon.

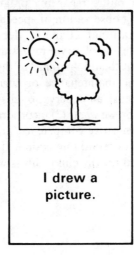

I drew a
picture.

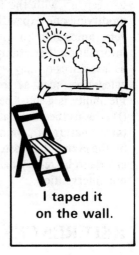

I taped it
on the wall.

the speaker's mind and know the identity of "this." The peer was also Roger's conversational partner for scene descriptions using actual activities, such as lunch in the cafeteria, as well as pictures of meaningful events.

At the end of 12 sessions Roger increased his functional communicative acts to 85% during his interactions (Fig. 5-8). His responsiveness to peers increased and the number of verbally self-directed communicative acts decreased (Fig. 5-7).

CONCLUSION

In the effort to provide an easy way to analyze children's communicative interactions in the classroom, we developed the Environmental Communication Profile. Our original intent was to document the classroom events that fostered functional communication for social and academic purposes and then increase these language uses during therapeutic intervention. In addition, we learned about the student's behaviors that were not contributing to classroom success (e.g., Sherry's *need* to ask questions). By using the ECP, we also were able to document progress and carryover of therapeutic efforts into the classroom. Perhaps most importantly, the data allowed us to give objective feedback to teachers and parents about the growth of their children in the use of language for specific purposes.

An added benefit is the flexibility of the ECP. This system allows us to keep up with the literature regarding pragmatic behaviors, thereby modifying and expanding observation of speech acts. It is designed to be very amenable to situational changes, depending on the desired information. For example, the observer may want to note gestures as well as utterances or may want to add "parent" to the cue category. Discourse categories, such as topic maintenance or turn-taking, can be added. Flexibility is a must because an observational system is usable only if it (1) gives us the information we want, (2) incorporates new research findings on the nature of communicative competence, and (3) places an emphasis on the events that foster or retard interaction. If we want our therapeutic efforts to be reality-based for the child, this is where we must begin with our intervention.

REFERENCES

Coggins, T. E., and Carpenter, R. L. (1981). The communicative intention inventory: A system for observing and coding children's early intentional communication. *Applied Psycholinguistics, 2,* 235–251.

Creaghead, N., and Margulies, C. (1982). Evaluating pragmatic skills of verbal and nonverbal children. *Journal of Communicative Disorders, 7,* 73–86.

Dore, I. (1978). Requestive systems in nursery school conversations: Analysis of talk in its social context, in R. Campbell and P. Smith (Eds.), *Recent advances in the psychology of language: Language development and mother-child interactions.* New York: Plenum Press.

Frankel, R. (1982). Autism for all practical purposes: A micro-interactional view. *Topics in Language Disorders, 3* (1), December, 33–42.

Gallagher, T., and Darnton, B. (1978). Conversational aspects of the speech of language disordered children: Revision behaviors. *Journal of Speech and Hearing Research, 21,* 118–135.

Goodglass, H. (1972). *The assessment of aphasia and related disorders: Stimulus cards.* Philadelphia: Lea and Febiger.

Halliday, M. A. K. (1977). *Learning how to mean: Explorations in the development of language.* New York: Elsevier North-Holland.

Kunze, L., Lockhart, S., Didow, S., and Caterson, M. (1983). Interactive model for the assessment and treatment of the young child, in H. Winitz (Ed.), *Treating language disorders.* Baltimore: University Park Press.

Lucas, E. (1980). *Semantic and pragmatic language disorders: Assessment and remediation.* Rockville, MD: Aspen.

Lund, N., and Duchan, J. (1983). *Assessing children's language in naturalistic contexts.* Englewood Cliffs, NJ: Prentice-Hall.

Miller, J. (1981). *Assessing language production in children.* Baltimore: University Park Press.

Musselwhite, C. R., St. Louis, K. O., and Penich, P. B. (1980). A communicative interaction analysis system for language-disordered children. *Journal of Communication Disorders, 13,* 315–324.

Newhoff, M., Silverman, L., and Millet, A. (1980). Linguistic differences in parents' speech to normal and language disordered children, in *Proceedings of the Symposium on Research in Child Language Disorders.* Madison: University of Wisconsin.

Newhoff, M., and Wilcox, M. J. (1981). Language intervention from a socio-communicative perspective. Short course presented to the American Speech-Language-Hearing Association, Los Angeles.

Prutting, C., and Kirchner, D. (1983). Applied pragmatics, in T. Gallagher and C. Prutting (Eds.), *Pragmatic assessment and intervention issues in language.* San Diego, CA: College-Hill Press.

Schwartz, R. (1983). Recent advances in pragmatics: Assessment and remediation for young language-impaired children. A workshop presented at Children's Hospital National Medical Center, Washington, DC.

Simon, C. (1979). *Communicative competence: A functional-pragmatic approach to language therapy.* Communication Skill Builders.

Tough, J. (1976). *Listening to children talking.* London: Ward Lock Educational.

Wiig, E., and Bray, C. (1983). *Let's talk for children.* Columbus, OH: Charles Merrill.

Wollner, S., and Geller, E. (1982). Methods of assessing pragmatic abilities, in J. Irwin (Ed.), *Pragmatics: The role in language development.* La Verne, CA: Fox Point Publishing, 1982.

Yoder, D. E., and Reichle, J. E. (1977). In P. Mittler (Ed.), *Research to practice in mental retardation* (Vol. 2).

Yorkston, K., and Beukelman, D. (1980). An analysis of connected speech samples of aphasic and normal speakers. *Journal of Speech and Hearing Disorders, 45,* 27–36.

APPENDIX 5-1

CHILDREN'S HEARING AND SPEECH CENTER
ENVIRONMENTAL COMMUNICATION PROFILE
Mary Balfour Calvert/Sharon L. Murray

CHILD'S NAME: _____

DATE: _____ CA: _____

ACTIVITY: _____ TIME: _____

RECORDER: _____

CHILD'S COMMUNICATIVE INTERACTIONS

VERBAL:
- DECLARATIVE/COMMAND
- QUESTION
- ECHOLALIA
- PERSEVERATIVE
- OTHER (jargon, loud vocal behavior)

NON-VERBAL:
- TACTILE
- ACTION/GESTURE
- FACIAL EXPRESSION
- EYE CONTACT
- NO RESPONSE

ENVIRONMENTAL EVENTS

VERBAL:

TEACHER:
- QUESTION
- DECLARATIVE/COMMAND
- DECLARATIVE/COMMAND TO OTHER CHILD

PEER:
- QUESTION
- DECLARATIVE/COMMAND
- DECLARATIVE/COMMAND TO OTHER CHILD

SELF:
- SELF-DIRECTED
- CHILD INITIATED TO TEACHER
- CHILD INITIATED TO PEER

NON-VERBAL:

TEACHER:
- EYE CONTACT
- ACTION/GESTURE
- FACIAL EXPRESSION
- NO RESPONSE

PEER:
- EYE CONTACT
- ACTION/GESTURE
- FACIAL EXPRESSION
- NO RESPONSE
- NOISE/ENVIRONMENT

TRANSITIONAL NOTE

Evaluation of communication skill adequacy can be done on an informal or formal basis and within naturalistic settings as well as within a more clinical setting. Realistically, a combination of procedures produces the most comprehensive picture of an individual's cognitive-linguistic-communicative abilities.

Chapter 6, by Damico, describes a more clinical approach (as contrasted to Calvert and Murray's environmental approach). Once identified as having a communication problem, the student's communication behaviors are subjected to in-depth analysis. Analysis of behavior is based on observations made during a conversation between the student and the clinician. Clinical discourse analysis permits the clinician to systematically observe the percentage of time that certain behaviors occur that either enhance or detract from the student's "communicator profile."

Damico also demonstrates how closely theory and practice are intertwined. He has engaged in a clinical application of Grice's description of the "cooperative principle" involved in discourse. In other words, conversation (or discourse) is possible only through a cooperative effort between participants. This cooperation is based on a "conversation scenario," or set of rules that govern speaker-listener behavior during the exchange of information. When the rules are violated, there is a breakdown in the quality of discourse. Damico has taken this theoretical model and used it as a framework for documenting why a student appears to be inept during conversation. Baseline data can be used to establish programming objectives as well as subsequently measure growth in the development of more productive communication behaviors.

CHAPTER 6

Clinical Discourse Analysis: A Functional Approach to Language Assessment

Jack S. Damico

"If you just listen to him, he seems to have a problem. He's hard to follow and the other kids don't really like to interact with him. His teachers say that he isn't a very good student . . . but I can't seem to find any specific problems according to my diagnostic battery." Many speech-language pathologists have made similar statements, especially in reference to older children with suspected language difficulties. The professional's clinical judgment and informal observations indicate problems, but the objective assessment tools do not support these impressions. Why not?

At least part of the explanation may be found in the assessment procedures commonly used. The tools that make up our diagnostic batteries are not sensitive to some of the functional aspects of communication, especially those that are affected in older language impaired individuals. This chapter discusses a procedure, entitled Clinical Discourse Analysis, that has been designed to assess functions of language. It is useful for identifying language impairments in school-age children. The chapter discussion is intended both to tell part of the story behind the development of Clinical Discourse Analysis and to explain what it is.

BACKGROUND

In the fall of 1976, I was faced with a situation experienced by most speech-language pathologists. I left the protection of a university graduate program and entered the "real world." Specifically, I was hired as a speech-language pathologist for the Albuquerque Public Schools. A number of realizations were forced upon me at that time, but none more unsettling than the fact that my training in language assessment was inadequate.

This realization was made clear after I convinced the teachers in my school that, as a language specialist, I could help them. I had conducted an in-service designed to generate language referrals on the basis of poor academic performance. In my presentation, I said that many academically delayed school children had language difficulties. I reasoned, therefore, that if teachers referred these children to me, I would diagnose their problems, initiate remediation procedures, and become a contributing member of the school faculty. The in-service session was successful, and a number of children were referred. Indeed, nearly a dozen names were submitted from the third, fourth, fifth, and sixth grade teachers. It was at this point that the problems began. First, I realized that the majority of assessment tools available were designed for students below the age of eight years. Second, I found that those tests that were less restrictive in terms of age range did not identify the students referred as language disordered. This seemed illogical because these individuals *were* academically poor students, and many had significant socialization problems. Additionally, even though I could talk with these students and get an impression of difficulty, I could not find an assessment tool to support my impressions.

I took a look at the tests and found two reasons for their inadequacies: (1) they seemed to overemphasize superficial aspects of language structure, and (2) they tended to fragment those aspects into many separate components.

The focus on the superficial aspects of language structure was largely due to the influence that the schools of structural linguistics and transformational grammar had on the development of our field (Hubbell, 1981; Leonard, 1972; Muma, 1978). Both of these schools stressed superficial language structures above other aspects. To be consistent with these prevailing linguistic schools, therefore, our field had become very surface structure–oriented, and test designers accordingly restricted the scope of language assessment. When our prototypical tests (e.g., Berko, 1958; Lee, 1966; Lerea, 1958; Templin, 1943) were created, they focused on directly observable elements of language structure, excluding less observable aspects of structure and meaning. While this resulted in a more empirically oriented methodology (Bloomfield, 1933), it also advanced the practice of viewing language as a list or lists of superficial structural elements. The fact that language is much more than this was generally ignored or given only passing mention (Carrow, 1974; Darley, 1964; Minifie, Darley, and Sherman, 1963; Weiner, 1967).

This orientation resulted in several practical problems for the school-based clinician. First, the majority of surface level structural elements included in our language tests were morphological units that were learned at an early age. By the age of six or seven years, these structures are used by a majority of children—both normal and disordered (Brown, 1973; Clark and Clark, 1977; Cromer, 1974; Karmiloff-Smith, 1979; Menyuk, 1964). Consequently, the structural tests were not usually normed beyond the age of eight years. Therefore, when an older child was tested, the norms were usually based more on acquired knowledge or academic abilities than on oral language skills. As a function of this testing procedure, these older children were classified according to a different set of guidelines and were labeled as having learning disorders rather than language disorders. They were, in effect, taken out of our professional domain.

The second problem with this structural orientation was that it tended to distort our field in the direction of highly prescriptionistic practices—especially in assessment (Damico, 1981; Drake, 1976). As a result, we were less able to validly diagnose speakers of minority dialects who exhibited atypical surface level syntactical abilities. While sociolinguists such as Fasold and Wolfram (1970), Labov (1970), and Shuy (1972) demonstrated that minority speakers presented language deficits, our structural tests were not designed to deal with such linguistic variation. This resulted in a number of testing abuses in our field (Arnold and Reed, 1976; Damico, Oller, and Storey, 1983; Omark and Erickson, 1983; Smitherman, 1981; Vaughn-Cooke, 1979). The structural tests were simply less appropriate for speakers of minority dialects.

The second major reason for the inadequacies of the tests in 1976 was the practice of fragmentation. The intent was to increase validity by breaking language down into subcomponents (Carrow, 1968; Harris, 1951; Lee, 1966). The actual result, however, was that a distorted view of language emerged—one stressing artificially separated parts or components of language rather than language as a functioning whole (Danwitz, 1981; Leonard, Prutting, Perozzi, and Berkeley, 1978; Oller, 1973). Something less than the full range of language ability was measured by these "discrete point" tests and to this extent the test scores were misleading (Rees and Shulman, 1978). Over the past several years, this "discrete point" approach to language assessment has been reviewed and criticized because it strips the essential qualities of intentionality and synergy from language (Bachman and Palmer, 1981; Muma, 1978; Oller, 1979; Prutting, 1982; Rees, 1978; Sommers, Erdige, and Peterson, 1978.

Fragmentation also led to problems with construct validity. For example, frequently inconsistencies were found between tests that purported to measure the same language abilities. There were also inconsistencies between what was observed in the formal testing situation and what children could do in actual conversation. Both of these problems have been documented through the work of Oller (1979, 1981, 1983) and his colleagues in the general field of testing and through the work of Prutting and her colleagues (Millen and Prutting, 1979; Prutting, Gallagher, and Mulac, 1975) in our specific field.

As the validity problem became clear, I tried to conceive of an approach to testing that would take a deeper look at language abilities. It seemed certain that what was needed was an approach to assessment that would reach beyond superficial categories and inventories and that would examine the functional effectiveness of individuals' attempts to communicate. I believed that we needed a rather different sort of assessment procedure. At the time I was learning about ongoing advances in discourse theory (Cole and Morgan, 1975; Halliday, 1975) and related developments in our field's movement toward communicative competence (Abkarian, 1977; Muma, 1975). Most importantly, however, was the theoretical and personal influence of John W. Oller, Jr., a professor of Linguistics at the University of New Mexico. His work encouraged me to believe that an assessment procedure that looked deeper into discourse processes would have a greater chance of revealing the kinds of language disorders likely to result in problems throughout the development of children from early childhood to adolescence and beyond.

CLINICAL DISCOURSE ANALYSIS

A research project was begun with the ultimate aim of creating a language assessment procedure that would avoid the difficulties inherent in the available tests and would allow for the assessment of language abilities in older school-age children. The procedure would have to analyze language from a functional rather than a structural viewpoint, to handle linguistic data holistically rather than as discrete and unrelated elements, and to sample communicative interaction rather than responses to artificial tasks related only minimally to social interaction. The developmental phase involved the integration of three related approaches: discourse analysis, error analysis, and clinical observation.

From the outset, discourse analysis was judged relevant because a functional perspective would have to focus on language behavior above the level of the sentence. Coulthard (1977) strengthened this belief when he stated that discourse analysis was primarily involved with the study of language function and suprasentential structure. Language use frequently relates to suprasentential structures and meanings and cannot be circumscribed by a grammatical rule system that operates exclusively at the sentence level. Instead, the constraints for language use are governed by such variables as speaker intent, physical setting, verbal context, social context, style, and apparently universal principles of communication, such as the need for cooperation. It was essential, therefore, that the behaviors to be analyzed be taken from a situation involving real discourse. This would allow for the analysis of a wide variety of language behaviors—both sentential and suprasentential—closely linked to interactional variables.

Error analysis was also judged relevant, since the procedure would need to be applied to the assessment of language disorders. Since errors are, by definition, deviant forms, their analysis seemed essential. While description of communicative strengths is important, the primary function of the speech-language pathologist is to discover difficulties that interfere with communication. The question always asked in diagnosis is, "What language errors mark this individual as disordered?"

The application of error analysis is also essential in the remediation process. Without a description of deficit areas, language therapy is inadequate (Leonard, 1972; Muma and Pierce, 1981; Rees, 1978; Simon, 1979). Error analysis met the requirements of clinical assessment and therapy planning. The major aim, therefore, was the identification of errors most apt to interefere with discourse.

Finally, in order to make the assessment as pragmatic as possible, the behaviors selected for analysis had to have clinical relevance. The tendency for researchers and test designers to arbitrarily identify language errors or assessment parameters without reference to actual data frequently results in artificiality and inappropriate intervention (Gould, 1981; Philips, 1972). Instead of molding the data to fit preconceived ideas and biases, the reverse should be the case. The use of clinical observation and data collection enabled us to avoid this difficulty. Behaviors selected for assessment were obtained directly from language samples.

A general approach to assessment was developed, building on discourse analysis as the procedural focus, error analysis as the primary aim for its development, and clinical observation and reliance on data as the method for development. The purpose of this chapter is to provide a sufficiently complete description of Clinical Discourse Analysis so that clinicians understand its purpose and potential as a tool to be used in designing individualized communication development programs. A more detailed version (i.e., an assessment manual) will be available at a later date.

A Strategy for Observing Communication Deficits

Language Sampling. In identifying problematic behaviors that affect the functionality of communication, it was necessary to collect data in communicative interactions that could be realistically monitored by clinicians. If the procedure was to have practical application, it had to be based on a practical method of data collection and analysis. Given this concern, the method selected was clinical language sampling. There were several reasons for this decision.

First, language sampling allows for holistic evaluation rather than viewing language as consisting of discrete and isolated units, and it preserves the intentionality of the communicative situation. Second, language samples are obtained in relatively open communicative settings. This tends to ensure the necessary range of data parameters because of the relatively unconstrained setting for data collection. This point is important in light of Bloom and Lahey's (1978) comments on the absence of language usage tests. They suggested that a major reason for this lack was the fact that standardized tests placed such severe constraints on the range of data obtained. These constraints acted to eliminate true communication and its functional qualities. Third, language sampling is a procedure that has been widely used in applied linguistic research and discourse analysis over the past 20 years (Bloom, 1973; Brown, 1973; Coulthard, 1977; Duncan, 1973).

Finally, it was not a new idea that "a clinical procedure such as the analysis of a speech sample may yield more useful information to the clinician than does traditional testing" (Lee and Canter, 1971, p. 316). Language sampling was, even in the late 1970s, a tool familiar to practicing clinicians. Therefore, for all of these reasons, the method of collecting and identifying functional language errors was language sampling.

Identification of Specific Problem Behaviors. The next process was the identification of error behaviors (or trouble spots) that impede functional discourse. This process was carried out in three steps: the identification of difficulties, selection of those problem behaviors most critical to interaction, and checks on the psychological reality of the selected behaviors.

The first phase of the process, the identification of problem behaviors, was accomplished through the analysis of language samples from 38 language disordered individuals. The subjects ranged from 6 years 7 months to 22 years 3 months of age and were diagnosed as having language disorders on the basis of three criteria: (1) each had been identified as having a language disorder as the result of a complete language evaluation conducted by a certified speech-language pathologist, (2) each was functioning at least one year below age level academically, and (3) each exhibited poor social skills as determined by the teacher or counselor.

Approximately 30 minutes of spontaneous language interaction was audiorecorded and transcribed for each individual. The researcher then analyzed the samples to identify behavior patterns that interfered with the successful completion of each interactive dyad. Twenty-seven problem behaviors were identified.

Phase two involved the reduction of these 27 problem behaviors to a set of reliable categories for further investigation and empirical validation. It was noted immediately that some of them were difficult to define and were highly variable. Therefore, the following criteria were established to reduce the total set of 27 behaviors to a manageably smaller number and more reliable set. The behaviors had to (1) be explicit (clearly definable); (2) occur in more than a single individual; (3) relate to language function in a discernible way; and (4) have demonstrable psychological reality (i.e., have a real impact on language processing). Based on these criteria, the 27 behaviors were reduced to 17. These 17 behaviors were retained as the basic core of observational components to be utilized in structuring the discourse assessment procedure. (These will be listed and discussed on subsequent pages).

Phase three in the selection of problem behaviors addressed validation. It overlapped the second phase because it involved an empirical check on the fourth criterion—the demonstration of the psychological reality of each problem behavior pattern. Not only was it necessary for the identified behaviors to be patterns interfering with discourse processing, but in addition they needed to be readily identifiable by professionals. That is, to be reliable indices of functional language difficulty they would also have to have psychological reality in the most practical sense. Clinicians would have to be able to spot them.

To ensure this outcome, I first searched the literature in language development, discourse analysis, and language disorders in an attempt to determine if any of the behaviors had been identified by other researchers. If a developmental basis could be established for any of the behaviors, or if any of the behaviors were considered significant for study by other researchers, such evidence was interpreted as an indication of psychological reality. Also, a set of informed judges (linguists and speech-language pathologists) were asked to listen to a set of tapes, which included language samples containing all of the problem behaviors. While listening to these tapes, the judges were asked to indicate utterances or behaviors that were suggestive of discourse difficulties. This procedure was suggested by Dr. Bruce Porch, who used a similar technique in the construction of the Porch Index of Communicative Ability (1967). It was reasoned that if these judges could reliably choose the utterances with the previously identified error behaviors, this would be another indication of psychological reality. Finally, seven of the most explicit behaviors were used in two empirical studies comparing their effectiveness with the effectiveness of more traditional categories employed as diagnostic indicators by speech-language pathologists.

In the first study (Damico and Oller, 1980), the two sets of behaviors were used as referral criteria. These sets of criteria were given to two matched groups of elementary school teachers. The first group of teachers received a training session using traditional surface-oriented elements, such as tense markers, plural formations, and pronoun case and gender as referral criteria. The second set of teachers received a similar training session, except that their referral criteria were the seven pragmatic behaviors (linguistic nonfluency, revisions, delays before responding, use of nonspecific vocabulary, inappropriate responses, poor topic maintenance, and need for repetition). The teachers were expected to observe and refer children for language evaluations on the basis of their particular set of criteria. Over a period of one academic year the teachers followed this procedure. The results of this study indicated that the pragmatic criteria were more effective in aiding teachers to accurately identify communication disordered children as compared with those who made dialectal or grammatical errors. The teachers using the pragmatic criteria referred significantly more children for testing ($P < 0.03$), and the accuracy of their referrals was significantly greater ($P < 0.001$). These results indicated an advantage of focusing on pragmatic or discourse behaviors instead of surface-oriented behaviors. This was taken as an indication of psychological reality.

The second study (Damico et al., 1983), used the same two sets of behaviors as predictors of language-based academic problems in Spanish-English bilingual children. Ten children were selected for this case study on the basis of criteria designed to identify Spanish speakers in the early stages of learning English through an immersion process. The two sets of behaviors were used to analyze language samples in both Spanish and English. Based upon these analyses, the children were classified as either having a language disorder or simply going through the process of learning English as a second language in a normal fashion. The objective was to determine if either set of behaviors could differentiate a language disordered student from an English as a Second Language (ESL) student. The results indicated that the pragmatic behaviors were more effective indices of language learning difficulties (as measured by academic and social progress over an academic year). These findings were further support for the psychological reality of these seven behaviors as they contributed to a descriptive profile of children with communication deficits.

Selection of a Theoretical Framework

Once these 17 behaviors were isolated as key variables in describing a communication-disordered child, the next step was to organize the behaviors on the basis of some suitable theoretical framework (Krashen, 1983). The framework selected was that of Grice's "cooperative principle" (1975).

Grice's Cooperative Principle. Grice's work characterizes the conditions governing conversation irrespective of the subject matter. Grice contended that conversation is accomplished only by a cooperative effort between participants to achieve transmission of meaning. The cooperation is based on a mutual and usually implicit adherence to a set of conversational postulates; if participants fail to do this, communication tends to break down and meaning is lost. Grice used four categories in defining his cooperative principle:

The Quantity Category
> This involves the amount of information that is provided during the interaction. The speaker should be as concise as possible to achieve the purpose of the interaction. Grice states two maxims here:
>
> - Make your contribution to the interaction as informative as is required.
> - Do not make your contribution more informative than is required.

The Quality Category
> Quality, in Grice's view, is concerned with the truth value of a contribution. As far as possible, each contribution must be believed to be true and based on adequate evidence. Therefore, the maxims could be:
>
> - Do not say what you believe to be false.
> - Do not say anything for which you lack adequate evidence.

The Relation Category
> This category is what is usually called "relevance." The contribution should be appropriate to the immediate needs of the conversation at each stage of the interaction. In other words, the maxim is:
>
> - Be relevant.

The Manner Category
   According to Grice, this category concerns not what you say but
how you say it. The supermaxim here is "be perspicuous." Specific
maxims related to this are:

- Avoid obscurity of expression.
- Avoid ambiguity.
- Be brief.
- Be orderly.

Grice's theoretical framework offered a number of advantages. His
whole framework is stated at a level of analysis that seemed easily adapted
to the task of classifying problem language behaviors (i.e., "errors"). Grice's
categories are general and reasonably explicit. They were designed to
account for underlying conditions of discourse irrespective of the
intentionality. His maxims, therefore, can easily accommodate the use of
clinical language sampling on the variety of speech acts produced. Also,
his framework was designed to deal with conversational functioning at a
level approaching and encompassing adult competence (i.e., it is criterion-
referenced). This means that an analysis procedure based on this framework
could be utilized over a wide range of ages. The framework is also happily
consistent with the current trend in speech-language pathology toward
synergy. That is, in order to apply these conversational postulates
successfully, the participants in an interaction must utilize language at all
levels along with contextual information, and they must be able to
incorporate inferential knowledge into their interactions. For example, it
is necessary to know the relationship and habits of two individuals in order
to realize that they are engaging in bantering behavior when they "insult"
one another.
   With Grice's theoretical framework in hand, the 17 problem behaviors
could be categorized within it. This was accomplished through the use of
informed judges. Consistent with Porch's procedures (1967), each of Grice's
categories was defined (as listed earlier), and the definitions were placed
on index cards. Similarly, the 17 behaviors were listed on cards with a
definition and an example of the behavior. A set of 20 judges (speech-
language pathologists and linguists) were asked to read the 17 error
behaviors and place each one under one of Grice's four categories. The
result was the completed descriptive analysis procedure, designed through
the collection of actual discourse errors and organized into a theoretical
framework according to the informed judgment of professionals. A
discussion of the actual analysis procedure and the list of problem behaviors
according to Grice's framework follows.

Table 6–1. The Organization of Problem Behaviors Under Grice's Categories in Clinical Discourse Analysis

Quantity Category
  Failure to provide significant information to listeners
  Use of nonspecific vocabulary
  Informational redundancy
  Need for repetition

Quality Category
  Message inaccuracy

Relation Category
  Poor topic maintenance
  Inappropriate response
  Failure to ask relevant questions
  Situational inappropriateness
  Inappropriate speech style

Manner Category
  Linguistic nonfluency
  Revision
  Delays before responding
  Failure to structure discourse
  Turn-taking difficulty
  Gaze inefficiency
  Inappropriate intonational contour

Description of the Completed Procedure

The procedure was organized according to the four categories described by Grice. While the division of these behaviors into one of the four categories is clinically relevant to the concept of error analysis, it should be noted that this is not an all-exclusive division. Just as Grice believed that there was some overlap between the four major categories of his "cooperative principle," some of these behaviors can overlap into one of the other categories. They are organized under the category that appears to be the most descriptive according to the informed judgments of professionals. Each of the problem behaviors appears under the pertinent category according to Grice. Table 6-1 summarizes this organization.

QUANTITY CATEGORY

Failure to Provide Significant Information to the Listener

The speaker does not provide the amount or type of information needed by the listener.

> *Example*   Examiner: So, how would I get to your house from here?
> "Turn right there where we play baseball and my house is down a little bit."

In the analysis of the language sample, this problem type can be most easily observed when the child spontaneously provides instructions or directions or when the examiner asks the child for specific information. The individual's verbalizations should be scrutinized for relevant, specific information that accomplishes the purpose of informing the listener.

The Use of Nonspecific Vocabulary

The speaker uses deictic terms such as "this," "that," "then," "there," pronominals, proper nouns, and possessives when no antecedent or referent is available in the verbal or nonverbal context. The listener has no way of knowing what is being referenced. Individuals displaying this difficulty also tend to overuse generic terms such as "thing" and "stuff" when more specific information is required.

> *Example*   Examiner: Well then, what is your favorite toy?
> "My favorite thing is . . . oh, stuff."

It should be emphasized that, when noting the use of generic terms, many are appropriate and should not be considered error behaviors. It is a common practice to use a generic term such as "stuff" to gloss over a communicative interaction in an appropriate manner. For example, if asked what you did over the weekend, you might respond, "Oh, we went to the baseball game and did some other stuff." In this situation, the use of the term is not inappropriate. The speaker answers the question—giving one specific bit of information—then glosses over the less important activities. This is *not* considered a case of the problem use of nonspecific vocabulary. Similarly, if an individual utilizes nonverbal or *shared* contextual information when speaking, nonspecific terms are acceptable. For example, an individual might say, "Hand me that thing" and point to a specific object. This is the major difference between the problem behavior in question and what the British psychologist Basil Bernstein described as the "restrictive code" (1960). Bernstein noted that users of "restrictive code" provide adequate information for comprehension, but they just rely more heavily on contextual and nonverbal cueing. In these cases, the nonlinguistic information provides the point of reference. In order for the use of nonspecific vocabulary to be identified as a problem behavior, the listener must not have any way of knowing what is being referred to.

Informational Redundancy

This involves the continued and inappropriate fixation on a proposition. The speaker will continue to stress a point or relate a fact even when the listener has acknowledged its reception.

> *Example* Examiner: . . . anyway, I'm glad you enjoyed the fair. Let's talk about something else. How do—
> "Did you ever see the bicentennial state fair?"
>
> Examiner: No, I didn't see that one. Hey, how do you like your teacher?
> "She's really O.K. She lets me work on my bulletin board . . . .She also lets me play with the cars."
>
> Examiner: The cars? Which cars are those?
> "The model cars in the state fair exhibit. How much do you really like the state fair?"

Several of the individuals who have exhibited this type of difficulty operate with limited topic repertoires. One student had five topics that he continually tried to work into the conversation. Another frequently tried to dominate an interaction with discussions of Mars, tektites, or the house of a friend. This problem behavior is different from the first two listed under the quantity category. Rather than too little information, this is a problem of overidentification—redundancy to fault. When this problem occurs, the speaker may be considered mentally ill at worst and boring at best (Coulthard, 1977). It should be emphasized that this error behavior involves *propositional* redundancy rather than *grammatical* redundancy, which has been discussed in light of Creole languages, minority dialects, and surface syntactical deviations (Labov, 1970; Scherer and Giles, 1979; Todd, 1974). For example, the child who uses double comparatives (e.g., "This is more better than that one") would not be described as exhibiting informational redundancy. This is a grammatical redundancy that is frequently associated with regional dialects.

Need for Repetition. Repetition is required prior to any indication of comprehension in spite of the fact that the material is not apparently difficult.

Example Examiner: What did the little boy do then?
". . . . ." (No response)
Examiner: What did the boy do then?
". . . . Wha . . . . What?"
Examiner: When he saw this (points to picture) what did the boy do?
"He ran."

This behavior relates to the individual's ability to function as the receiver of information rather than the sender. It is still, however, a problem with the quantity of information provided. In other words, we need to observe performance in both the listener and speaker roles during discourse. The individual needs additional information even when the message sent to him or her is adequate and the environment is free of interference from extraneous noise or other conflicting factors. As with the other behavior, this error may have many possible causes. Clinical experience suggests that this problem may be due to semantic difficulties, neurological processing, lack of presuppositional knowledge, or a learned pattern of simply asking for a repetition rather than attending initially.

QUALITY CATEGORY

Message Inaccuracy

An attempted communication involves the relating of not quite accurate information. This problem behavior is only indirectly linked to moral issues. It is not intended as a gauge of moral integrity, although the association is probably inevitable even if undesirable. It is recognized that there are many reasons why inaccurate information is transmitted. Although the purpose or cause of violating the quality maxims may not be apparent, the important point is that the inaccuracy be discovered. The effects of this type of problem are significant. If undiscovered, the result is misinformation. If discovered, the result will be a loss of credibility for the speaker. Everyone knows someone who "talks out of both sides of the mouth," or who "doesn't know what he's talking about." Indeed, one characteristic of behavior disorders in children is persistent exaggeration (Erickson, 1978). However, contextually obvious or intentional violations of the quality maxim for various reasons are not considered models of message inaccuracy. These behaviors (e.g., indirect speech acts, bantering, ritualized insults) are noted in their contexts and are often, perhaps usually, interpreted correctly.

RELATION CATEGORY
Poor Topic Maintenance

The speaker makes rapid and inappropriate changes in the topic without providing transitional cues to the listener.

> *Example* ". . . but I missed it [an early TV program] 'cuz I went to bed."
> Examiner: That early? You must have had a hard day.
> "Yeah."
> Examiner: What made it such a hard day?
> "The raking."
> Examiner: That's hard work isn't it?
> "Our teacher said, uh . . . whoever wins in checkers—I won—goes to McDonald's."

This problem behavior frequently causes disequilibrium. The receiver is "swept off of his verbal feet," and the thrust of the interaction is lost. When a topic is not maintained, two considerations are possible. First, the individual may be exhibiting error behavior. The second consideration is that the individual may be utilizing a communicative strategy to avoid the interaction or topic. Clinical experience suggests that this use of topic switching is accompanied by loss of eye contact or defensive posturing by individuals, and if pressed on the topic, they will exhibit even more reluctance to interact.

Inappropriate Response

The individual makes turns that indicate radically unpredictable interpretations of meaning. It is as though the individual were operating on an independent discourse agenda.

> *Example* Examiner: How do you like school?
> "I don't know him yet."

This particular behavior is easy to spot but difficult to explain. The individual does not provide relevant answers to the questions asked, so the attempt to secure information must be restated or it fails to get through. As in the example cited above, the individual's interpretation of meaning may be so unpredictable that it gives the appearance of a complete topical shift. The child, however, understood the word "school" to be a proper noun. While it is a relation problem, just as poor topic maintenance, it is a different error type.

Failure to Ask Relevant Questions

The individual does not seek clarification of information that is unclear. Consequently, there is little or no "verbal play" (Muma, 1975) if the message received from the speaker is unclear or too difficult for the individual to comprehend. Communication breaks down. A failure to ask questions will greatly increase language difficulties owing to a lack of compensation for comprehension problems. The result is usually an inappropriate response or no response at all. Consequently, this problem behavior pattern is noted by determining the number of occasions of inappropriate responding or nonresponding without questioning when the context demanded this behavior for a productive communicative interaction.

Situational Inappropriateness

This behavior tends to account for a generalized lack of relevance. The speaker's utterance is not only irrelevant to the discourse or the question asked, but it also occurs in an inappropriate social or interactional situation.

> *Example*   Examiner: Come in and sit down,_____.
>   It's nice to meet you.
>   "Why does twenty years go by so fast?"
>   Examiner: Pardon, what did you say?
>   "Why does twenty years go by so fast?"
>   Examiner: . . . Why do you ask that question?
>   "I don't know. . .do you always blink your eyes like that?"

In this example, the individual committed two different error types. First, he asked a question that was abrupt and unexpected in a greeting exchange. Second, he violated several politeness conventions when he drew attention to the examiner's nervous tic. Such violations of social conventions or politeness constraints are reacted to adversely in our society, and the individual may be perceived as rude or boorish.

Inappropriate Speech Style

The speaker does not change the structural, lexical, or prosodic form of his utterances according to the needs of the listeners.

Example   Examiner: O.K. Bill, leave the tape recorder alone.
"But I want to play with it. You're not fair" (in a whiny voice).

The ability to change speech style to accommodate one's listener is one of the most studied areas in child language acquisition. Research shows that this ability is acquired at an early age (Maratsos, 1974). When this problem behavior arises, there is a communicative breakdown due to incomprehensibility or an adverse reaction as a result of being "talked down to." A commonly observed example is a child who whines persistently as a manipulative ploy. Lack of code switching behaviors involving minority dialects or slang at inappropriate junctures are also examples of this problem (Poplack, 1982).

MANNER CATEGORY

Linguistic Nonfluency

The speaker's production is disrupted by repetitions, unusual pauses, and hesitation phenomena.

Example   "Sh. . .uh . . .she . .um. . .she comes at dinner."

This behavior has commonly been noted (Dechert and Raupach, 1980; Goldman-Eisler, 1958; James, 1973; Loban, 1963; Muma, 1971). It is indicative of a temporal mapping problem. That is, the speaker has difficulty rapidly and efficiently fitting a verbal sequence into an experiential context. Consequently, he or she stalls or delays while attempting to map the utterance forms into the situation, and there is a rather jerky quality apparent as the individual searches for words and appropriate syntax to code a thought. It should be noted that this behavior occasionally occurs in the speech of normal language users. Ochs (1979) and Chafe (1975) have described similar behaviors as functions of normal discourse usage. The difference, however, is one of degree. Although normal language users have some infrequent mapping problems, language disordered individuals exhibit persistent difficulty. Indeed, the research with Clinical Discourse Analysis indicates that frequent occurrence of this behavior is an index of a language proficiency problem that underlies both interactional and academic difficulties.

Revision

The speaker seems to come to dead ends in a maze, as if starting off in a certain direction, then coming back to a starting point and beginning anew after each attempt. There are many false starts and self-interruptions.

Example "Well, you see. . .if you want—sometimes when you ca— . . .
a lot of times when you can't go out, you can just play with
your twin brothers."

This behavior may seem the same as linguistic nonfluency at first, and in fact both are temporal mapping problems. However, nonfluencies are distinct from revisions. In the former the child never seems to get going without difficulty but in the latter (a deeper problem, it seems) the child gets going but arrives nowhere only to start again in a different, usually unproductive direction. There are some children who have this problem but rarely show linguistic nonfluencies.

Delays Before Responding

Communicative exchanges initiated by others are followed by pauses of inordinate length at turn-switching points.

Example Examiner: Well, what did you do at recess?
". . .played tag."

This behavior is the third temporal mapping problem identified in this procedure. It is different from the first two, however, in that it involves input. Such pauses tend to affect the natural flow of conversation and are usually disruptive to the interaction. Just as with the other two temporal mapping difficulties, this problem is one of degree. The frequency of occurrence is important, as is the length of the interval between taking a turn as a listener versus that of a speaker. In order to determine natural and unnatural temporal delays, a pilot study was conducted involving listener judgments of videotaped discourse. Results indicated that delays longer than 2.3 seconds *when not preceded by an open ended question requiring a thoughtful pause,* were judged unnatural approximately 92% of the time.

Failure to Structure Discourse

This problem behavior is the most global of the 17. It occurs when the discourse of the speaker lacks forethought and organizational planning. As a result of this characteristic, the discourse is confusion—even if all of the propositional content is present. It is not enough simply to provide all the essential information. It must be presented in a logical and temporally sequential format for maximum comprehensibility (Oller, in press). Levy (1979) is one of the few professionals to have thus far addressed this behavior.

Turn-Taking Difficulty

The participant in a conversational interaction does not attend to the cues necessary for the appropriate exchange of conversational turns. This results in one of two possible outcomes. First, the individual does not allow others to add information. This is characterized by interruptions or consistent and inappropriate bids for the turn.

> *Example* Examiner: Well, I think that the be—
> "I like the green one best."
> Examiner: Yes, that's a nice one. How about the red one?
> Do you wa—
> "Can we find more like this one?"

The second possibility involves an opposite reaction. Rather than always bidding for the turn, this individual does not read the switching cues appropriately and, therefore, does not hold up his part of the interaction.

> Examiner: Not over, no, it's not.
> "What do you mean by that?"
> Examiner: Well, most of the year is gone. . .but not all of it.
> You know?
> ". . . . ." (No response.)

This behavior is different from the need for repetition because it occurs during turn switching and a specific response to a question is not required. The tagging by the speaker is simply one type of cue to give the turn away. There are, in fact, many cues that act as turn taking signals in English. Duncan (1973) lists six types frequently used in our culture: intonation, paralanguage, body motion, sociocentric sequences, pitch, and syntax. Appropriate turn taking is learned early in an individual's language development (Bruner, 1975; Coulthard, 1977), and it is considered one of the principal rules for interaction (Sachs, Schegloff, Jefferson, 1974). When inappropriate turn taking occurs it interferes with the quality of the interaction.

Gaze Inefficiency

The individual's use of eye contact is inconsistent or absent. The attempts to "color" communication with gaze are inappropriate. Eye contact is an essential component of discourse. Kendon (1967) observed definite gaze changes according to the interaction and numerous studies have emphasized the importance of gaze (Allen and Guy, 1977; Argyle, Ingram, Alkema, and McCallin, 1973; Beattie, 1978). Although the use of gaze is variable between cultures, it is an important discourse tool, and the inefficiency and inappropriate use of it affects the thrust of communication and the attitudes toward the person exhibiting the inefficiency (Dunaway and Damico, no date).

Inappropriate Intonational Contour

The speaker's ability to embellish or "color" his or her meaning through the use of linguistic suprasegmentals, such as pitch levels, vocal intensity, and other inflectional contours is poor. This often results in misinterpretation of the speaker's intent. Additionally, listeners frequently attempt to make sincerity judgments on the basis of a speaker's verbal output according to intonational signals.

Once the behaviors utilized in Clinical Discourse Analysis are described, the next step is to detail the analysis procedure.

CLINICAL APPLICATION

Clinical Discourse Analysis, as noted, is a descriptive approach designed for the analysis of spontaneous language samples. The focus of the assessment is on the functionality of discourse regardless of the underlying cause. For example, the individual assessed may exhibit linguistic nonfluencies as a result of a number of factors. He or she may have a set of inaccurate syntactical rules or may exhibit a difficulty with his or her semantic rule system. Both of these problem areas, however, will adversely affect temporal mapping and will interfere with discourse.

The following list is a set of procedures to follow when using Clinical Discourse Analysis:

1. A spontaneous language sample is collected over two sessions and consists of approximately 180 utterances. This sample should be collected during conversational interaction rather than in simple picture description activities. This is essential in order to analyze the individual's discourse abilities.

2. The sample should be transcribed as soon as possible. This will aid in the recall of situational cues not observable through the use of audiotape.

3. When transcribing, it is essential to preserve the speaker-listener dyad, the nonlinguistic context, the intonational contour, and all verbal segments, such as pauses or false starts. All of this information is necessary for analysis.

4. The segmentation of utterances is accomplished through a modification of the procedure recommended by Barrie-Blackley, Musselwhite, and Rogister (1978). Specifically, we place more emphasis on their Communication Unit for segmentation purposes than on the Phonological Unit, and we do not omit verbal segments, such as false starts, mazes, or hesitation phenomena. These behaviors are obviously important

to our analysis. (For example, "Thi. . .this girl jumped him." We would not omit the "Thi. . ."; it is a linguistic nonfluency.)

5. Once the language sample has been transcribed, the sample should be read through while listening to the tape. This will aid in placing the correct intonational contour on the transcription and in correcting any transcription errors.

6. Next, we proceed by analyzing each conversational turn and marking any of the described error behaviors *and* any other discourse errors that occur. It is important that this step involve only the identification of these behaviors and not interpretation. All problem behaviors should be identified and marked *before* determining if the occurrences are within normal limits.

7. Then we count the number of utterances with one or more discourse errors and determine the frequency of occurrence of each of the behaviors. This will aid in our description of the individual's communicative abilities.

8. It is important to note the number of single word utterances and nonverbal responses. Many individuals with discourse difficulties may compensate by using short utterances or nonverbal communication. Although this may be acceptable in some situations, it tends to hide difficulties that affect the range of possible interactions. When a large number of single word utterances are noted, we analyze the language with and without these utterances. If there is a significant difference between the two analyses, the individual may be shielding difficulties.

9. It should be emphasized that Clinical Discourse Analysis is a descriptive approach and should be treated as such. Although there are some figures on a partial counting procedure (which will not be dealt with in this chapter), this tool was not designed for quantification. Additionally, this procedure should not be used as the sole basis for labeling an individual as having a communication disorder. Numerous other factors, such as academic and social abilities, the informed judgments of teachers and peers, and other valid assessment procedures should be used in making this determination.

Now that the procedure has been described and a set of guidelines has been provided for its use, it may be beneficial to provide an actual example.

CASE STUDY

Thad is a 10 year 3 month old boy who had transferred into his present school nearly four months before the examiner saw him. His teacher referred him to the special education department for possible placement in a classroom for the emotionally disturbed. At the time of the referral, she expressed concern over his inability to attend to tasks and his poor social skills. When tested by an educational diagnostician, Thad performed within normal limits on the Wechsler Intelligence Scale for Children—Revised (WISC-R) (Wechsler, 1974), but he earned scores approximately two years below his grade level on the tests of academic achievement. As a portion of his complete evaluation, he was referred to the school-based speech-language pathologist.

Thad's initial language evaluation consisted of the administration of four different tests. On the Peabody Picture Vocabulary Test–Revised (Dunn and Dunn, 1981), Thad's score placed him at the 58th percentile. This is equivalent to a "vocabulary age" of 10.8. The Clinical Evaluation of Language Functions (CELF) (Semel and Wiig, 1980) also showed him to be functioning at age level. His scores placed him at the 61st percentile on the processing section and at the 46th percentile on the production section. In addition, he did not experience any difficulty on the individual subtests. When the speech-language pathologist performed an informal syntactic analysis on an 89 utterance language sample, she found no significant error patterns. Thad's performance on the Word Test (Jorgensen, Barrett, Hinsingh, and Zachman, 1981), however, was different. His overall score placed him at the 28th percentile and he exhibited difficulty on two of the subtests. On the Semantic Absurdities subtest, he scored at the 15th percentile, and his score on the Multiple Definitions subtest placed him at the 5th percentile. Owing to the inconsistency of test scores and "a hunch" that he had more problems, another speech-language pathologist was consulted.

Upon request, additional language samples were collected, transcribed, and analyzed using Clinical Discourse Analysis. The transcript of this analysis is partially reproduced in Appendix 6–1. The results of the analysis may be found in Table 6–2.

Based on this analysis procedure, Thad does exhibit discourse difficulties. His spontaneous interactions contain one or more problem discourse behaviors in 104 utterances, or in 49.05% of his 212 utterances. This is a high percentage of occurrence and will adversely affect his communicative abilities. The general impression that one forms when talking to Thad bears out this fact. His interactive partner is unsure of his meaning much of the time, and there is the impression that Thad is greatly confused. In addition, there does not appear to be much content in what he is saying. It is little wonder that his teacher described him as "bizarre." A breakdown of the problem patterns according to Clinical Discourse Analysis, however, allows for a more detailed and descriptive explanation.

Table 6–2. Clinical Discourse Analysis Worksheet for Thad

CLINICAL DISCOURSE ANALYSIS

Quantity	43
Insufficient information	20
Nonspecific vocabulary	18
Informational redundancy	—
Need for repetition	5
Quality	2
Message inaccuracy	2
Relation	14
Poor topic maintenance	9
Inappropriate response	4
Failure to ask relevant questions	STRONG ABILITY
Situational inappropriateness	—
Inappropriate speech style	1
Manner	168
Linguistic nonfluency	97
Revision	52
Delay before responding	2
Failure to structure discourse	14
Turn-taking difficulty	—
Gaze inefficiency	—
Inappropriate intonational contour	3

Total Utterances	212
Total Discourse Problem Behaviors	222
Total Utterances with These Behaviors	104
Percentage of Utterances with Problem Behaviors	49.05%

Thad's main difficulties are in the Manner and Quantity categories. Although problems in either category would diminish his conversational effectiveness, the combination of the two error types is especially pernicious. Not only is he failing to provide enough information for effective meaning transmission, but in addition he is not able to present what little information he does have in an efficient and organized manner. This is the major reason for the impression of confusion on the listener's part. Thad also presents nine occurrences of poor topic maintenance, which add even more confusion.

Looking at the individual behavior types, Thad exhibits the greatest difficulties with temporal mapping. His large number of linguistic nonfluencies (97 instances) and revisions (52 instances) suggest that he has a problem fitting verbal sequences into a conversational context. This inefficient mapping process is indicative of deeper language proficiency problems, which should affect both his interactive and his academic language skills. The two year delay in academic achievement appears to support this contention. It is interesting to note that he did not exhibit many delays before responding (i.e., receptive temporal mapping problems). His mapping difficulties were largely restricted to production. There are several possible explanations for this observation. The most likely, however, may be that he is able to utilize contextual information to a greater extent receptively as an aid to this linguistic mapping. This could also explain the absence of many mapping problems on selected subtests of the CELF. The CELF subtests of Producing Model Sentences and Producing Formulated Sentences provided specific contextual information, which limited the need for mapping alternatives. Hence, he exhibited few nonfluent instances on these tasks.

Thad also exhibited a pattern of failure to structure discourse (14 global instances)—another Manner difficulty. His difficulties with this behavior appeared to be due to two different problems. The first involves temporal sequencing (see utterances 89 to 99). Regardless of the cause, the problem behavior caused confusion, even if all the prepositional content was present. Thad's teacher's comment about his inability to attend to tasks may be another indication of this problem with the appropriate sequencing of experience (Oller, in press).

Analysis of the Quantity difficulties indicate problems in supplying adequate information. Thad exhibited 20 instances of a failure to provide significant information and 18 instances of the inappropriate use of nonspecific vocabulary. These problem behaviors are likely to be responsible for the impression of a general lack of content. It may also be a reason for his poor social skills. Interactional confusion caused by such Quantity difficulties results in negative reactions when meaning transmission fails and causes others to be reluctant to engage in conversational interaction with Thad.

In summary, Thad exhibited numerous discourse difficulties characterized by Manner and Quantity violations. Although he also exhibited strength in his receptive abilities and in willingness to ask relevant questions for clarification purposes, his problem behaviors result in frequent conversational breakdowns. When the results of Clinical Discourse Analysis are considered in light of Thad's delayed academic skills, his poor social interactions, and his negative teacher evaluations, he does appear to have a significant language disorder.

Early educational objectives for Thad would be as follows:

1. Reduce Thad's instances of linguistic nonfluency and revision behaviors by structuring language input at his level of comprehension.

2. Increase his ability to determine and transmit important aspects of verbal messages—particularly in giving directions.

3. Increase Thad's awareness of the need to provide specific referents rather than nonspecific terms during conversation.

4. Increase Thad's ability and willingness to plan discourse—or message formulation—before speaking.

SUMMARY

A new language assessment tool, Clinical Discourse Analysis, is provided that is consistent with the movement of our profession toward applied pragmatics (Gallagher and Prutting, 1983). The procedure analyzes the functionality of language discourse in a holistic fashion, focusing on language in conversational interaction. It has been used with over 600 individuals ranging in age from 6 years 3 months to 74 years 3 months. Clinical Discourse Analysis offers help in certain problem cases, especially in diagnosing language disorders in older children.

REFERENCES

Abkarian, G. G. (1977). The changing face of a discipline: Isn't it "romantic"? *Journal of Speech and Hearing Disorders, 42*, 422–435.

Allen, D. E., and Guy, R. F. (1977). Ocular breaks and verbal output. *Sociometry, 40*, 90–96.

Argyle, M., Ingram, R., Alkema, F., and McCallin, M. (1973). The different functions of gaze. *Semiotica, 7*, 19–31.

Arnold, K. S., and Reed, L. (1976). The grammatic closure subtest of the ITPA: A comparative study of black and white children. *Journal of Speech and Hearing Disorders, 41*, 477–486.

Bachman, L., and Palmer, A. (1981). The construct validity of the FSI oral interview. *Language Learning, 31*, 67–86.

Barrie-Blackley, S., Musselwhite, C. R., and Rogister, S. H. (1978). *Clinical oral language sampling: A handbook for students and clinicians.* Danville, IL: Interstate Printers and Publishers.

Beattie, G. W. (1978). Sequential temporal patterns of speech and gaze in dialogue. *Semiotica, 23,* 29–52.

Berko, J. (1958). The child's learning of English morphology. *Word, 14,* 150–177.

Bernstein, B. (1960). Language and social class. *British Journal of Sociology, 11,* 271–276.

Bloom, L. M. (1973). *One word at a time: The use of single word utterances before syntax.* The Hague, Netherlands: Mouton.

Bloom, L. M., and Lahey, M. (1978). *Language development and language disorders.* New York: J. Wiley and Sons.

Bloomfield, L. (1933). *Language.* New York: Holt, Rinehart and Winston.

Brown, R. (1973). *A first language: The early stages.* Cambridge, MA: Harvard University Press.

Bruner, J. S. (1975). From communication to language—a psychological perspective. *Cognition, 3,* 255–288.

Carrow, M. A. (1968). The development of auditory comprehension of language structure in children. *Journal of Speech and Hearing Disorders, 33,* 99–111.

Carrow, E. (1974). Assessment of speech and language in children, in J. McLean, D. Yoder, and R. Schiefelbusch (Eds.), *Language intervention with the retarded.* Baltimore: University Park Press, pp. 52–88.

Chafe, W. (1975). Creativity in verbalization and its implications for the nature of stored knowledge, in P. Cole and J. H. Morgan (Eds.), *Studies in syntax and semantics: Speech acts* (Vol. 3). New York: Academic Press.

Clark, H. H., and Clark, E. V. (1977). *Psychology and language.* New York: Harcourt Brace Jovanovich.

Cole, P., and Morgan, J. H. (Eds.). (1975). *Syntax and semantics: Speech acts* (Vol. 3). New York: Academic Press.

Coulthard, M. (1977). *An introduction to discourse analysis.* London: Longman Group Limited.

Cromer, R. F. (1974). Receptive language in the mentally retarded: Processes and diagnostic distinctions, in R. L. Schiefelbusch and L. L. Lloyd (Eds.), *Language perspectives— acquisition, retardation and intervention.* Baltimore: University Park Press.

Damico, J. S. (1981). Beware the new prescriptionist: One description of linguistic research. *Hearsay, 2,* 3–8.

Damico, J. S., and Oller, J. W., Jr. (1980). Pragmatic versus morphological/syntactic criteria for language referrals. *Language, Speech and Hearing Services in Schools, 11,* 85–94.

Damico, J. S., Oller, J. W., Jr., and Storey, M. E. (1983). The diagnosis of language disorders in bilingual children: Pragmatic and surface-oriented criteria. *Journal of Speech and Hearing Disorders, 48,* 385–394.

Danwitz, Sister M. W. (1981). Formal versus informal assessment: Fragmentation versus holism. *Topics in Language Disorders, 1,* 95–106.

Darley, F. L. (1964). *Diagnosis and appraisal of communication disorders.* Englewood Cliffs, NJ: Prentice-Hall.

Dechert, H. W., and Raupach, M. (Eds.). (1980). *Temporal variables in speech: Studies in honour of Frieda Goldman-Eisler.* The Hague, Netherlands: Mouton.

Drake, G. F. (1976). LSA Report: The source of American linguistic prescriptionism. *TESOL Newsletter, 10,* 9.

Dunaway, D. K., and Damico, J. S. (no date). *Black English and teachers.* Unpublished manuscript.

Duncan, S. (1973). Towards a grammar for dyadic conversation. *Semiotica, 9,* 29–46.

Dunn, L. M., and Dunn, L. M. (1981). *Peabody picture vocabulary test—revised.* Circle Pines, MN: American Guidance Service.

Erickson, M. T. (1978). *Child psychopathology*. Englewood Cliffs, NJ: Prentice-Hall.

Fasold, R. W., and Wolfram, W. (1970). Some linguistic features of Negro dialect, in R. W. Fasold and R. W. Shrug (Eds.), *Teaching standard English in the inner city*. Washington, DC: Center for Applied Linguistics.

Gallagher, T. M., and Prutting, C. A. (1983). *Pragmatic assessment and intervention issues in language*. San Diego, CA: College-Hill Press.

Goldman-Eisler, F. (1958). The predictability of words in context and the length of pauses in speech. *Language and Speech, 1,* 853–860.

Gould, S. J. (1981). *The mismeasure of man*. New York: W. W. Norton.

Grice, H. P. (1975). Logic and conversation, in P. Cole and J. Morgan (Eds.), *Studies in syntax and semantics: Speech acts* (Vol. 3). New York: Academic Press.

Halliday, M. A. K. (1975). *Learning how to mean: Explorations in the development of language*. Amsterdam: Elsevier–North Holland.

Harris, Z. (1951). *Methods in structural linguistics*. Chicago, IL: University of Chicago Press.

Hubbell, R. D. (1981). *Children's language disorders*. Englewood Cliffs, NJ: Prentice-Hall.

James, D. (1973). Another look at, say, some grammatical constraints on, oh, interjections and hesitations. In *Papers from the Ninth Regional Meeting, Chicago Linguistic Society,* pp. 242–251.

Jorgensen, C., Barrett, M., Hinsingh, R., and Zachman, L. (1981). *The Word Test*. Moline, IL: LinguiSystems.

Karmiloff-Smith, A. (1979). Language development after five, in P. Fletcher and M. Garman (Eds.), *Language acquisition*. Cambridge, MA: Cambridge University Press.

Kendon, A. (1967). Some functions of gaze direction in social interaction. *Acta Psychologica, 26,* 22–63.

Krashen, S. D. (1983). Second language acquisition theory and the preparation of teachers: Toward a rationale. Paper presented at the 34th Annual Georgetown University Round Table on Language and Linguistics. Washington, DC, March, 1983.

Labov, W. (1970). The logic of nonstandard English, in F. Williams (Ed.), *Language and poverty: Perspectives on a theme*. Chicago: Markham Publishing Company.

Lee, L. L. (1966). Developmental sentence types: A method for comparing normal and deviant syntactic development. *Journal of Speech and Hearing Disorders, 31,* 311–330.

Lee, L. L., and Canter, S. (1971). Developmental sentence scoring: A clinical procedure for estimating syntactic development in children's spontaneous speech. *Journal of Speech and Hearing Disorders, 36,* 315–340.

Leonard, L. (1972). What is deviant language? *Journal of Speech and Hearing Disorders, 37,* 427–446.

Leonard, L., Prutting, C., Perozzi, J., and Berkeley, R. (1978). Nonstandardized approaches to the assessment of language behavior. *ASHA, 20,* 371–379.

Lerea, L. (1958). Assessing language development. *Journal of Speech and Hearing Research, 1,* 75–85.

Levy, D. (1979). Communicative goals and strategies: Between discourse and syntax. In T. Givon (Ed.), *Studies in syntax and semantics: Discourse and syntax,* (Vol. 12). New York: Academic Press.

Loban, W. D. (1963). *The language of elementary school children*. Champaign, IL: National Council of Teachers of English.

Maratsos, M. P. (1974). Preschool children's use of definite and indefinite articles. *Child Development, 45,* 446–455.

Menyuk, P. (1964). Syntactic rules used by children from pre-school through first grade. *Child Development, 35,* 533–546.

Millen, C. E., and Prutting, C. A. (1979). Inconsistencies across three language comprehension tests for specific grammatical features. *Language, Speech and Hearing Services in Schools, 10,* 162–170.

Minifie, F. D., Darley, F. L., and Sherman, D. (1963). Temporal reliability of seven language measures. *Journal of Speech and Hearing Research, 6,* 139–148.

Muma, J. R. (1971). Syntax of preschool fluent and dysfluent speech: A transformational analysis. *Journal of Speech and Hearing Research, 14,* 428–441.

Muma, J. R. (1975). The communication game: Dump and play. *Journal of Speech and Hearing Disorders, 40,* 296–309.

Muma, J. R. (1978). *Language handbook: Concepts, assessment, intervention.* Englewood Cliffs, NJ: Prentice-Hall.

Muma, J. R., and Pierce, S. (1981). Language intervention: Data of evidence. *Topics in Learning and Learning Disabilities,* July, 1–11.

Ochs, E. (1979). Planned and unplanned discourse, in T. Givon (Ed.), *Studies in syntax and semantics: Discourse and syntax* (Vol. 12). New York: Academic Press.

Oller, J. W., Jr. (1973). Pragmatic language testing. *Language Sciences, 28,* 7–12.

Oller, J. W., Jr. (1979). *Language tests at school: A pragmatic approach.* London: Longman Group Limited.

Oller, J. W., Jr. (1981). How do we tell when tests are the same or different? Paper presented at the Second International Language Testing Symposium, Darmstadt, Germany, May, 1980.

Oller, J. W., Jr. (1983). *Issues in language testing research.* Rowley, MA: Newbury House.

Oller, J. W., Jr. (in press). Episodic organization and language acquisition, in S. Williams (Ed.), *Proceedings of the Fourth Delaware Symposium on Language Studies: Linguistics, humanism, and computers.* Norwood, NJ: Ablex.

Omark, D. R., and Erickson, J. G. (Eds.). (1983). *The bilingual exceptional child.* San Diego, CA: College-Hill Press.

Philips, S. U. (1972). Acquisition of rules for appropriate speech usage, in C. B. Cazden, V. P. John, and D. Hymes (Eds.), *The functions of language in the classroom.* New York: Teachers College Press.

Poplack, S. (1982). Bilingualism and the vernacular, in B. Hartford, A. Valdman, and C. R. Foster (Eds.), *Issues in international bilingual education.* New York: Plenum Press.

Porch, B. E. (1967). Porch index of communicative ability: *Theory and development* (Vol. 1). Palo Alto, CA: Consulting Psychologists Press.

Prutting, C. A. (1982). Pragmatics as social competence. *Journal of Speech and Hearing Disorders, 47,* 123–133.

Prutting, C. A., Gallagher, T. M., and Mulac, A. (1975). The expressive portion of the NSST compared to a language sample. *Journal of Speech and Hearing Disorders, 40,* 40–48.

Rees, N. S. (1978). Pragmatics of language, in R. L. Schiefelbusch (Ed.), *Bases of language intervention.* Baltimore: University Park Press.

Rees, N. S., and Shulman, M. (1978). I don't understand what you mean by comprehension. *Journal of Speech and Hearing Disorders, 43,* 208–219.

Sachs, H., Schegloff, E., and Jefferson, G. (1974). A simplest systematics for the organization of turn-taking for conversation. *Language, 50,* 696–735.

Scherer, K. R., and Giles, H. (1979). *Social Markers in Speech.* Cambridge: Cambridge University Press.

Semel, E. M., and Wiig, E. H. (1980). *Clinical Evaluation of Language Functions.* Columbus: OH: Charles Merrill.

Shuy, R. (1972). Some more things that reading teachers need to know about language, in H. Klein (Ed.), *The quest for competency in teaching reading.* Newark, NJ: International Reading Association.

Simon, C. S. (1979). *Communicative competence: A functional-pragmatic approach to language therapy.* Tucson, AZ: Communication Skill Builders.

Smitherman, G. (1981). "What go round come round": King in perspective. *Harvard Educational Review, 51,* 40–56.

Sommers, R. K., Erdige, S., and Peterson, M. K. (1978). How valid are children's language tests? *Journal of Special Education, 12,* 393–407.

Templin, M. (1943). A study of sound discrimination ability of elementary school pupils. *Journal of Speech Disorders, 8,* 127–132.

Todd, L. (1974). *Pidgins and creoles.* Boston: Routledge and Keegan Paul.

Vaughn-Cooke, A. F. (1979). Evaluating language assessment procedures: An examination of linguistics guidelines and Public Law 94-142 guidelines. *Georgetown University Round Table on Languages and Linguistics,* pp. 231–257.

Wechsler, D. (1974). *Manual for the Wechsler Intelligence Scale for Children—Revised.* New York: Psychological Corporation.

Weiner, P. S. (1967). Auditory discrimination and articulation. *Journal of Speech and Hearing Disorders, 32,* 19–28.

APPENDIX 6-1
Sample Transcript (Partial)

Name: <u>Thad</u>   School: _____   Teacher: _____

Age: <u>10-3</u>   Date: <u>2-19-82</u>   Evaluator: <u>J.S. Damico</u>

Key:

FSI	=	Failure to provide information	DR = Delays before responding
NSV	=	Nonspecific vocabulary	DS = Failure to structure discourse
RED	=	Informational redundancy	TTD = Turn taking difficulty
NR	=	Need for repetition	GI = Gaze inefficiency
MI	=	Message inaccuracy	IIC = Inappropriate intonational contour
PTM	=	Poor topic maintenance	: : = Pause longer than 2.3 seconds
IR	=	Inappropriate response	( ) = Parenthetical comment
FRQ	=	Failure to ask relevant question	◜ = Intonational contour
SI	=	Situational inappropriateness	= = Stress for emphasis
ISS	=	Inappropriate speech style	◖⌐ = Thoughtful pause
LNF	=	Linguistic nonfluency	/ = Interruption
R	=	Revision	

First meeting of the client and the clinician. Both are sitting at a round table on the same side in the resource room. The interaction is informal and the two are just conversing. The client is eating sunflower seeds. The conversation picks up where it left off during the walk over to the room.

Clinician

Gee..it's almost the end of the month isn't it?

Client

1. Right (laughs and nods).

2. We have uh. . .guy that's going away.
   ^{LNF}

3. His name is Ronnie.

Where is Ronnie going?

   ④ He goin. . .he's gonna move to uh. . .Los ^{R} ^{LNF} Lunas.

Why would someone want to move to Los Lunas?

   5. . . .I don't know (shrugs and laughs).

Can you give me any idea?

   ⑥ Any idea? ^{NR} (asked relevant Q)

Yeah, why would he want to move to Los Lunas. . . or does he want to move to Los Lunas?

   ⑦ Cause uhm. . .cause uhm. . .his parents and ^{LNF} ^{LNF} and him. . .his brother — whole family had ^{R} planned. ^{FSI}

Had planned to what?

   8. Move to Los Lunas. (Got up and walked to trash can.)

Alright. Well, tell me a little about yourself, Thaddeus. ----- Have a seat.

   9. O.K. There's one thing that I like.

O.K.

   ⑩ There's one thing that I have. . .about me. ^{LNF}

   11. I like cars.

   ⑫ I like to play with them and. . . . ^{FSI}

   13. Let's see what I do with them.

   ⑭ Sometimes my sister bothers me. ^{PTM}

When you play with them?

   15. Play with what? (Relevant Q)

   16. No, at school she does.

The cars.

   17. Not with the cars.

Oh. . . . Well, tell me about how she bothers you.

18. Last night uh.^{LNF} .I made a uh. . . ^{LNF} a. . . little project.

19. It's called a.^{LNF} ..it's called a trailer.

20. See I had the trailer part and the hook up part to put together.

Yeah.

21. But I only had to find one.^{FSI}

One what?

22. Wheel to put on.

Did you find it?

23. Yeah.

24. (and) uh.^{LNF} . . and then I had --after I had uhm.^{LNF} .. had cleaned my room up. ^{LNF} . . . I had put the thing on.^{NSV}

What whole thing on?

25. The trailer.

26. The dresser.

Oh. . . .what did you put it on, Thad?

27. I hooked it. ^{LNF} up. . . I hooked ^R I. ^{LNF}. I knew I had a jeep somewhere around my room that has a hook.

Uh huh.

28. I left to find it.

29. I wanted to find it. . . I looked in my room . . .but no.

30. And then⌊. . .⌉I looked in there and my sister, Naomi. ^{LNF} . . my sister.^{FSI} . . .

Uh huh.

What was gone?

(31.) I came back and saw mine and they were gone. [NSV]

Wait a minute, you were talking about the trailer and suddenly you're talking about cars. . . . What's going on? . . . What are we talking about?

32. My cars.

33. They were gone!

What cars are you talking about

Oh? They were gone?

(34.) . . . . (15 sec.) [NR]

(35.) About my little . . [LNF] Hot Wheel cars.

36. Yeah, they were gone (shrugs shoulders and waves hands). [LNF]

Gone. Hmmm. What happened to them?

37. See, I knew that my sister was playing with them but she didn't have my permission to. [LNF]

From where, Thad?

(38.) And then uhm. . [LNF] . and then uhm. . . [LNF] [FSI] I came back.

39. Probably from school.

(40.) (and) then my my little Hot Wheel cars were gone. [LNF]

Yeah. . . . They were gone, huh?

What happened to them, do you think?

(41.) I knew I had uhm. . [LNF] .lined 'em all up on my dresser. [LNF] [FSI]

42. Um hm (nods head).

(43.) I found out that uhm Naomi---She told me. . [LNF] [R] [LNF] the truth. [FSI]

44. She said she was playing with 'em and she stuck
    'em in her little bag.

Oh. . . . Thad, what was the truth?

45. She has a little bag.

46. It's where she puts her little dishes and all that.

47. (and then) she had stuck the cars in there.
    LNF

Uh huh. I figured that one out.

(48.) (and then) I went into the garage see see if I
    could find. . . my cars.
    LNF

Yeah.

Ah!

(49.) They were they were. . . . .
    FSI

50. Uh huh. They were there.

They were there?

51. My sister put 'em in the bag (laughs).

How did they get out there?

52. Maybe she wanted to play a little trick on me.

Why'd she do that?

53. . . . I really wasn't mad.
    LNF

(54.) I was surprised. . .that that that I hadn't seen 'em.
    LNF   R

I see. . . . What did you think of that?

(55.) (and then) I -- one day -- that day after I
    R
    got home from school see uh. . .my sister she
    R
    was in taking a nap.
    LNF

(56.) And uh. . .then. . .and then Naomi uh -- I said
    R
    "Naomi, the next time you do this without my
    permission I'm going to turn you around -- put
    R
    you in your room, turn you around and spank
    you,"

57. and then then she she knew that I uhm[LNF] could do that.[LNF]

Uh huh. What would your mother do, though, if you did do that?

58. She knows that some --[R] I I'm her boss.[LNF][NSV]

59. I'm the boss of my whole thing my own thing, when she's in my room.[NSV]

Who knows that?

60. Them.[NSV]

Who, Thad?

61. My mom and dad do.

62. They know I'm bigger than her.[LNF]

63. and one morning my sister she uh. .she tried to turn the TV on and then I grabbed her by the arm.[PTM][LNF]

64. I put her in her in her room.[LNF]

65. Just to stop her.

Why'd you do that?

66. Not just -- so she wouldn't get into trouble.[R]

O.K. . . . What types of things do you do when you get home in the afternoon, Thaddeus?

67. Huh [. . .] after I get home I show my mom and dad my report.[FSI]

68. Even though . . . that my dad has a uhm -- has the whole week off.[PTM][R]

69. See, he has the whole week off.

Oh. . . . How about your afternoon activities, Thad?

(70). Oh.⌊. .⌉uhm what else⌊. .⌉uhm and then then [LNF]
I then I do my work.

What work?

(71). The usual. [FSI]

What *is* that work, though?

72. Oh, homework.

73. After I do that I get my mom to correct it and
I uhm uhm -- after I do that I say goodbye to [LNF]
my mom.

Does she leave in the afternoon?

74. Yeah, she goes to work and stuff.

75. and after I done that I just watch TV.

You rascal! You watch television, huh?

76. Uh huh (laughs).

What do you watch on TV?

77. I watch⌊uhm. . .⌉on Mondays I watch Private
Benjamin, on Tuesdays I watch Happy Days,
on Wednesdays I watch the Greatest American
Hero.

What's that about?

78. . .uh. . .uhm. . .sometimes I like to uh. . . [IR] [DR]
watch TV a lot. [LNF]

79. uh. . . the Greatest American Hero? [NR] (RELEVANT Q)

What's the Greatest American Hero about?

80. It's about⌊uh. . .⌉this guy named Ralph.

81. He fights all the bad guys. [R]

(nods yes)

(82). and and at the ending he uh -- and then and [LNF]
then uh the police comes and takes him to jail. [NSV]

Takes Ralph to jail?

83. No, takes the bad guys he hadda fight.

84. That he hadda get rid of.

Oh. . .I see.

85. Uh. . . it's fun.

It is, huh?

86. Yeah?

87. I still watch it.

Do you?

88. Yes, I still watch it on Wednesdays.

Pardon?

(89) PTM IIC Like my dad?

(90) Well uh.. .on Wednesdays my dad hadda tried
    to. . .tried to reach my mom on the CB cause
    my mom -- I knew I knew all about this uhm
    . . .this uhm. . .CB that my dad bought my
    mother.

(91) 'Cuz uh. . .'cuz I I had looked in to see when
    uh -- after I got home I go, "Did you buy any-
    thing for mom?"
    and then and then my dad says, "Yeah."

(92)(93) Like uh like if I go in the garage.

94. I see something that's really for -- that's really
    not for me and Naomi or my Dad . . . . .

Uh huh.

95. Then it's really for my mom.

96. I know that that's for my mom.

97. My my dad he had already put aa uhm put the CB in there. [LNF] [NSV]

98. (and) uhm..uhm and then my daddy he hooked the CB up in the car. [LNF]

    Uh huh.

99. There's a big antenna cause my uh daddy -- see my daddy's. . .friend — (his name's Ozzie) — he had gave -- given my daddy this this CB. [LNF] [R] [R]

    Yeah.

100. Well, the CB died out on him.

    Uh huh.

101. so my daddy/ (GOOD TURN-TAKING)

    Why did it die out?

102. [. . .]I don't know.

103. I don't even know why. [LNF R]

104. but then uh my uh -- one day my mom and dad -- not my mom and dad but my grand-mother and grandfather were gone -- was gone my uh -- see my da my dad he usually uses my mom and da -- my grandfather and grand-mother's CB. [R] [R] [LNF] [R]

    He uses their CB?

105. So so it's ---- and also uhm one job that he has -- he works for uh Downtown Inn. [LNF] [PTM] [R] [NSV]

    Who?

106. My dad.

Yeah?

(107.) 'Cuz they 'cuz -- it used to be uhm . . . the Ramada Inn Downtown.

Why did they change the name?

108. Now it's the Downtown Inn.

109. I don't know.

Have you ever been down there where your dad works, Thad?

(110.) Sometimes, he lets me watch with him at the the desk.

I used to do that myself when I was in school.

It was not always much fun.

111. Tell me.

(112.) I really get tired and want to leave but I -- but my dad won't won't won't let me.

Hmmm. That's tough. . . . Thad, how do you like school here?

113. It's alright.

(114.) I liked Kent.

Who is that?

115. . . .who is -- uh? (ASKS RELEVANT Q)

You said you liked Kent, who is he?

116. That's the place I went before.

Oh, your last school?

117. Yeah.

(118.) I wonder if he's there yet?

Who are you talking about?

(119.) The the man coming to our room.

TRANSITIONAL NOTE

Damico expresses a concern of many speech-language pathologists who are required to identify the underlying reasons for a student's poor image as a communicator: Short answers to standardized test questions do not tax cognitive organization and formulation skills to the degree that classroom and social encounters frequently demand. The use of a language sample appears to be one of the more sensitive procedures for observing, in an in-depth manner, those behaviors that make a student appear incompetent during communicative interactions. Second, a systematic analytical procedure is necessary that permits quantification of observations and pinpoints disruptive patterns, which is what Damico presents.

In the past, analysis procedures applied to language samples have focused primarily on language structure (or syntax). The value of Damico's approach is that structure is placed in proper perspective. There is little argument among communication specialists that without adequate structural knowledge, communication attempts will be disjointed or perhaps incoherent; pragmatic variables, however, are of equal importance when considering an individual's communication profile. By isolating 17 problem behaviors and computing the percentage of occurrence of each, it is possible to describe to educators why a student appears to be incompetent as a communicator. Through such description, educators become more cognizant of the nature of the communication process and behaviors that interfere with the sending and receiving of messages. This awareness helps them become more observant, which in turn, results in better future referrals to speech-language services.

A language sample provides an estimate of expressive language skill. It is also necessary to engage in probes of language processing skills and cognitive organization. In Chapter 7, Chappell provides a description of certain problem areas observable in young adolescent language-learning disabled students and suggests a battery of tests that will probe each of the areas he isolates. As Chappell points out, it is necessary to view the interaction of "mental operations and language levels" to ascertain at what point the student begins to experience frustration and then breakdown in the ability to cope with the demands of a cognitive-linguistic task. Because standardized test scores are required by PL 94-142 for the identification and placement of special education students, Chappell's guidelines permit the clinician to zero in on particular problem areas, select an appropriate and descriptive test, and use the results to fulfill state and federal assessment guidelines.

Once again, the reader has an opportunity to view the interaction of theory and practice. Chappell uses Guilford's Structure of the Intellect model as the framework to systematically probe cognitive-linguistic interactions.

CHAPTER 7

Description and Assessment of Language Disabilities of Junior High School Students

Gerald E. Chappell

This chapter considers the nature and assessment of language disabilities experienced by young adolescents from the perspective and organization of the Guilford's (1967) Structure of the Intellect model. The segment of Guilford's model that considers semantic content involves all information in the form of meanings to which words commonly become attached, hence this segment is most notable in verbal thinking and in verbal tests, where things signified by words must be known. The language disabilities evident in test performance are presented in this chapter. These disabilities interrupt and limit the communication performance of middle school students during their interaction and learning in the social and educational contexts of home, school, and community.

The semantic segment of Guilford's Structure of the Intellect model (Fig. 7–1) provides a theoretical reference for observing five mental operations (comprehension, evaluation, memory, convergent production, and divergent production) and five language levels (basic vocabulary, superordinate classification, language systems, information transformation, and information implication). Specific deficit behaviors observable in language disabled adolescents are presented at those five language levels. Assessment options and a clinical battery are suggested for measurement of the five mental operations at each language level.

By viewing the interaction of these mental operations and language levels, it is possible to better understand the communicative and language processing difficulties that students experience daily in their educational and social interactions. It is impossible to separate cognitive from linguistic operations; thinking, reasoning, and problem solving are involved in

Figure 7-1. The Structure of Intellect model, with three parameters (other parameters may need to be added). From Guilford, J. P. (1976). *The nature of human intelligence.* **New York, McGraw-Hill Book Company, p. 63. Reprinted with permission.**

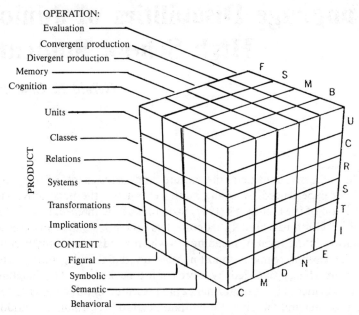

communication acts, such as inquiring, informing, regulating, and imagining. Mental operation, then, is an integral part of communicative functioning as the student takes both the listener and speaker roles in use of language in educational and social contexts.

It is critical when considering deficits at each language level, to be sensitive to the possibility that the language level deficits will be evident to a greater or lesser degree depending upon the mental operation through which the testing is completed. It is also critical to be sensitive to the possibility that breakdown occurs predominantly in a mental operation regardless of the language level at which information is being processed, e.g., the basic vocabulary or transformation levels. Finally, it is important to realize that a mental operation deficit may be coupled with a language level deficit to further confound the complexity of the interruption in communication performance. For example, the evaluator might find a basic vocabulary referencing problem plus a sentence forming system problem in a high level autistic adolescent who has a marked evaluative operation problem.

The first section of this chapter addresses the nature of the mental operations involved in communicative interactions. Mental operations are defined as mental acts that process and use information in the thinking, reasoning, and problem solving of life's daily transactions. The second section addresses various language levels at which students may experience deficits and considers the functional breakdown at each level. Language levels are defined as the distinct structural forms in which linguistic data and their meanings are organized.

DESCRIPTION OF THE MENTAL OPERATIONS

Guilford (1967) theorized that five mental operations exist: comprehension, evaluation, memory, convergent production, and divergent production. This section interprets the nature of each and offers exemplary tests that show how a specific task, involving a particular level of linguistic information, does engage the specific operation.

Comprehension Operation

The comprehension operation pertains to the receptive decoding and understanding of linguistic information previously learned or the discovery of the meaning in linguistic stimuli as they are presented. This operation incorporates an awareness, cognition, and recognition of all meaning that underlies linguistic reference (Guilford, 1967; Meeker, 1969). For example, a junior high school student must adequately comprehend the teacher's instruction, the commercial educational materials (instructional and test), and peer and parent speaker information and messages.

When performing on a comprehension task or interaction, the student's response demonstrates and reflects the extent to which the meaning of the linguistic stimuli has been decoded and understood. The Reading and Vocabulary Subtest of the *Test of Adolescent Language* (Hammill, Brown, Larsen, and Wiederholt, 1980) is a reading test of the comprehension operation. This subtest presents three related written stimuli (words) of a concept class and requires the student to comprehend two other terms of the same class from another set of four words. For example, the student is given a set such as miserable—forlorn—tragic and then asked to identify two words within this set (parcel—massacre—*dismal—pitiful)* that have a similar meaning. The comprehension operation is basic to and involved in all other operations to greater or lesser degree.

Evaluation Operation

The evaluation operation is involved in assessment of the accuracy or pertinence and appropriateness of linguistic meaning. Both the listener-reader and the speaker-writer must evaluate or judge the correctness, suitability, and desirability of information (e.g., whether or not a misread word "fits" the semantic and syntactical context of the rest of a sentence). Skill in using the evaluative operation implies having a sensitivity to linguistic error or to any discrepancy between expected and presented information. Evaluation is always made in terms of known standards, organization rules, and relationships. For example, the middle school adolescent needs to self-evaluate how well his or her discourse abides by the conversational postulates (e.g., due truthfulness, clarity, completeness, organization, etc.) as he or she considers listener feedback for signs of miscomprehension and need to revise the message.

A good example of a subtest that requires use of the evaluation operation is the Processing Relationships and Ambiguities Subtest of the Clinical Evaluation of Language Functions Test (CELF) (Semel and Wiig, 1980). The student performs in an evaluator role, making a yes-no decision as to the correctness or incorrectness of a proverb interpretation (e.g., Still water runs deep. Does this mean: the water is deep in some places?), a statement of familial relationship (e.g., If David had an uncle, could David's uncle be called David's father's brother?), and a statement of temporal-sequential relationships (e.g., Does Wednesday come between Tuesday and Thursday?). As both speaker and listener, an adolescent must engage in this cognitive operation called evaluation, through which he or she will monitor the completeness and accuracy of information being communicated.

Memory Operation

The memory operation pertains to the short-term and long-term storing and recalling of linguistic information. Short-term memory must be adequately supportive of the comprehension and evaluation operations by holding all requisite linguistic information long enough for decoding and evaluation. Long-term memory must be intact enough to store all forms of linguistic reference that will be converged upon or diverged from during the convergent and divergent production operations (discussed in the next paragraphs). Memory will be taxed in some degree in almost all instructional, test, and communicative interactions, so observation of memory can be done informally.

Convergent Production Operation

The convergent production operation involves generating new linguistic information in response to a specific linguistic constraint or demand of the presented stimuli. Convergent operation requires the adolescent to use semantic, organizational rules that have been acquired through experience to converge upon a most appropriate answer. For example, this operation is utilized when completing a verbal analogy (e.g., superordinate-subordinate classification comparisons, as in "Shirt is to clothing as chair is to _____ " requires a select single answer, furniture).

A second example is the highly restrictive opposition constraint imposed in the Verbal Opposites Subtest of the Detroit Tests of Learning Aptitude (Baker and Leland, 1967) (e.g., lost—found, victory—loss, difficult—easy). The Writing and Vocabulary Subtest of the Test of Adolescent Language (Hammill et al., 1980), as a third example, requests the student to demonstrate his or her knowledge of a word's meaning by placing it into a sentence or composing a sentence (e.g., using a word like *episode, briskly,* or *obtain* in a sentence). Tests that involve defining words are also included under the convergent production operation.

Divergent Production Operation

The divergent production operation requires producing multiple linguistic answers within reasonably flexible boundaries through use of orderly rules or principles. When engaging in the divergent operation, the adolescent can be more fluent, flexible, elaborate, and original; he or she is asked to produce multiple logical answers from that larger repertoire of acceptable answers.

The Verbal Expression Subtest of the Illinois Test of Psycholinguistic Abilities (Kirk, McCarthy, and Kirk, (1968) is a good example of a divergent production task for an upper elementary child. The student is encouraged to present multiple semantic features (all of which are scoreable, such as composition, function, and user), yet he or she remains bound to report only features that are semantically relevant. A second example is the Multiple Definitions Task (F) of the Word Test (Jorgensen, Barrett, Huisingh, and Zachman, 1981). In this task the student has to offer at least two meanings for a word, such as *pound.* He or she is at liberty to select any two of the four possibilities (money, weight, place, or action) to pass the item.

The immediate contrast between convergent and divergent production is the differences between "zeroing in" in the former, and "expanding out" in the latter (Meeker, 1969).

THE LANGUAGE LEVELS: DESCRIPTION, DISABILITIES, AND ASSESSMENT

The junior high student's mental operation capability must proficiently comprehend, remember, evaluate, or convergently or divergently comprehend or produce linguistic information at five organizational levels. At any given moment of educational instruction or interpersonal conversation, for example, the student may be required to use one or more mental operations to process incoming linguistic information at one or more linguistic levels. The Synonyms Task (B) of the Word Test (Jorgensen et al., 1981) requires the student to engage in convergent mental operation as he or she listens to a stimulus word such as *journey* and is asked to provide another word (basic vocabulary language level that has a similar meaning (e.g., trip).

While Guilford's (1967) Structure of the Intellect model offers organization for six levels of linguistic information, only five have been adapted for use in this chapter: a basic vocabulary level, a classification level, a language system level, an information transformation level, and an information implication level. Because of curricular demands, the junior high school student uses each of these kinds of information and meaning. When disabilities are involved, communication and learning may be interrupted.

This section addresses five of Guilford's linguistic organizational levels, provides examples of deficit behavior at each level, and presents recommended assessment instruments for testing for and identifying such deficits in each language level.

Basic Vocabulary Level

Guilford's (1967) "unit products" (core or basic vocabulary concepts, such as nouns) and "relations products" (concepts such as the comparative word *longer* or the directional word *over*) are forms of vocabulary having semantic meaning fields. This level includes all single word vocabularies, inclusive of such abstract concepts as *rapid, migration,* and *interaction.*

Included in the vocabulary data of a concrete object concept's semantic field (such as a baseball) are intraconcept relations such as name (baseball), size (small), shape (round), composition (leather), function (hit-throw-catch), color (white), weight (light), texture (smooth), and so forth, and interconcept relations such as user (catcher-pitcher-hitter-fielder), place of use (diamond or field), time of use (day or night games), and associative concepts (bat-mitt-plate). Each concept and its word symbol, whether a noun, verb, adjective, adverb, pronoun-preposition, or conjunction, involves a semantic field of pertinent meaning elements and definitive concept boundaries.

Any task or mental operation (comprehension, memory, evaluation, production), that focuses on single concept meaning such as defining, comparing, contrasting, drawing analogy, citing opposites, or placing a word in a sentence, entertains linguistic information at the basic vocabulary level.

Deficit Behaviors

Deficits in Word Knowledge and Usage

Failure to know concepts or word meanings. Adolescents with language disabilities often have not learned the meaning of words such as agile, expedient, or ironic that their peers have learned in home or school context. When these words are referenced by the teacher in instruction, or friends in conversation, the student fails to comprehend their meaning. Additionally, when presented with definitions and asked to provide the vocabulary word such as, "What is a person who writes music called? (composer), convergent production is impossible and the student responds with, "I don't know." Unknown words will not be recognized by the student in receptive tasks either (e.g., on the Peabody Picture Vocabulary Test). Expressively, at moments when it would be opportune to use such vocabulary, the words are not available.

Substitution of inaccurate words. The junior high school student with language disabilities often experiences semantic limitation and imprecision. When he or she performs in picture naming, describing past experiences, defining, comparing or conversing (Wiig and Semel, 1980) he or she unwittingly substitutes words that are close in meaning to other words within the same class (e.g., "fire at me," for "shoot at me") or is imprecise and to a degree inaccurate in the words he or she substitutes (e.g., "he slid" for "he slipped"). The errors may be of three types, which, at any given moment of performance, may be difficult to differentiate:

1. In-class substitutions. Perhaps the most severe misreference is the substitution that is within the semantic class membership, e.g., intersubstitutions such as *lemon* for *orange,* or *coffee* for *tea.*

2. Imprecise substitutions. This is the substitution of a very general or common word (thing) for the required specific one (book), or the substitution of a word that covers only an element of the intended meaning (use of *sport* for *hobby).* Occasionally word opposites (brother for sister), and words having phonological similarity (except for accept) may also be offered (Wiig and Semel, 1980).

3. Restrictive multiple meanings for words. The child evidences a concreteness, narrowness, or inflexibility (Wiig and Semel, 1976, 1980) in his or her word knowledge. The cognitive-linguistic operation sputters for the child fails to understand and use words for dual and multiple meanings because he or she is restricted to common (denotative), concrete meanings. The student is susceptible to receptive miscomprehension (e.g., miscomprehending "He accidentally sat on his glasses and broke them," as sitting on several drinking glasses instead of eyeglasses) and expressive limitation. The adolescent may know and use "run" in the sense of "The jogger is running three miles," and "The car engine is running," but not in the sense of "His thoughts are running in circles," "His nose is running," or "The water is running down the sidewalk." A second example of grammatical usage that might cause comprehension problems would be the word "strike" as it changes grammatical classes from a verb (I saw him s..._e her), to a noun (They went on strike), to an adjective (She is a striking person) or to an adverb (He got his way strikingly fast).

Wiig and Semel (1980) suggest, that the above-mentioned kind of comprehension problems may result from (a) failure to shift to alternate meanings (e.g., from drinking to seeing glasses), (b) failure to differentiate abstract from concrete meanings (e.g., fell in love versus fell down), or (c) failure to differentiate grammatical class meanings (e.g., "The horse is running" [verb] from "She has a run in her stocking" [noun]).

The attainment of full concept closure remains most problematic for students, perhaps because our instructional techniques poorly define meaning or are poorly explicit. The individual learner often has to use his or her intuition and context to "guesstimate" concept denotative essence, feature boundaries, and any legitimate extensions in connotative meaning. The above kinds of errors (word substitutions) are usually committed without the student's awareness of the substitution.

Paucity of verbal report for individual concepts. An additional problem experienced by the language disabled adolescent is that he or she often offers limited information in verbal accounts or reports. The problem is most evident in divergent production tasks such as responding in free association, engaging in concept definition, and specifying concept comparison and contrast. The student offers a limited quantity and diversity of information (very few meaning elements) in his or her response and thus the response is incomplete. He or she may do relatively well in single-answer convergent production tasks but fall short in the multiple response divergent tasks. Analysis may show that critical meaning relations are absent from the repertoire of features he or she offers. For example, asked to tell about a pencil sharpener in a vocabulary definition task, the student may provide name, color, and function and then be at loss to offer more salient data about the item. When asked to compare the pencil sharpener with a knife, he or she may remark that "you use both of them" and have little more to say. Definitions, comparisons, and other kinds of expressive accounts that pertain to the meaning of the single word are never fully adequate. Schwartz and Solot (1980) refer to this problem as "paucity of expression," with the child often relying on the listener to start communication, prod, encourage, or otherwise cue a response.

Word Finding Problems and Associated Behavior. In their discussion of disorders of auditory expressive language, Johnson and Myklebust (1967) included a word-finding difficulty they termed "anomia." They viewed anomia to be a word auditorization, selection, and retrieval problem, as they emphasized poor evocation of name, quality, and relationship vocabulary.

Wiig and Semel (1976) use "dysnomia" to label word-finding disability. They emphasize the reduction in accuracy and speed of verbal associations and the availability of verbal labels in convergent production tasks, wherein tight linguistic constraints request specific vocabulary (e.g., verbal opposites and analogy tasks). They suggest that the dysnomic student tends to give wrong names phonetically and to substitute words that are in some way semantically related to the target word (e.g., telephone for stethoscope). Wiig and Semel (1980) further comment that the dysnomic child with learning disability may have difficulties in recalling and retrieving specific words (as requested by tight linguistic constraints) accurately and speedily when asked to name pictures or objects, find proper names, or describe past experiences or events, or take part in spontaneous conversation. The problem may also show up in free verbal association when the student is asked to name as many concepts from a class as he or she can in a short predetermined time. The student may be slow, repeat words, get stuck after the first few, or show a very restricted range of available words (Wiig and Semel, 1980).

The word finding difficulties of learning disabled children and adolescents (Wiig and Semel, 1980) appear to cross input modalities. These individuals may have trouble naming objects or events; naming objects to be identified by touch; and naming during reading. Their problems also seem to encompass both the recall and retrieval of proper names for objects, animals, actions, attributes, and other characteristics. The problems occur even when the words they are trying to recall and retrieve are familiar to them and easily recognized on picture vocabulary tests. In rapid conversation, the continuous search for specific words may cause idiosyncratic patterns of expression. Pragmatic proficiency in use of language suffers.

German (1979) found that eight to eleven year old learning disabled subjects (achieving at least 1.5 grade levels below the matched normals in reading recognition, spelling, and mathematics) evidenced word finding difficulties. They were not inferior in finding high frequency words in any task, but the area in which they did respond significantly more slowly was in finding low frequency names in two stimulus conditions: naming to open-ended sentences (e.g., You part your hair with a _____[comb]), and naming to description (What is something you use to part your hair, has teeth, and may be made of plastic? _____ [comb]). The author felt that her subjects did not do well on the former task because of the cloze procedure's automatic nature, which may have prohibited inhibition of incorrect responses. In turn, the request to synthesize the descriptions in the latter task may have significantly interfered with the subjects' word finding process, putting greater demands on word retrieval than either picture naming or the open-ended sentence condition. German speculates that such auditory conditions may be far more challenging to the retrieval process than the traditional picture-naming context. She implies that in order to attain a complete profile, the clinician should therefore assess for word finding deficits in both intrasensory auditory and intersensory visual-to-auditory tasks.

Wiig and Semel (1980) comment that untrained parents and teachers may not recognize the idiosyncratic reactions and habits (such as substitutions) a child may establish when he or she has word finding problems. The pressure and frustration felt when the student is obliged to produce a response but cannot find the word to express his or her ideas or answer a question may have detrimental effects. After repeated frustrations, the student may find refuge in silence. The following behavioral patterns (Schwartz and Solot, 1980; Wiig and Semel, 1980) may accompany word finding problems.

Undue hesitancy and dysfluency

1. Excessive prolonged pauses, searching, groping, delayed retrieval—for example, I went to the. . .(pause). . .store to buy some. . .(pause). . .delicious. . .(pause). . .food.

2. Overuse of meaningless fillers—for example, starters to begin comments, *And then* I went to the store. . .*and then*. . .I bought something. . .*well*. . .*well*. . .that was delicious; or stereotyped interjections and place holders—for example, *You know*. . .I would like. . .*uh well*. . .*er*. . .*you know*. . .a coke.

3. Perseverative repetitions of words and phrases—for example, I'm going to have cream. . .ice *cream*. . .vanilla *ice cream*.

Undue overuse of dysnomic word substitution patterns

1. Indefinites—for example, . . .*somehow,* I went to. . .that place. . .*somewhere* to buy. . .*something* delicious.

2. Synonyms (German, 1982)—for example, He wears a cloak (for cape).

3. General or imprecise words lacking specificity—for example, I went to this *place* to buy. . .*stuff* and got some. . .*junk* that tasted. . .good.

4. Circumlocutions—for example, I went to this place. . .*where you buy things to eat* and ordered a plate of that *long, wormlike stuff.*

5. In-class responses—for example, She drank out of a. . .*cup* (for glass). German (1982) found her learning disabled group often offered a concept with similar function (e.g., vacuum for broom), or a semantically related reference—for example, It goes with knife (fork), and some verb substitutions—It's my beat (heart).

6. Stereotyped or borrowed phrases or terms—for example, You see I went to the. . .*whatchamacallit* store to get a. . .*thingamajig.*

7. Indiscriminate use of pronouns—for example, substituting pronouns when proper names are needed, as in In this story. . .*they* chase. . .*him* until. . .*he* tells where. . .*she* lives.

8. Inconsistency in retrieval—for example (at one moment): It's a. . .Oh, I can't think of the word that names that picture. You put ashes in it. (Yet, a moment later): My Mom has a fancy *ashtray* in the kitchen.

Deficits in Simultaneous Analysis and Seeing Logical Relationships. The student experiences difficulty in the simultaneous analysis of all the components within a sentence, or he or she fails to see the logical relation that is inherent in the structure of the sentence or in the relationship between elements. These problems involve basic vocabulary and their meanings and meaning interrelationships. Examples of items that would be difficult include the following:

The comparative, e.g., Are water melons *larger* than basketballs?

The familial, e.g., Is my *cousin* Joe my uncle's son?

The temporal, e.g., Does December come *before* November?

The passive, e.g., Was the boy *brought* by the woman?

The spatial, e.g., Is the Kangaroo's pouch *below* its arms?

The analogous, e.g., *Is* a key to a door *as* a dial *is* to a phone?

The polar opposite, e.g., Is huge the *opposite* of tiny?

Wiig and Semel (1980) attribute such problems to faulty simultaneous analysis of all the critical words, deficits in imagery or failure to revisualize the relationships, deficits in retention and recall of critical word order, or failure to see the critical meaning relationship.

Assessment Recommendations: Basic Vocabulary Level

Since the knowledge of basic vocabulary, and the ability to flexibly use such meaning, is so crucial to advancement in the educational program and success in interpersonal social discourse, the assessment battery first of all places heavy priority in test emphasis at this level through a select group of six discrete item subtests. As Figure 7–2 reveals, convergent production is emphasized in four of the tasks, evaluation in the fifth, and divergent production in the sixth, under the rationale that production tasks are the more demanding operation-based tasks and hence are those most likely to uncover disability features.

The first recommended set of subtests for measurement at the vocabulary level is the evaluative Processing Relationships and Ambiguities Subtest of the Clinical Evaluation of Language Function Test (Semel and Wiig, 1980), and the convergent production Auditory Association Subtest of the Illinois Test of Psycholinguistic Abilities (Kirk, McCarthy, and Kirk, 1968). The former requires the adolescent to respond with yes-no evaluation of the accuracy of 24 concept meanings as they have been correctly or incorrectly used in the context of six logical relationships: four familial (e.g., aunt, uncle), four passive (e.g., chosen, pulled), four comparative (e.g., older, heavier), four spatial (e.g., between, middle), four temporal-sequential (e.g., after, between), and four analogous (e.g., big to little). The Auditory Association subtest, although having a 10 year ceiling, can still identify inconsistency in an older junior high school student's discernment of the underlying logical relationship upon which the stimulus analogies are based. Verbal analogies have as their meaning-base the same semantic features or relations upon which vocabulary is based (e.g., color, composition, place, user, parts). The linguistic constraint of the analogy task requires a convergence upon each item's three stated elements to discern the logical relationship of the elements and to produce the missing, or fourth, element (e.g., *Snow is to white, as blood is to red* = color). The convergent producer must generate words that fit the specified comparison linguistic constraint of the diverse set of analogies. An examiner may first pretest the student's analogy-drawing ability by presenting the traditional format (i.e., A _____ is to _____ as a _____ is to _____). The reason for this is that the structure phrase of the Auditory Association subtest gives helping cues by stating the stimulus items as attributes—for example, A dog *has* hair; a fish *has* (scales). Another suggestion is to add about six analogies based upon superordinate or subordinate classification e.g., Train is to vehicle as shirt is to (clothing).

These subtests help to identify problems in forming logical relationships, difficulty in the simultaneous analysis of multiple concepts, misinterpretation of word meaning, imprecise word usage, and dysnomic behavior.

As Figure 7–2 reveals, a trio of three subtests is recommended to test the adolescent's basic vocabulary production ability. The General Information Subtest of the Peabody Individual Achievement Test (Dunn

Figure 7-2. Recommended assessment battery. CELF, Clinical Evaluation of Language Functions (Semel and Wiig, 1980); WT, The Word Test (Jorgensen et al., 1981); PIAT, Peabody Inividual Achievement Test (Dunn and Markwardt, 1970); ITPA, Illinois Test of Psycholinguistic Abilities (Kirk et al., 1968); TOAL, Tests of Adolescent Language (Hammill et al., 1980); TOWL, Test of Written Language (Hammill and Larson, 1978); DTLA, Detroit Tests of Learning Aptitude (Baker and Leland, 1967).

	Comprehension	Evaluation	Convergent Production	Divergent Production
		Cognitive – Linguistic Operations		
Basic Vocabulary		CELF:Processing Relationships (& Ambiguities)	WT:Synonyms PIAT:General Information ITPA:Auditory Association TOAL:Speaking/Vocabulary	WT:Multiple Definitions
Classification			WT:Associations	
System	TOAL:Reading/Grammar CELF:Processing Word & Sentence Structure		TOWL:Thematic Maturity Chappell Story Reformation	
Transformation		CELF:Processing (Relationships) & Ambiguities		
Implications			DTLA:Social Adjustment A	

Levels / Product / Linguistic

and Markwardt, 1970) requires the student to converge upon information offered in definitions and questions to produce the word that labels various noun and verb educational concepts. The following are examples of items that the eight and ninth graders have to confront: By what means does one attempt to revive a person who has almost drowned (artificial respiration)? By what process does the government obtain money from its people (taxation)? What is the process called when water is turned into steam (evaporation)? In the Word Test (Jorgensen et al., 1981), Synonym Task (B), the student must produce a word having similar meaning for each of 16 concepts such as donate, quarrel, and vacant. On the Multiple Definitions Task (F) of the Word Test (Jorgensen et al., 1981) the junior high school student must shift into divergent production. The task direction is as follows: "The next words have more than one meaning. Tell me what _____ means. Tell me something else it means." The 14 items have two or more common meanings, such as *tip* (point, gratuity, hint, action) or *train* (locomotive, teach, part of dress).

As a group this trio of tests helps identify deficits in word knowledge, imprecise word usage, dysnomic problems, and limitation in multiple meanings.

Finally the Speaking/Vocabulary Subtest of the Test of Adolescent Language (Hammill et al., 1980) requires the student to place abstract words, such as hindrance, excavate, and morbid, into sentences. This demonstrates knowledge of the word meaning through use of each word in an original sentence.

Failure in word knowledge, imprecision, dysfluency, and overuse of word substitution patterns may be evident in a student's performance on this subtest.

The Classification Level

Classification refers to categories of superordinate abstractions, such as clothing or furniture, into which multiple related concepts can be grouped. Each superordinate category has its own respective subordinate membership of basic vocabulary terms (clothing: shirt-pants-coat; furniture: chair-table-couch). The classification level of information is involved if the student is asked to engage in convergent thinking and identify the category term appropriate for a stimulus subordinate set (e.g., appliance, when presented with washing machine, stove, refrigerator). A divergent task might ask the student for two legitimate examples of items within a particular category (such as bus, train, car, boat when presented with a superordinate term, vehicle).

Deficit Behaviors

Although the proof remains sparse at present, the speculation is that junior high school students with language disabilities will often fail to use superordinate terms and relationships in the following manner:

1. Failure to produce verbal classificatory terms in convergent production, e.g., inability to specify that "gun-sword-knife" are weapons.

2. Adequate verbal production of superordinate classifying terms but failure to use such facilitatory organizational structure when giving verbal account of concepts, in concept definition, in concept comparison-contrast, and in the drawing of analogies. This is a failure to effectively utilize classification in divergent production when it would be an efficient cognitive strategy.

Language disabilities at the classification level have not been well delineated in the literature. Wiig and Semel (1976) report that inability to name superordinate (class members) when given a superordinate such as "fruit" constitutes one aspect of disability, as does that inability to name the superordinate when given names of class members. Semel and Wiig (1980) developed a subtest (Producing Word Associations) for testing knowledge of foods and animals for their Clinical Evaluation of Language Function Test because they had observed that learning disabled children produced significantly fewer names of foods during a 60 second time limit than did achieving students. The responses of the students with learning disabilities also indicated that they did not employ obvious grouping or associative clustering strategies. They named foods at random, shifting from one food category to another, perhaps naming first a type of meat, then a type of dessert, and frequently repeating items; there was no cognitive organization guiding their responses. The clustering strategies of the academically achieving group, on the other hand, proceeded systematically through categories such as fruits, vegetables, meats, and desserts, naming as many in each category as they could think of.

Assessment Recommendations: Classification Level

Because there are few tests available for measuring language performance at the classification level, it is recommended that one formal test be used along with several informal investigations. The recommended commercial test is the Association Task (A) of the Word Test (Jorgensen et al., 1981), in which the student must "provide a reason" for rejecting one word from a group of four. For example, if the student deleted "hair" from the stimulus set of "bush, *hair*, tree, grass," he or she would need to provide a rationale for doing so, such as the remaining trio of items are all plants. The scoring protocol does not require superordinate terms in all instances. For example, functional (they can cut) and descriptive (all green) terms are also appropriate answers. It is recommended that as an informal probe, the examiner push the student for the most appropriate classification (or superordinate term) for these latter types of items to ascertain if the student is capable of doing this.

Another informal probe during the testing of analogies is to ask the student to provide the category that is the basis of the comparison (e.g., grass is to green as sugar is to *white* = color). Another informal measurement is to have the adolescent define classifiable concepts (such as guitar) to see if a mature Aristotelian definition format (Litowitz, 1977) is used. Syntactically, this means that the student embeds the classification reference into a formal sentence—e.g., A *guitar* is a *musical instrument* with strings upon which a musician plays songs.

This workup should reveal whether or not the adolescent knows the classification terms and uses the organization inherent to superordinate classification to succeed in other linguistic tasks.

The Language System Level

Guilford (1967) explains that the system level involves complexes, patterns, organizations, or structured aggregates of interdependent or interacting parts, such as a verbally stated outline, plan, or program. The morphosyntactical system of English inflections is considered an example, wherein a set of affixes mark specific meanings for derivation, plurality, tense, and so forth. When the full system is understood, all inflections will be used in their obligatory context. A second example would be the discourse rules. These conversational postulates represent a pragmatic system of interpersonal communication rules that regulate speaker-listener participation and topic switching. A final example is linguistic systems, which serve to organize, interrelate, and integrate basic vocabulary concepts.

Although the following subtests were not included in the recommended battery of assessment instruments listed in Figure 7-2 they are discussed here as examples of test instruments that measure language performance at the system level. the Listening/Grammar Subtest of the Test of Adolescent Language (Hammill et al., 1980) is viewed as a sentence level system test because it requires the student to listen to a set of three sentences and then identify the two that have the same meaning, even though their linguistic structure varies. For example, (1) Neither will be speaking to the other, (2) They plan never to speak to each other, (3) Either one or the other will be speaking. In this case, sentences one and two convey the same meaning.

The Writing/Grammar Subtest of the Test of Adolescent Language (Hammill et al., 1980) is a variation of this format. The student is asked to read from three to six sentences and then combine them into a single sentence by using deletion, combination, or placing elements into clauses. For example, the student must place the following short sentences into one long sentence: "He had dreamed. He dreamed of money. He dreamed of excitement. He dreamed of adventure." To be successful at this task the student must understand higher features of transformation grammar.

Deficit Behavior

Seven patterns of deficit behavior have been identified at the complex system level. Although each is reported as a distinct set of features, the features and feature patterns do overlap.

Failure to Comprehend Complex Linguistic Structure. The adolescent with language disabilities often fails to comprehend the meaning of linguistic information that is presented in complex sentence structure, both auditorily and during reading. The comprehension breakdown may be evidenced indirectly by low performance in the classroom or directly on comprehension tests. The linguistic complexity of the teacher's instruction. the educational program's commercial materials for academic subjects, and even parental directives may present problems. For example, on formal tests, such as the Processing Words and Sentence Structure Subtest of the Clinical Evaluation of Language Function Test (Semel and Wiig, 1980) the student may experience the following difficulties:

1. Failure to comprehend sentences stated in passive, questions, negative structures, or complex combinations thereof. The student would reveal these comprehension problems when asked to identify the picture that goes with "The boy is being followed by the dog" or "The girl doesn't have a big, black and white, striped dog."

2. Failure to comprehend meaning interrelationships coded in complexly embedded sentences. In such a case, the student would not fully understand all aspects of "The woman who is standing by the stove mixing batter to bake a cake dropped an egg on the floor."

This type of comprehension problem may be indirectly reflected when a student offers a paucity of modification (e.g., an absence of adjectival transforms, relative clauses, participial constructions, nonexpanded verb phrases, and so forth) during reformulation of complex information presented in a story narrative. In such a reformulation type of narrative task, the adolescent may also fail to reiterate obligatory interrelationships (e.g., temporal, cause and effect, conditional) because he or she did not grasp their meanings during the receptive processing; his or her comprehension skill could not handle complex systemic relationships. Any suspicion that a comprehension deficit is present calls for a direct administration of a comprehension test.

Faulty Semantic Referencing. This system-based deficit is an extension of, and often the explanation for, inaccurate word usage at the basic vocabulary level. When an adolescent's semantic language system is weak, he or she fails to make fine differentiations among concepts or words that are close in meaning. The failure is evidenced by in-class substitutions and substitutions of imprecise or common concepts for specific ones (Wiig and Semel, 1980). Examples are as follows:

1. Weak concept formation or differentiation among similar concepts of a verb group such as *stumbling, tumbling, tripping, slipping, sliding,* and *falling,* as evident by inaccurate word substitutions (e.g., He *tumbled* for *stumbled)* on his way down the stairs.

2. Weak concept formation or differentiation among a related group of words, such as evaluative adjectival concepts (excellent, good, superior, tremendous, fantastic) or descriptions of size (huge, mammoth, giant, large, massive).

3. Weak concept formation or differentiation among a group of concepts that provide reference for coordination and class inclusion or exclusion (e.g., *either-or, all-some, all-except)* (Wiig and Semel, 1980), as is evident by inaccuracy in word selection. For example, *"Neither* (instead of *either)* you do it or I'll tell Mom."

4. Inaccurate pronoun reflexivization, as evidenced by errors such as hisself-himself and theirselfs-themselves.

5. Inaccurate or imprecise spatial reference (e.g., *between, close to, next to,)* or temporal-sequential reference (e.g., *before, while, after, until).*

6. Undue failure to specify agents or events by proper name designation or description before shifting into anaphoric pronoun reference, which results in confusing pronoun usage (e.g., *She* tore *his* clothes before *they* came).

Grammatical ¬naccuracy. These are persevering failures that the adolescent with language disabilities may face in mastering the use of markers and word form changes—deficits in mastery of the rules or features of the subsystems of the English morphosyntactical system. These problems may linger throughout the elementary school years in oral form and then continue to be most problematic in written expression at the junior high school level. Examples include the following:

1. Omission or inaccuracy in use of the markers and word forms of the tense system, such as overregularization of the past tense irregular forms (caughted) and modal auxiliary confusion due to a lack of clear distinctions among the terms within the modal system, such as the semantic nuances carried by could, would, most, might, or should.

2. Omission or inaccuracy in use of derived words such as the irregular comparative forms (using "good-gooder-goodest" for "good-better-best"), or failure to master the -ist suffix as in pian*ist,* and substituting a phrase such as "he is the *piano man."*

3. Failure to incorporate the exceptions (e.g., men, children, mice) to the regular rules for pluralizing.

Grammatical Simplicity Due to Formulation Limitation. Grammatical simplicity and lack of structural flexibility are frequently evident in the adolescent's overuse of short sentences, excessive use of such linking coordinators as "and" and "so," and failure to incorporate obligatory connectors or subordinators that tie clausal elements together into complex sentences (Schwartz and Solot, 1980). Examples are as follows:

1. Limited ability to generate complex combinatorial structure (inclusive of obligatory clausal cojoinings or embeddings of the relative, noun, and subordinate clauses) that are necessary to express critical semantic interrelationships such as cause-effect, reason, and conditionality. For example, instead of using more complex combinatorial structure to generate a sentence, such as "The lady decided *that she would give her money to her son* because she wanted to live, and, *since he was a specialist,* he was the one *who could cure her,"* the student offers a series of simple sentences that do not code the complete thought: "The lady gave money to her son. And she wanted to live. And he was a specialist."

2. Failure to generate expansions of the subject-verb-object phrase components of complex sentences through the use of adjectival, adverbial, participial, or relative clauses to elaborate upon features such as character mood and intention. For example, rather than saying "The rich old lady who had cancer should have given the money from her will to her faithful secretary Jenny," the student offers, "The lady with cancer didn't give money to Jenny." Story reformulation tasks (Chappell, 1980) present an opportunity to observe this reduction in complexity and modification (see Appendix 7-1).

Paucity of Report Across System Information. The young adolescent who shows evidence of paucity of report at the system level displays a relatively consistent pattern of insufficiency. His or her responses are rarely satisfactory because of content incompleteness. Examples include the following:

1. When initially generating an oral or written sequence of information (such as segments of a story he is asked to create, a narrative account of a recent vacation experience, or the sequence of steps in planning a high school dance), he offers far less information than would be considered adequate from a listener's point of view. For example, "My family camped. We were attacked. No one was hurt."

2. When engaged in a descriptive recount of a sequence of information, verbal or written (e.g., a story, historical account, or report of a science project), the student is remarkably brief and insufficient. For example, "There's water and heat. It boils."

Disorganization. Schwartz and Solot (1980) suggest that when the student demonstrates poor organization and sequencing of information he or she may display (1) rambling, (2) disjointed phrases, and (3) repetition, rewording, and circumlocution.

1. The adolescent may display disorganization in the presentation of sequenced, interrelated multiple-event accounts through undue interjection of starters, place holders, perseverative repetition, and incomplete sentences or misordering of events. The problem appears to be more one of conceptual organization than one of linguistic organization and proficiency. Although the student may formulate some rather complex ideas in complex language structure, he or she still remains disorganized. For example,

> "Well. . .to fix a tire. . .or your wheel. . .you gotta take the tire off. . .you gotta lift up. . .you jack up the car and use this thing. . .its square metal wrench. . .to loosen the bolts. . .you know the nuts. . .then you take the wheel off the axes. First you ask the guy at the garage if he will fix the tire. You lock up the car so it won't. . .you put the car in gear so it stays put."

2. In story reformulation or discourse tasks the youth may use excessive interjections and incomplete sentences, may incoherently omit critical events or insert irrelevant ones, may be inaccurate or confused relative to others, or may misorder his or her presentation of the events. Johnston (1981) comments that there is a place in evaluation and intervention for use of narrative story structure. She suggests using the technique of Stein and Glenn (1979), which considers the categories, combinatorial rules, and suprasentential grammar of stories. Individuals with language disability may exhibit developmental problems in narrative formation. They may not do well in providing story setting, may give initiating events without following with consequential events, and may not incorporate adequately complex episode structure.

3. Although their population was one of psychotic adolescents, Yudkovitz, Lewison, and Rottersman (1976) report many features that can be expected in more subtle form in persons with language disabilities who have problems in system organization. For example, in discourse, topic introduction may be inadequately covered so that the listener remains unsure of what is being talked about, or there is no closure of the topic, so the listener is not sure when it is finished. Once into the account, the speaker may display lack of topical organization resulting in incoherence and inadequate or confused sequencing of events and steps. There may be fragmentation, incompleteness, and disjointedness.

Pragmatic Insensitivity. A confounding variable relative to the system deficit patterns cited above is the possibility that a pragmatic breakdown could explain the presence of grammatical simplicity or inaccuracy, paucity of report, inaccuracy of reference, and degree of organization. These features may appear because of the adolescent's faulty presupposition (or assumptions) of how explicit he or she must be in order for the listener to comprehend what he or she says. Thus, the young adolescent may be able to successfully comprehend all that is said to him or her (as could be proved on a comprehension test), may have the linguistic proficiency to generate very mature and sophisticated linguistic structures (as might be evident when he or she is asked to place individual words into sentences), and yet, because of pragmatic insensitivity, may formulate nonexplicit or disorganized messages because he or she fails to tune into the listener's needs with respect to how semantic data (or information to be shared) must be organized and placed into complex linguistic structures. Examples include the following:

1. The adolescent may use general words (e.g., "thing" or "stuff") and overuse pronouns because he or she inaccurately assumes that semantic referencing can be very vague and still be understood. Pragmatically, he or she may be insensitive to the listener's confusion when he or she is imprecise through reliance on indefinite pronouns or general, "empty " words.

2. The adolescent may also fail to realize that certain semantic interrelationships will not be drawn and comprehended by the listener unless they are made explicit by the speaker. He or she fails to see the need to use select obligatory linguistic features (such as the subordinator *because* to form a clause, which would make it clear what caused the reported effect or temporal condition). He or she fails to incorporate such features because of faulty presupposition that they are not necessary.

3. Some students may show a "pragmatic wandering" when formulating-reformulating semantic events as they fabricate untrue and irrelevant events. For example,

> "Well, this old woman decided she was going to make her son into a nice playboy. . .so she hires a bunny. The bunny Jenny turns the doctor into a real charmer. Then Mom pays for them to go to California and get married. Mom took me to California last year."

When pragmatic insensitivity is a prevailing problem, there will probably be much inconsistency in the accuracy of referencing, the degree of organization, or the complexity of formulating. The student might be able to demonstrate capability in each of these areas during structured tasks or when pinned down to do so through a stringent feedback from a listener.

Assessment Recommendations: Language System Level

As Figure 7-2 reveals, the following quartet of diagnostic subtests (two comprehension tests and two production tests) is recommended to best assess performance at the language system level.

The Processing Words and Sentence Structure Subtest of the Clinical Evaluation of Language Function (Semel and Wiig, 1980) requires the student to process multiple segments of information within sentences. Special attention is focused on measuring comprehension of tense markers, wh-questions, and clausal embedding. Sample sentences include the following: The boy *who is sitting under the big tree* is eating a banana; The woman asked, How much does this apple cost? On each subtest item the student has to find the picture within an array that matches the stimulus sentence.

The Reading/Grammar Subtest of the Test of Adolescent Language (Hammill et al., 1980) requires the young adolescent to read, comprehend, and find two sentences from an array of six sentences with the same meaning (but phrased differently). An example of two such sentences would be as follows: *The girl has finished drawing her picture,* and *The picture drawn by the girl is finished.* Students with basic literacy can be guided to perform on this test and can be given corrective help until they accurately read each sentence out loud and thereafter use the written text in their comparison of sentential meanings.

The above subtests will survey for deficits in basic auditory comprehension of complex sentences and for ability to see optional ways to say messages.

The Story Reformulation Procedure (Chappell, 1980) requires convergent reproduction of a complexly integrated and interrelated system of events. The interplay between the syntactic, semantic, and pragmatic aspects of the oral language performance of fourth through eighth graders can be considered at a system level. Appendix 7-1 presents an analysis procedure that is simpler to use and score than the one in the 1980 article.

The Thematic Maturity Subtest of the Test of Written Language (Hammill and Larsen, 1978) directs the student to look at three pictures projecting an outer space theme and write a complete story about them. A point is offered for each of 20 possible specified features that the student incorporates into his or her story creation. This author has found that inclusion of any seven of the following features matches seventh grade expectancy level, and any eight reach eighth grade level.

Writes in paragraphs.
Names pictured objects.
Gives personal names to main characters.
Gives proper names to robots, planets, animals, etc.
Explains why environment is hostile.
Includes all three pictures.
Has a definite ending.
Offers a new life story.
Includes dialogue.

This combination of tests surveys for deficits in grammatical accuracy, referencing, paucity of report, noninclusion of critical details, and organization (including sequencing, relevance, and coherence) at the language system level.

Language Transformation Level

Guilford (1967) uses transformation to refer to changes, revisions, redefinitions, or modifications by which any linguistic information in one state is transformed into another state. Transformation would include, for example, any literal form that can also have a figurative meaning, such as proverbs (beauty is only skin deep), idioms (the cat's got your tongue), homonym riddles (what has wheels and flies? A garbage truck), metaphors (the ship plows the seas), and similes (she has cheeks like roses). Some poets frequently use such transformations to alter meaning creatively and more richly convey their ideas. The junior high school English teacher requires students to comprehend transformations as they appear in the literature and to master the altered meaning. This type of educational task requires sophisticated metalinguistic skill—i.e., ability to explain the nature of our language and its transformations. In addition, peer groups adopt new metaphoric terms for "in group" interaction that demand quick transformation of meaning. Members failing to transform with the rest suffer in peer group social interactions.

Deficit Behaviors

Adolescents who are experiencing language disabilities at the transformation level will demonstrate the following problems:

Problems in Comprehending, Using, and Explaining Transformed Meaning. They will experience difficulty in interpreting the figurative level of idioms, proverbs, riddles, fables, puns, similes, and the subtle transformations of meaning that characterize poetry.

Wiig and Semel (1976) report cognitive problems in processing words having multiple meanings, idioms, puns, metaphors, and proverbs, as well as in formulating alternative titles to a story. These authors further comment (1980) that, typically, learning disabled children perceive and interpret only the literal, concrete meaning of words when they encounter idioms such as "He hit the roof," or "I'm all tied up at the office." When they limit their interpretation of metaphors and similes to the literal and concrete meaning of each word they are confused about representational meaning. The abstract and generalized meaning of proverbs may also continue to elude them as they remain at the concrete level of interpretation and fail to understand why people bother to tell them something so obvious as "You can't cross a bridge until you come to it."

General Metalinguistic Ignorance. There appears to be little insight into the nature of language and how it serves and is used by speakers. Miller (1979) reported the behavior of some pragmatically disordered language children (several at the 8, 9, 10, and 11 year levels). Her subjects were weak in their metalinguistic understanding of language—their ability to talk about language and tell how to use it. For example, they had little or no grasp of how one can play with language. They tended to see and give only a concrete response (airplane) to riddles such as "What has four wheels and flies?" and did not comprehend a nonsensical, amusing response (garbage truck) that is based on a pun. Explanation of what a riddle is and why it is funny was limited to "a joke." In the second research task, in which they were asked to retell the riddle (after a short break), only one subject even attempted to do so. The subjects failed completely in their attempt to explain 10 idioms, usually giving a literal meaning or description (e.g., "He's on edge" = "He's on a cliff"). The subjects were also unable to explain the meaning of compound words such as "showboat."

Assessment Recommendations: Language Transformation Level

Very few commercial tests are available for measurement at this level. Since the explanation of transformed information is a relatively difficult task for middle school adolescents, the preferred assessment mode is to ask the student to determine the accurate meaning of a proverb from choices provided by the examiner. The Processing Relationships and Ambiguities Subtest of the Clinical Evaluation of Language Function (Semel and Wiig, 1980) uses this format. It is recommended at the basic vocabulary level (Fig. 7–2) but performance on the eight item proverb and idiom set can be considered separately for evaluation of the transformation level. To do this, informally examine whether or not the student passes, or misses, more than half of the items. This behavioral profile demonstrates a predominant success or a predominant failure on the task. The student who fails over 50% of the eight items can be asked for explanations on both the items failed and those correctly answered to pin down the adequacy of his or her perspective on such transformation of meaning.

Language Implication Level

Guilford (1967) defines implication as additional linguistic information that can be expected, anticipated, or predicted from given linguistic information. There is an intimate connection or interrelationship between the expected and the given that is of a cause-effect, conditional, or inferential nature. The junior high school student, in his or her relations with family and with peers, teachers, and many others, must discern linguistic implication for successful problem solving and adjustment in many facets of the educational program and society in general; not everything that is expected to be known is explicity stated. An individual is expected to make logical inferences on occasion.

The answering of "What if. . .?" questions is a good example of a divergent production task at this level, if alternative solutions are sought. On other tasks the student is required to give a single answer to explain why a certain prescribed happening or course of action must be so. For example, Why are criminals locked up? In a task such as this, the student must express rather specific implication about expectant societal and personal responsibilities. A third example is where the student has to formulate a viable solution for problematic situations (e.g., What would you do if you found a broken glass on the sidewalk?).

Deficit Behaviors

The observable difficulties at this level included the following:

Problems in Discerning and Explaining Implications. This deficit area includes problems involving causes, effects, concomitant conditions, and solutions.

1. Social imperception in adolescence (Wiig and Semel, 1976) often ends in social maladjustment and patterns of antisocial behavior that are not foreign to the descriptive account of the psychosocial character of many students with language disabilities. This social behavior is probably closely tied to deficits in problem solving that result in faulty interpersonal relationships.

2. Wiig and Semel (1976) remark that youngsters with learning disability frequently have impaired cognition of semantic implications;

they are often unaware of possible causes, effects, and concomitant conditions relative to problematic past and future personal interactions. This population also experiences problems in explaining cause-effect relationships and in completing stories wherein they must verbalize the implications of actions.

2. Bruno (1981) in the Test of Social Inference looked at the ability of learning disabled students (ages 9 to 11.6 years) to draw inferences by making an inductive leap from visible cues in 14 stimulus pictures to what they could most reasonably imply. He found that the learning disability students showed subtle social perceptual deficits by responding to details that were irrelevant to the interpretation of the inference or by being illogical. They more frequently failed to predict consequences, and the quality of their responses lacked the richness shown by the normal subjects.

Faulty Presupposition of Intended Meaning and Inference in Discourse. During conversation the participant misreads the other participant's meanings. In addition, he or she is inaccurate in presupposing what the other person will be able to infer from his or her message as it is presented. He or she violates many of the rules of conversation that deal with clarity, truthfulness, and relevance of information.

Many of the social perceptual problems of young adolescents with language disabilities probably arise from faulty presuppositions about what is said, or is not said, to them during interpersonal discourse and about what they say, or do not say, to others. They misinterpret what is meant by the comments of others and either may say too much or say too little in their verbal report to others. They fail to be duly succinct and pertinent; much of their content is repetitious and therefore useless to the listener. Because of the word finding problems and word substitution patterns, they may lack clarity, precision, and explicitness. They may not appreciate, pragmatically, what must be reported explicitly in their interpretations of verbal absurdities in talking about nature of language (metalinguistic comments), and in their explanation of the problematic situations within their environments, such as causes, potential consequences, and alternative solutions.

Assessment Recommendations: Language Implication Level

There is also a paucity of formal tests available at this level of language for measurement of performance integrity. Administration of the Social Adjustment Subtest A of the Detroit Test of Learning Aptitude (Baker and Leland, 1967) can be useful. The task has many "What could you do if...?" social and emergency type problems for use in surveying ability to analyze and express implication (e.g., What would you do if you find the house across the street is on fire?). The student has to identify the problematic situations and formulate viable solutions. Each item should be graded very stringently, with the student being expected not only to tell what to do to solve the problem but also to give a good reason for the suggested solution. The responses should be self-protective and also show social responsibility for the welfare of others. As the task requires both comprehension and convergent production, it can be sensitive to deficits in social perception and understanding of life-saving responsibilities.

This chapter has drawn upon Guilford's (1967) Structure of the Intellect model to describe cognitive-linguistic deficits observed in language-learning disabled adolescents.

SUMMARY

Twenty of the cells in Guilford's (1967) semantic segment are included in Figure 7-2 with each assessment instrument placed in the cell that it best measures. All subtests in the suggested battery are available commercially. The administration of all 12 subtests is viewed essential to obtain a reasonable measurement of the complex language performance displayed by the young adolescent. When considering all available other similar commercial subtests, most tests were selected because of the following features: (1) they were viewed to be the "best of the group" as far as the time it takes to give them, (2) they showed good fit of mental operation or language level aspects of the modified version of the semantic section of the Structure of the Intellect model (Guilford, 1967), (3) their age range was appropriate for adolescents, (4) there is relative ease of scoring and interpreting, and (5) each has the potential for allowing the student to demonstrate language disabilities in the respective area. The battery had to be selectively limited, priority-wise, in the number of subtests involved. Undoubtedly the recommended battery will quickly change as more appropriate subtests surface commercially. When the teacher or multidisciplinary team description of the student's cognitive and communication deficits is specific as far as level of disability, then only the appropriate subcomponents of the full battery need to be given.

REFERENCES

Baker, H. J., and Leland, B. (1967). *Detroit tests of learning aptitude.* Indianapolis, Ind: Bobbs-Merrill.

Bruno, R. M. (1981). Interpretation of pictorially presented social situations by learning disabled and normal children. *Journal of Learning Disabilities, 14,* 350–352.

Chappell, G. E. (1980). Oral language performance of upper elementary school students obtained via story reformulation. *Language, Speech, and Hearing Services in Schools, 11,* 236–251.

Dunn, L. M. (1959). *Peabody picture vocabulary test.* Circle Pines, MN: American Guidance Service.

Dunn, L. M., and Markwardt, F. C. (1970). *Peabody Individual Achievement Test.* Circle Pines, MN: American Guidance Service.

Freeman, M. (1981). Is mainstreaming working in the middle school? Unpublished independent study project, University of Wisconsin at Stevens Point.

German, D. J. (1979). Word-finding skills in children with learning disabilities. *Journal of Learning Disabilities 12,* 43–48.

German, D. J. (1982). Word finding substitutions in children with learning disabilities. *Language, Speech, and Hearing Services in the Schools, 13,* 223–230.

Gorham, D. R. (1954). *Proverbs test.* Missoula, MT: Psychological Test Specialists.

Guilford, J. P. (1967). *The nature of human intelligence.* New York: McGraw-Hill Book Company.

Hammill, D. D., Brown, V. L., Larsen, S. C., and Wiederholt, J.L. (1980). *Tests of adolescent language: A multidimensional approach to assessment.* Austin, TX: Services for Professional Educators.

Hammill, D. D., and Larsen, S. C. (1978). *Test of written language.* Austin, TX: Services for Professional Educators.

Johnson, D. J., and Myklebust, H. R. (1967). *Learning disabilities.* New York: Grune & Stratton.

Johnston, J. R. (1981). Words for the moment. Presentation at Wisconsin Speech and Hearing Conference, 1981.

Jorgensen, C., Barrett, M., Huisingh, R., and Zachman, L. (1981). *The Word Test: A test of expressive vocabulary and semantics.* Moline, IL: Lingui-Systems, Inc.

Kirk, S. A., McCarthy, J. J., and Kirk, W. D. (1968). *Examiner's manual: Illinois test of psycholinguistic abilities.* Chicago: University of Illinois Press.

Kellner, M., Flood, C., and Yoder, D. E. (1977). *Language assessment tasks.* Madison, WI.

La Greca, A. M., and Mesibov, G. B. (1981). Facilitating interpersonal functioning with peers in learning disabled children. *Journal of Learning Disabilities, 14,* 197–199.

Litowitz, G. (1977). Learning to make definitions. *Journal of Child Language, 4,* 289–304.

Meeker, M. N. (1969). *The structure of intellect: Its interpretations and uses.* Columbus, OH: Charles E. Merrill.

Miller, L. (1979). Pragmatics and analysis of school age language disorders. Paper presented at the Atlanta Convention of the American Speech and Hearing Association.

McArthur, D. S., and Roberts, G. E. (1982). *Roberts apperception test for children.* Los Angeles: Western Psychological Services.

Muma, J. R. (1973). Language assessment: The co-occurring and restricted structure procedure. *Acta Symbolica, 4,* 12–29.

Schwartz, E. R., and Solot, C. B. (1980). Response pattern characteristic of verbal disorders. *Language, Speech and Hearing Services in the Schools, 11,* 139–144.

Semel, E. M., and Wiig, E. H. (1980). *Clinical evaluation of language functions.* Columbus, OH: Charles E. Merrill.

Shewan, C. M. (1979). *Auditory comprehension test for sentences.* Biolinguistics Clinical Institutes.

Soenksen, P. A., Flagg, C. L., and Schmits, D. W. (1981). Social communication in learning disabled students: A pragmatic analysis. *Journal of Learning Disabilities, 14,* 283–286.

Stein, N., and Glenn, C. (1979). An analysis of story comprehension in elementary school children. In R. Freedle (Ed.), *New directions in discourse processing.* Norwood, NJ: Ablex.

Wechsler, D. (1949). *Wechsler intelligence scale for children.* New York: The Psychological Corporation.

Wentland, T. J. (1970). *A test of conceptual categorization.* Stevens Point, WI: Unpublished manuscript.

Westby, C. E. (1980). Childrens' narrative development—cognitive and linguistic aspects. Prepared for Conference on Language, Learning, and Reading Disabilities: A New Decade.

Wiig, E. H., and Semel, E. M. (1976). *Language disabilities in children and adolescents.* Columbus, OH: Charles E. Merrill.

Wiig, E. H., and Semel, E. M. (1980). *Language assessment and intervention for the learning disabled.* Columbus, OH: Charles E. Merrill.

Yudkovitz, E., Lewison, N., and Rottersman, J. (1976). *Communication therapy in childhood schizophrenia: An auditory monitoring approach.* New York: Grune & Stratton.

APPENDIX 7-1

THE STORY REFORMULATION ANALYSIS PROCEDURE

Summary of the Research Project and Application to Adolescent Population

Previous comparisons had found the story reformulation performance of fourth graders to be competitive with that of fifth, sixth, and seventh graders in turn. Thus the story reformulation performance of only fourth graders was investigated to consider the usefulness of this analysis procedure. Most fourth graders could be accurate and adequate in their semantic referencing of some of the critical story features and plot interrelationships, and in their organization and use of grammatical text.

The following analysis procedure, therefore, is viewed as useful for adolescents. Each component represents a significant cognitive-semantic facet of the story and thus as each in turn is passed or failed it serves as a measurement of reformulation skills. Since the four story components are critical to effective story narration, measurement of how well these components have or have not been met provides a rich sample of ability-disability. As the number of components failed increases, the likelihood of problems in semantic accuracy and completeness, undue grammatical simplicity, or organization also increases. Students who fail all components seem to do so for a variety of combined reasons. Usually each excessively omits semantic detail and critical elements of script specification and each evidences a concerning semantic inaccuracy. Incoherence, incompleteness, and disorganization will destroy their story's integrity. Most students offer one or more complete sentences throughout their stories, but often do not do so at the points where they need to draw critical event interrelationships. The rest of the time, and in a more characteristic manner, many of them narrate their stories in a series of short sentences coordinated by excessive use of "and."

The Story Reformulation Analysis Procedure

Instructions: This is a language screening exercise to see how well you can understand and retell a story. I want you to listen carefully to this story so that you can retell it in your own words. First listen to the first half of the story as I read it, and then you retell that half. Then listen to and retell the second half of the story. Tell the story as completely as you can so that a listener who does not know the story could fully understand it.

Audiotape and record each segment as the subject retells it. If the subject is nervous, cannot concentrate or forgets, or if a distraction interrupts, resulting in only one or two statements about the story, let him or her relisten and begin the reformulation again.

The Story: The Rich Woman Solves a Problem

First Half. There was a rich old woman who was sick because she had cancer. She planned to will all of her money to her faithful secretary, Jenny, instead of her son, Bill, because he had been mean to her. But then Bill, who was a cancer specialist, promised to cure her if she gave him all the money. Since she did want to live, she decided that she would give him all the money provided that he marry Jenny and cure the cancer. However, her problem was that she knew that Jenny would refuse to marry Bill inasmuch as he was very nasty and did not love her.

Second Half. Since the sick old lady knew that she had to change her son from a nasty person to a nice doctor, she ordered her bank to buy a medical building with an office and clinic for him. She told Bill that he could have the building for free, provided that he hire the secretary and under the condition that he develop a good bedside manner while he was curing her cancer. Well the story ended OK in that as Bill gradually worked with Jenny he fell in love with her and changed into a warm, loving person. Therefore, all the mother's wishes came true because, one, Bill married Jenny; two, he found a cure for Mom's cancer; and three, they all lived happily together in Mom's big house and spent her money.

The Analysis Scheme and Procedure

General Criteria. Using a tape recorder with an instant "pause" mechanism on it, advance the student's tape through his or her expression of each story event or component under test in turn. Listen carefully to the accuracy and completeness of what is said as you compare it with the scoring criteria for each component below and use the scoring sheet to check only the features that are passed or the criteria that are met. In addition to the specific pass-fail criteria delineated below in the description of the individual components, do not pass or check an item if any of the following are true of the student's performance:

a. Do not score or accept references that are inaccurate semantically, e.g., the student reports a kinship other than son for Bill, such as brother, husband, or some guy or man; or the relationship of the secretary Jenny is inaccurately cited to be that of a sister or a daughter; or the student reports complete fabrications, such as "and the woman died," "so they lived in Florida," or "the doctor operated on her liver."

b. Do not score exophoric references (i.e., immediately referring to the character as *he* or *she* or *they* without having first named who was under reference, e.g., the old lady, Bill, etc.). This error relates especially to the introductory comment or report for either the first or second segment of the story, i.e., failure to first designate (or redesignate) Mom, the son, or the secretary as *she* or *he* is immediately used.

c. Do not score references wherein there is pronoun confusion or intersubstitution (i.e., an inaccurate interchange of *he* for *she*, or vice versa) in references to the male-female character(s) for a specific event. This error is often the first or second anaphoric reference in sentences beyond the sentence that designates (or redesignates) the characters, e.g., then he (for she—the Mom) promised to give her (for him—the son) all the money.

d. Do not score points *b* or *c* unless the student expresses efficient obligatory structures that make the cause-effect reasons or conditional stipulation fully explicit. In most cases this has to be the expression of a linking subordinator such as *because* or *if*, which clearly ties two clausal events together in particular interrelationship.

Generally components *a*, *c*, and *d* focus upon critical details of the setting, shifting, and concluding of the plot and script to sample the student's degree of coverage or inclusion of story data and episodes (essential events, characterization, organization). The *b* and *c* sequence emphasizes cause-effect and conditional interrelations that are viewed to be critical to proficient progression of story meaning and integrity.

Specific Scoring Criteria

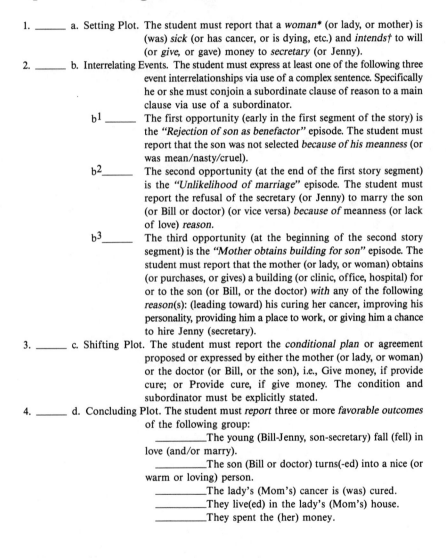

1. _____ a. Setting Plot. The student must report that a *woman** (or lady, or mother) is (was) *sick* (or has cancer, or is dying, etc.) and *intends†* to will (or *give*, or gave) money to *secretary* (or Jenny).

2. _____ b. Interrelating Events. The student must express at least one of the following three event interrelationships via use of a complex sentence. Specifically he or she must conjoin a subordinate clause of reason to a main clause via use of a subordinator.

   b¹ _____ The first opportunity (early in the first segment of the story) is the *"Rejection of son as benefactor"* episode. The student must report that the son was not selected *because of his meanness* (or was mean/nasty/cruel).

   b² _____ The second opportunity (at the end of the first story segment) is the *"Unlikelihood of marriage"* episode. The student must report the refusal of the secretary (or Jenny) to marry the son (or Bill or doctor) (or vice versa) *because of* meanness (or lack of love) *reason.*

   b³ _____ The third opportunity (at the beginning of the second story segment) is the *"Mother obtains building for son"* episode. The student must report that the mother (or lady, or woman) obtains (or purchases, or gives) a building (or clinic, office, hospital) for or to the son (or Bill, or the doctor) *with* any of the following *reason*(s): (leading toward) his curing her cancer, improving his personality, providing him a place to work, or giving him a chance to hire Jenny (secretary).

3. _____ c. Shifting Plot. The student must report the *conditional plan* or agreement proposed or expressed by either the mother (or lady, or woman) or the doctor (or Bill, or the son), i.e., Give money, if provide cure; or Provide cure, if give money. The condition and subordinator must be explicitly stated.

4. _____ d. Concluding Plot. The student must *report* three or more *favorable outcomes* of the following group:

   _____The young (Bill-Jenny, son-secretary) fall (fell) in love (and/or marry).

   _____The son (Bill or doctor) turns(-ed) into a nice (or warm or loving) person.

   _____The lady's (Mom's) cancer is (was) cured.

   _____They live(ed) in the lady's (Mom's) house.

   _____They spent the (her) money.

*Features in parentheses are alternative possibilities.

†The italicized concepts are the critical essense of the component that must be passed or reported.

TRANSITIONAL NOTE

A clinician should always know why a particular test is being administered. There should be specific reasons for acquiring the type of information that the test yields and an understanding of how the acquisition of this information will lead directly to programming objectives. This rationale is usually based on an operational definition of "communication disorder."

Chappell's assessment battery, described in Chapter 7, evolved from a conceptual model that focused on the interaction of cognitive and linguistic skills and the types of communication deficits that could be observed, depending upon the level of that interaction. Guilford's Structure of the Intellect model provided the framework for the general procedural rationale. Chappell also gives a specific rationale for the use of each recommended test within the battery by describing the deviant behaviors that could be observed systematically. He provides a justification for the test he selected—over other tests available—that would best identify deviant cognitive-linguistic skills.

Tests are not perfect. Researchers, being aware of this, frequently subject tests to empirical scrutiny as they study a test's reliability, validity, time-efficiency, and clinical usefulness in describing deviant behaviors. The Token Test by DeRenzi and Vignolo is one of those assessment tools that clinical intuition has suggested is very useful in describing memory and linguistic processing problems. Research has probed the degree to which clinical intuition has been accurate. In Chapter 8, Murray describes a study completed at Children's Hospital in Washington, DC, that examined the sensitivity of DeSimoni's adaption of the DeRenzi and Vignolo procedure in describing language processing problems in preschool children as well as school-age children.

The study by Murray, Feinstein, and Blouin is another example of how research is directly related to clinical practice. It is important to investigate the usefulness of tests that are frequently relied upon by clinicians. Research findings can help modify or support clinical intuition about the usefulness of a certain procedure.

CHAPTER 8

The Token Test for Children: Diagnostic Patterns and Programming Implications

Sharon L. Murray,
Carl B. Feinstein,
and
Arthur G. A. Blouin

No single test or series of specific tasks provide all the answers to behavior in children. Fortunately, this is widely accepted, and an evaluation usually consists of interviews, careful history-taking, observations, formal and informal tasks, and trial periods of intervention. Within this process we find that some tasks are consistently sensitive to particular kinds of behavior. In our clinical experience of evaluating over 2,000 children a year for speech, language, and learning problems at Children's Hospital in Washington, DC, we have gained an increasing appreciation of the information we are able to obtain from the Token Test format (DeRenzi and Vignolo, 1962). When the general format of this test was published by DiSimoni (1978), we designed an extensive study to compare the results we obtained from the Token Test for Children with general data on development, academic progress, and attention deficits presented by school programs and parents who brought children into our facility for evaluation.

Findings from this study will be presented and discussed in this chapter. Implications for assessment and programming in public schools for children who demonstrate auditory processing problems, in terms of attention, memory and comprehension will also be addressed.

The Token Test (DeRenzi and Vignolo, 1962) has been mentioned extensively in the literature as a measure of comprehension and auditory memory in adult aphasic individuals (Boller and Vignolo, 1966; Noll and Randolph, 1978; Orgass and Poeck, 1966; Swisher and Sarno, 1969; Wertz, Keith, and Custer, 1971; Wertz and Perkins, 1972). The test format also has been used widely with children, but little has been known regarding its predictability of language processing problems in school or in social interactions across age groups.

In 1975, Tallal reported findings of an investigation in which the Token Test (DeRenzi and Vignolo's version) was used to compare the performance of developmental dysphasic and matched control children, aged 6 years 9 months to 9 years 3 months. Tallal found a performance profile emerged with the dysphasic group which indicated that this group had more difficulty with Part 4 than with Part 5. This finding suggested that these children had greater problems with auditory retention (or verbal memory) than with grammatical complexity. (For example, an item in Part 4 is "Touch the small yellow circle and the large green square" and an item in Part 5 is "Put the red circle *on* the green square.") Also, the few errors made by the control subjects were predominantly on Part 4. Tallal's findings supported the potential strength of the Token Test as a discriminator between short-term auditory memory deficits (comprehension of six critical elements—small yellow circle and large green square) and grammatical comprehension deficits (*"Together with* the yellow circle *take* the blue square").

LaPointe (1975) reported that the Token Test (DeRenzi and Vignolo format) identified subtle receptive language deficits in learning disabled adolescents. Wiig and Semel (1976) found that the adolescent performance on the Token Test (DeRenzi and Vignolo format) correlated positively with performance on the Wiig-Semel Test of Linguistic Concepts (Wiig and Semel, 1976), thus supporting its validity as a measure of interpreting linguistic information. When Robb and Lass (1976) looked at children's performance on the Noll and Berry modification of the Token Test (1969) and compared the results with those of the Brenner Developmental Gestalt Test of School Readiness (Brenner, 1964) and the Basic Grammatical Concepts Test (Brenner, 1964), they found a significant correlation. These investigators suggested that the Token Test, therefore, could be included in preschool readiness batteries because it could predict success or failure in school.

These investigations suggested the possibility that the Token Test format might be effective as an indicator of potential or existing learning problems and as a discriminator between specific areas of difficulty with school-age children. However, before further statements could be made, a well-standardized version needed to be developed for children, since most of the previous investigations used adaptations of the adult version (DeRenzi and Vignolo, 1962) with a limited normative base.

In 1978, DiSimoni published the Token Test for Children (TTC), which provided norms for children ages 3 years 0 months through 12 years 5 months and was based on Noll's version (1970). The normative data for the broad age range allow wide application of TTC. Let us review the sections of TTC. The TTC consists of five parts, the first four of which introduce commands that increase in length but not in linguistic complexity. The fifth part consists of commands that vary in length, semantic, and structural complexity. Examples from each subtest are as follows:

Part 1: Touch the green circle (two to three critical elements)

Part 2: Touch the small green circle (three to four critical elements)

Part 3: Touch the green circle and the blue square (four to five critical elements

Part 4: Touch the small yellow circle and the large green square (six to seven critical elements)

Part 5: *Except for* the *green one, touch* the *circles* (four critical elements embedded in a complex syntactical construction)

The purpose of the present discussion is twofold: (1) to compare performance profiles of preschool and school-age children on the TTC; and (2) to investigate its use as an indicator of learning difficulties as well as a discriminator of specific areas of difficulty. The two aspects of the study will be presented separately.

PROCEDURE

The children who participated in this study were referred to our clinic for speech and language evaluations by a concerned parent or teacher. We divided the children into two groups according to age: preschool, 4 years 0 months to 6 years 6 months (N = 25) and school-age, 6 years 7 months to 11 years 11 months (N = 30). In the preschool group there were 18 boys, with a mean age of 5 years 3 months, and 7 girls, with a mean age of 4 years 7 months. In the school-age group there were 27 boys, with a mean age of 8 years 5 months, and 3 girls, with a mean age of 10 years 0 months. All children had normal hearing, and they were given a standard speech and language evaluation, which included standardized tests in addition to the TTC. The focus of our discussion in this chapter, however, will be on their performance according to the TTC.

In addition, the Preliminary School Report adapted from the Conners Teacher Questionnaire (Conners, 1973) was used to obtain teacher description of testing, grade placement, achievement in school subjects, classroom behavior, group participation, and attitude toward authority. For the purposes of this chapter, only the descriptions of grade placement, level of academic intervention (e.g., tutoring, special class), and achievement in school subjects will be used. Reporting of standardized testing was too sparse to be used as a basis for comparison.

RESULTS AND DISCUSSION

Part I. Profiles of Performance

We will consider the results for the school-age group first. As a result of the entire speech and language testing, including the TTC, we found 24 children with delays in language performance but normal speech development. There were six children with normal language test performance but a speech disorder. We separated these children to look at their TTC profile performances (Fig. 8–1). The resulting pattern for the speech-impaired children nearly mirrors that reported by Tallal (1975) for her control group—that is, a mild dip in performance with both Parts 4 and 5 but slightly more difficulty with Part 4.

The pattern for the children whom we will call "language impaired" was quite similar to Tallal's dysphasic group, although as a whole the children's profiles show equal difficulty with Parts 4 and 5.

We separated the preschool children into the same two categories: speech impaired but normal language and language impaired but normal speech. The four children in the speech impaired group demonstrated a profile similar to that of the older speech impaired group, with a slight dip in Part 4 (seven critical elements demanded of auditory memory) (Fig. 8–1). The profile that emerged for the 21 language impaired children was quite different from the profile of the school-age language impaired group. The preschool group's profile shows group means that are one to two standard deviations below the norm on all subtests.

When we compare the results of the preschool and school-age language impaired children, two distinct profiles emerge. The older group managed Parts 1, 2, and 3 with relative ease but had difficulty with Parts 4 and 5. The profile for the preschool group reflected neither Tallal's profiles nor that of the school-age group in this study. Part 1 emerged as the most significant indicator of possible learning difficulty. In other words, if the preschool child had difficulty with Part 1 (Touch the *red circle*), this was an indicator that language processing or concept acquisition was delayed.

The profile differences on the TTC between the age groups possibly can be explained as a function of the instrument itself. Part 1 is simple

Figure 8–1. TTC profiles for the school-aged group (6 years 7 months, to 11 years 11 months) and the preschool group (4 years 0 months to 6 years 6 months).

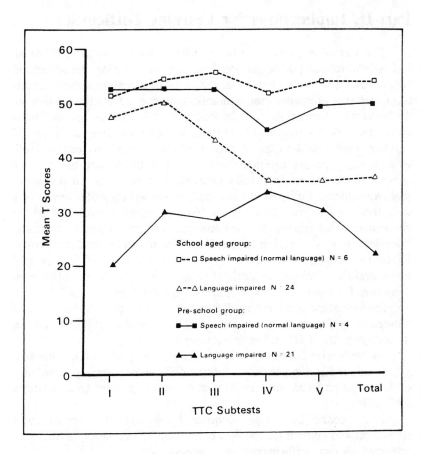

in terms of syntax, length, and semantic complexity (Touch the red circle); therefore, it sensitively identifies young children who have not yet mastered this level of developmental expectation. The younger children are not expected to do as well on the remaining four subtests according to DiSimoni's version of the test, which is based on the normative data. For school-age children, the first three subtests should not be a linguistic challenge, since they tap auditory memory of up to four or five critical elements. The difficulties older children encounter with Part 4 are most likely due to short-term memory or attentional deficits, since only the length and number of critical elements of the stimulus increase. Part 5 is sensitive to syntactic-semantic confusions as well as short-term memory or attentional deficits.

Part II. Implications for Learning Difficulties

The second issue we wish to consider is the use of the TTC as an indicator of learning difficulty. Further, we want to explore the suggestion that it could provide a differential diagnosis of attention deficits, short-term memory problems, and semantic-syntactic difficulties. When we analyzed the information from the Preliminary School Report completed by teachers for the school-age language impaired children, 23 of the 24 children were found to be at least one year behind in reading level. Additionally, spelling problems and writing abilities were noted to be commensurate with reading ability. One child had reading and mathematics levels appropriate for his grade, but spelling and writing skills were poorly developed, and he was failing in his general classroom work. All of the children received teacher descriptions such as "poor memory abilities," "problems paying attention in class," or "doesn't understand directions." Given this consistent relationship between reading difficulties and behavioral descriptions, we decided to look at the TTC for differential diagnoses for these nonachieving school-age children.

Individual patterns emerged from actual test performance, which allowed us to differentially diagnose why an individual child was having difficulty on the TTC and in the classroom.

To summarize our research data, three types of performance emerged:

1. One indicating pervasive learning difficulties affecting knowledge of language structure and content and including short-term memory difficulties.

2. A second indicating adequate knowledge of language form (structure) and content (semantics) but a short-term memory deficit that impacted on test performance and learning.

3. A third indicating adequate language and short-term memory abilities but attention difficulties.

The performance of three children in the school-age language impaired group are included as examples of the profiles which emerged.

Case 1: Sherrie

Sherrie was 8 years 6 months old. She was in a class for children with specific learning disabilities and was just mastering reading and mathematics skills equivalent to the beginning first grade level. The school was considering a change to a classroom for children with emotional disturbance owing to Sherrie's difficulties with social adjustment in class. Her performance on the TTC indicated three areas of deficit: (1) reduced short-term auditory memory capacity with problems in retaining detail beyond three to four critical elements as reflected on performance of Parts 1 to 3; (2) fluctuating attention, which was evident only for tasks that were auditorily stressful; and (3) suspected semantic base for terms referring to position in space and time, such as "away from," "between," "after," "before." Her TTC test profile (Fig. 8–2) showed the impact of these difficulties on this kind of task. Classroom performance could be easily predicted for an activity that requires sustained attention to and retention of lengthy verbal instructions.

Case 2: Henry

Henry was 8 years 2 months old. According to his teacher his reading and mathematics skills were at the first grade level. He was being considered for a language-learning disability classroom at the time that we saw him. He had been retained in first grade. In his current second grade placement he was receiving resource help for reading. The results of his performance on the TTC indicated good attention, a latent response style with a natural tendency to reauditorize, and a limited short-term auditory memory for linguistic detail (Fig. 8–3). As the commands increased in length, Henry could not retain specific detail (e.g., of critical elements).

Case 3: Brian

Brian was 10 years 2 months old. He was in the fourth grade and his teacher reported that his reading and mathematics skills were on grade level, but his day-to-day performance was poor. He had trouble paying attention, would forget assignments, and was beginning to distract others in class. Brian's performance on the TTC clearly indicated an "in-out" attention (Fig. 8–4). His performance fluctuated *within* each level rather than as a result of an increase in stimulus length or linguistic complexity. He also demonstrated an impulsive response style.

These three children performed quite differently on the TTC and their differences were clearly evidenced on the individual TTC profiles. Their individual differences, however, had similar results in the classroom—i.e., learning difficulties. The value of the TTC profiles was the help in determining *why* there were difficulties learning, which then allowed us to intervene appropriately in each individual case.

For Sherrie we strongly recommended a class for children with specific learning disabilities but with strategy changes. In addition to recommending individual language intervention, we suggested the following instructional strategies for the classroom, based on Sherrie's extremely limited short-term auditory memory and fluctuating attention:

1. Instructions should be given in single, discrete steps.
    a. Get a pencil
    b. Listen to the spelling words
    c. Write each word
2. Syntactic complexity should remain at a simple level without conjoiners, such as *"Match* the pictures to the words. Write the word for each picture. Give me your paper." Although the content is similar, consider the difference in syntactic complexity of this alternative: "After matching the pictures to the words, write the word for each picture and put your paper in the top right hand corner of your desk."
3. Present information at a slow rate.
4. Monitor her attention.
5. Reduce both visual and auditory distraction by: (a) use of a three-sided carrel at her desk, and (b) proximity to the teacher or person instructing.

Since Sherry was demonstrating an emerging strategy of rehearsal (or "reauditorization") we also recommended that this be encouraged as a strategy in the classroom.

For Henry we recommended the following:

1. A classroom for children with specific *language*-learning disabilities that would provide a small teacher-pupil ratio.
2. Redundancy of teaching.
3. Visual and content supports for assisting memory.

For Brian the possibility of an overall attention deficit disorder was indicated. This needed to be assessed medically while at the same time classroom strategies could be initiated to increase Brian's focused attention. The strategies we suggested were the following:

1. Preferential seating close to the speaker and away from distractions.
2. Gain his attention *before* presenting information or giving a direction—e.g., "Is everybody listening? Look at me and raise your hand."
3. Check for attention following a direction by asking Brian to restate the instruction.
4. List all key vocabulary for visual reference (on the board or on paper).
5. Use visual aids for instruction.

6. *Write* instruction in simple language for reference; for example, "Before opening your spelling books, be sure you have enough paper and a pencil" can be *written* simply as

    a. Get one pencil

    b. Use three sheets of paper

    c. Open your spelling book to page 3

7. Have Brian maintain an assignment book that must be checked at the end of each day for accuracy.

8. Provide quiet study areas.

9. Give praise.

In addition to these suggestions we recommended an academic tutor for Brian for two reasons: (1) to increase the redundancy of classroom learning, thereby avoiding impending failure; and (2) to relieve the parents of the need to assume the tutor role which had become a frustrating and negative experience.

CONCLUSION

Our findings indicate that the TTC is sensitive in describing several areas of difficulty: (1) problems with sustained attention when the context is somewhat abstract; (2) the development of color, shape, and size concepts; (3) short-term auditory memory capacity when a child's task is to go beyond rote recall (as in digit or sentence imitation tasks) and demonstrate understanding of a directive; and (4) manipulation of syntactic and semantic knowledge. In order to differentiate between these areas of difficulty when assessing the performance of a particular child, we must look at the individual test profile. In addition, as diagnosticians we should

1. Note performance of younger children on Part 1 as indicative of color and shape concepts.

2. Note performance of older children on Part 4 as indicative of short-term memory capacity for detail.

3. Watch for "in-out" focused attention.

4. Note a dependency on rehearsal strategies in order to carry out the directives.

5. Detect indications of impulsivity in response style, or a latent response style that may suggest internal rehearsal.

6. Determine the impact of short-term auditory memory capacity on the ability to understand a directive versus a poor syntactic-semantic base.

We then combine information on each student with the results from an entire evaluation to include history, observation, and informal testing in order to formulate appropriate educational recommendations.

REFERENCES

Boller, F., and Vignolo, L. (1966). Latent sensory aphasia in hemisphere-damaged patients: An experimental study with the Token Test. *Brain, 89,* 815–830.

Brenner, A. (1964). *Anton Brenner developmental gestalt test of school readiness.* Los Angeles, Western Psychological Services.

Conners, C. K. (1973). Rating scales for use in drug studies with children. *Psychopharmacology Bulletin* (Special Issue, Pharmacotherapy of Children), pp. 24–29.

DeRenzi, E., and Vignolo, L. (1962). The Token Test: A sensitive test to detect receptive disturbances in aphasics. *Brain, 85,* 665–678.

DiSimoni, F. (1978). The Token Test for children. Hingham, MA: Teaching Resources.

Lapointe, C. (1975). Token Test performances by learning disabled and academically achieving adolescents. Unpublished masters thesis, Boston University.

Noll, J. D. (1970). The use of the Token Test with children. Paper presented at the annual convention of the American Speech and Hearing Association, New York, November 1970.

Noll, J. D., and Berry, W. (1969). Some thoughts on the Token Test. *ASHA, 27,* 37–40.

Noll, J. D., and Randolph, S. R. (1978). Auditory semantic, syntactic, and retention errors made by aphasic subjects on the Token Test. *Journal of Communication Disorders, 11,* 543–553.

Orgass, B., and Poeck, K. (1966). Clinical validation of a new test for aphasia: An experimental study of the Token Test. *Cortex, 2,* 222–243.

Robb, E., and Lass, N. (1976). A correlational investigation of children's performance on the Token Test, the Brenner Developmental Gestalt Test of School Readiness, and a basic grammatical concepts test. *Journal of Auditory Research, 16,* 64–67.

Swisher, L., and Sarno, M. (1969). Token Test scores of three matched patient groups: Left brain-damaged with aphasia; right brain-damaged without aphasia; non-brain-damaged. *Cortex, 5,* 264–273.

Tallal, P. (1975). Perceptual and linguistic factors in the language impairment of develpmental dysphasics: An experimental investigation with the Token Test. *Cortex, 11,* 196–205.

Wertz, R., Keith, R., and Custer, D. (1971). Normal and aphasic behavior on a measure of auditory input and a measure of verbal output. Paper presented at the annual convention of the American Speech and Hearing Association, Chicago, 1971.

Wertz, R. T., and Perkins, M. P. (1972). Measures of auditory input and verbal output in children. *Journal of the Colorado Speech and Hearing Association, 5,* 11–18.

Wiig, E., and Semel, E. (1976). *Language disabilities in children and adolescents.* Columbus, OH: Charles Merrill.

TRANSITIONAL NOTE

Clinicians and educators continually try to locate standardized tests and informal observational procedures that can *document casual observations* of a student's difficulties in the classroom. There are numerous procedures available, each claiming to be the panacea. It is through research projects such as the one described in Chapter 8 that we begin to refine *our* evaluation of evaluation procedures.

When discussing implications of their research findings, Murray, Feinstein, and Blouin gave specific examples of how they shared assessment notations with classroom teachers. From these notations, specific modifications in programming were possible, with the result being a context in which the child had a better chance of reaching his or her potential.

Chapter 9 focuses in greater detail on the presentation of communication evaluation results to educators. Although the format for evaluation reports may differ from facility to facility, the over-all objective of a report should be a *description* of the cognitive-linguistic, pragmatic, and language processing behaviors that the student is currently using. As educators and staff members listen to an oral report during an multidisciplinary IEP conference or read a report on a student with whom they have had earlier interaction, a behavioral profile should emerge that explains the casual observations that "the student doesn't make sense," or "never understands an assignment." The purpose of Chapter 9 is to offer suggestions for how to organize and present evaluation data so that colleagues and parents better understand the nature of a student's communication difficulties.

CHAPTER 9

Presentation of Communication Evaluation Information

Charlann S. Simon
and
Cynthia L. Holway

"Please take a look at Joe for me. I think he has some speech problems. He talks in circles and he never listens to directions." With such a request, a teacher may ask the speech-language pathologist to analyze and then describe the student's communication problems. If the speech-language pathologist merely presents a series of scores on standardized tests when the testing results are shared, the teacher will probably not be encouraged to request future evaluations. Scores alone are sterile. The interested professional who seeks to better understand a student's communication deficits needs a *description* of problem areas and some recommendations for how the student can be helped either through skill-building activities or through compensatory strategies.

The way in which a clinician presents results of an evaluation reflects theoretical biases and definitions of adequate versus deviant communication behaviors. Team members at an IEP staffing will be able to understand the rationale for a student's program if the nature of the student's communication problem is clearly described by the clinician. It is necessary to describe deviant or ineffective communication or cognitive strategies and then relate programming recommendations to these observations.

The purpose of this chapter is to consider the nature of communication evaluation and to offer suggestions for how evaluation information can be effectively presented to teachers and administrators. The mode of presentation will vary depending on the purpose of sharing the information.

PHILOSOPHICAL BIASES REGARDING EVALUATION

Communication evaluation is at best an evolving phenomenon. Over the past decade it has become increasingly apparent that we have not always used the most sensitive types of evaluation tasks that would directly lead to effective programming. Through this critical analysis of conceptual frameworks underlying procedures and the procedures themselves, there has been an impetus to develop modes of observation that permit systematic analysis of deficits in those cognitive-linguistic skills that are required or highly esteemed for use within the educational system and for social interaction.

Traditional assessment formats, such as standardized test batteries, are still employed by some individuals and institutions. There is a growing awareness, however, that short responses on a series of predetermined items do not reflect *communicative* competence (Leonard, Prutting, Perozzi, and Berkley, 1978; Lucas, 1980; Muma, 1978; Siegel and Broen, 1976). What is needed is the combination of informal (clinician-constructed) probes into the quality of language processing and language use and the judicious use of standardized tests or subtests to meet federal guidelines in PL 94-142. The resulting information permits the clinician and educator to pinpoint specific areas of deficit, do so quickly, and develop an individualized set of programming objectives for the student that will promote better coping skills to meet communicative demands of the classroom and in social encounters.

Evaluation begins with an hypothesis about the nature of communication. In other words, we must ask, "What is the behavioral profile of the competent versus the incompetent communicator?" Those features of communication that are considered "competent" serve as programming objectives, and those that interfere with the transmission of information or social interactions are considered "incompetent." These incompetent behaviors serve as the focus for "awareness therapy," in which an individual becomes more cognizant of effective cognitive-linguistic strategies. An example of competent versus incompetent expressive language behaviors appears in Table 9–1. Clinicians "should have an intervention model that outlines needed information, enabling them to know where they stand in terms of what they know and need to know" (Muma, 1978, p. 217).

PRESENTATION OF EVALUATION INFORMATION

Judging from the literature, there is little interest in writing reports on learning and communication disorders. In fact, among the 4010 abstracts

Table 9-1. A Clinician's Model of Expressive Communicative Competence

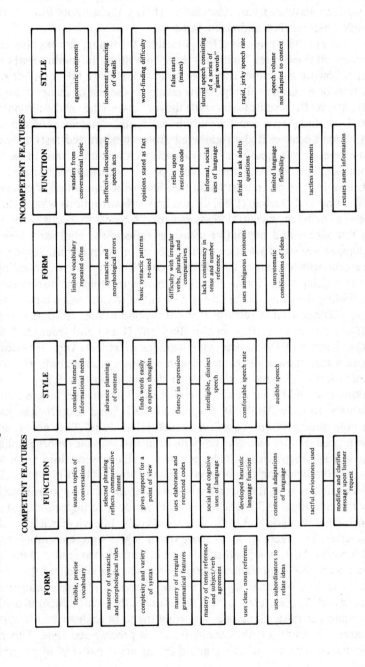

COMPETENT FEATURES

FORM	FUNCTION	STYLE
flexible, precise vocabulary	sustains topics of conversation	considers listener's informational needs
mastery of syntactic and morphological rules	selected phrasing reflects communicative intent	advance planning of content
complexity and variety of syntax	gives support for a point of view	finds words easily to express thoughts
mastery of irregular grammatical features	uses elaborated and restricted codes	fluency in expression
mastery of tense reference and subject/verb agreement	social and cognitive uses of language	intelligible, distinct speech
uses clear, noun referents	developed heuristic language function	comfortable speech rate
uses subordinators to relate ideas	contextual adaptations of language	audible speech
	tactful deviousness used	
	modifies and clarifies message upon listener request	

INCOMPETENT FEATURES

FORM	FUNCTION	STYLE
limited vocabulary repeated often	wanders from conversational topic	egocentric comments
syntactic and morphological errors	ineffective illocutionary speech acts	incoherent sequencing of details
basic syntactic patterns re-used	opinions stated as fact	word-finding difficulty
difficulty with irregular verbs, plurals, and comparatives	relies upon restricted code	false starts (mazes)
lacks consistency in tense and number reference	informal, social uses of language	slurred speech consisting of a series of "giant words"
uses ambiguous pronouns	afraid to ask adults questions	rapid, jerky speech rate
unsystematic combinations of ideas	limited language flexibility	speech volume not adapted to context
	tactless statements	
	restates same information	

From Simon, C. S. (1979). *Communicative competence: A functional-pragmatic approach to language therapy.* Copyright by Communication Skill Builders, Inc. Reprinted with permission.

presented in the 1971–80 Abstracted Bibliography published by the American Psychological Association (1982), the authors did not find a single abstract that addressed this topic.

Lucas (1980) presents a few guidelines for report writing plus sample reports on three cases. She states that "In writing the [evaluation] results, the following guidelines should be followed: (1) give the complete names of tests or measures; (2) report the results as the test or measure suggests; (3) interpret the results; (4) integrate the results with the child's chronological age level; and (5) put conclusions into a diagnostic statement or summary" (p. 125). Lucas uses data gathered from standardized tests as well as language sample measures. She suggests that it is important to recognize contradictions between these two types of information and use these observations in the report to tie the diagnostic evaluation together.

Lund and Duchan (1983) discuss how a report reflects what a clinician views as being most central to assessment. "A report that consists primarily of test scores and normative measures reflects the clinician's view that language assessment is documenting deviation from norms. Some reports are primarily extensive and detailed case history reviews, revealing the diagnostician's bias for an etiological model of language disorders—that is, finding the cause of the problem is central to their assessment. Reports that are organized in sections that correspond to areas of deficit identify the areas that are salient for the clinician" (Lund and Duchan, 1983, p. 313). Lund and Duchan provide samples of reports (pp. 314–316) that demonstrate how a difference in clinician perspective about the role of evaluation is reflected in the style of the report written. They do this by taking one child's data and presenting this information in two different formats. In their Appendix A (pp. 320–326), Lund and Duchan present sample clinical reports based on "structural analysis." They note that with the procedure they recommend (structural analysis) the report emphasizes the child's "regularities." "The goal is to make observations from which the child's behavior can be predicted and intervention planned. . . .The deficit area or areas that are described will depend on the patterns presented by the individual child. The report will include specific recommendations for further analysis and for intervention goals. Interviews with the child's caregivers are likely to focus more on the child's present status than on past events. History and other kinds of information are not excluded from the reports, but information is emphasized which is relevant to the question of the child's language regularities and relates to planning intervention" (Lund and Duchan, 1983, p. 313). Their use of the term "structural analysis" is somewhat misleading; they are using the term to describe the systemic characteristics of a child's communication process and style. This might include an analysis of the regularities of error patterns in pragmatics, syntax, disfluency, or articulation. They are not confining their analysis to language structure (syntax) alone.

When considering the reasons for the meager amount of information available on writing reports and sharing diagnostic information, several possible explanations seem reasonable. It might be assumed that everyone has learned a productive, professional format from a university training program or that guidelines are provided by one's employer. Another factor is the way in which a clinician's conceptual orientation to the nature of communication and the evaluation process will dictate both the format and content of a report. In view of these factors, it may be presumptuous to suggest guidelines for presenting evaluation findings. If the guidelines are too general, they may be useless, yet if they are too specific, they may be biased in terms of the author's clinical or operational model.

Appendix 9-1 makes it immediately apparent how the content of an evaluation procedure will dictate the content of a report. Appendix 9-1 provides a listing of 70 recommended ways to collect information on communication performance directly and indirectly. The type of observation as well as the analysis procedure for data collected will have a significant impact on any report. For example, some of the suggested observational formats focus on general development or classroom behavior, some on receptive or expressive language factors, and others on just one specific type of communication behavior (such as vocal abuse). In terms of specifying the severity of a problem, some procedures suggest yes-no responses, whereas others recommend descriptive comments and some provide guidelines for quantifying observations in terms of developmental level or percentage or occurrence of a particular behavior.

It is advisable to keep procedural options open to new theoretical insights and analytical strategies as they are developed.

> Clinicians must be constructively critical and open to new evidence and better prodecures. To do less is to be a technician rather than a professional. . . .There is no such thing as a definitive test in the behavioral sciences. Clinicians should think in terms of descriptive procedures rather than tests. Descriptive procedures. . .deal with the integration of events as an index of underlying systems. . . . There is a hierarchy in these [cognitive-linguistic-communicative] systems. If an individual does not show a cognitive basis for language, there is cause for question about carrying out an assessment of his linguistic systems. Similarly, an individual who is not yet verbal would have only rudimentary communicative skills. (Muma, 1978, pp. 219–220)

Regardless of the underlying philosophy about the nature of language, the product of an evaluation should be description. Although some of the procedures presented in Appendix 9-1 address only certain aspects of communication, it is possible to combine a variety of these procedures to create a comprehensive, descriptive evaluation report. This might include the results of checklists given to parents and teachers or the clinician's use of research questions to probe aspects of the student's behavior that have not been tapped by standardized tests. Obviously, the comprehensiveness of any evaluation procedure will depend upon time limitations, employer demands, and personal preferences. It is recommended, however, that the following factors be considered when selecting segments of an evaluation procedure:

1. The stimuli should be culture-free and age appropriate.

2. Relevant information should automatically flow from the procedure that will have a direct effect on intervention.

3. There should be an opportunity to observe cognitive organization; auditory processing of information that requires integration, memory, inference and evaluation; and expressive language form, content, function, and style by permitting the student to *communicate* rather than just *respond* with a simple yes or no or utterance of three to four words.

4. As much as is possible, evaluation tasks should simulate the listener, speaker, content, and context variables that the student must face within the academic setting or in social interactions.

5. When a choice among procedures must be made, choice should be dictated by the degree of descriptive information that will be obtained within the least amount of time and that can then be translated into therapy objectives.

The communication evaluation report, then, should "paint a picture" of a student's skills in the speaker and listener roles, and it should provide an indication of whether the student needs communication therapy. If the descriptive results indicate intervention, specific objectives should be stated. Although there may be additional background information and listing of tests administered, these segments should receive secondary consideration and be accompanied by interpretative remarks that show the relevance of the information to the student's diagnostic profile.

TYPICAL PURPOSES FOR REPORT WRITING

Within the public school setting, there are usually four types of contexts in which information is shared and some kind of written or oral report is required:

Notes for an IEP Staffing. Observations are shared with parents, teachers, and administrators as the child is entered into a special education program; initial IEP objectives are included.

Formal Diagnostic Report. This provides a formal description of the student's communication problem, test scores and their interpretation, and programming recommendations; PL 94–142 requires that this information be updated every three years.

Progress Reports. These can be of two types: (1) periodic progress notes sent to parents, and (2) comparative data in the child's file on test performance and behaviors observed during a language sample, to document advances that have been made.

Transfer Report. When a student transfers to another school system or an out-of-state school, it is advantageous to the student's programming for the former clinician to provide the new clinician with a description of the type of programming the student had been receiving (reflecting the philosophical biases of the clinician as well as the student's needs) and indicating the student's current level of functioning; with this detailed information, it is more likely that programming will experience transition rather than change.

In Chapter 5, Calvert and Murray presented a protocol for analyzing student communication behavior within the school setting. In Chapter 6, Damico described his application of Grice's (1975) discourse model to the analysis of an individual's communication behavior. Chappell, in Chapter 7, outlined a test battery that efficiently taps cognitive-linguistic skills of school-age children. Although each of these evaluation methods would produce a slightly different type of evaluation report format, the feature that each would share is the descriptive value of the information collected. The form in which this descriptive information could be shared for each of the four above stated purposes would vary. For the purpose of consistency, an additional evaluation procedure (Simon, 1984a; 1984b) will be discussed briefly and used as the basis for our suggestions on how to provide descriptive information when (1) sharing diagnostic notes at an IEP staffing, (2) preparing a formal diagnostic report, (3) demonstrating longitudinal performance, and (4) communicating with another speech-language pathologist about the nature of a student's past programming.

A FUNCTIONAL-PRAGMATIC EVALUATION PROCEDURE

The goal of a communication evaluation procedure is to gather descriptive data on a student's skill in the listener and speaker roles. Additionally, it is important to observe cognitive strategies utilized (Bransford, 1979; Kagan, 1965; Torgesen, 1982; Wong, 1982). Our philosophical perspective could be summarized as follows:

1. Receptively, it should be determined whether the student can integrate information within and among sentences and make inferences

Table 9-2. Clinical Outline for the Communicative Competence Evaluation Procedure

I. Introduction
   1. The interview
   2. Administer two subtests from standardized measures.
II. Auditory Tasks
   1. Indentification of absurdities in sentences
   2. Identification of absurdities in long sentences or paragraphs
   3. Integration of facts to solve a riddle
   4. Comprehension and memory for facts
   5. Comprehension of a paragraph
   6. Comprehension of directions
III. Expressive Tasks
   1. Sequential picture storytelling
   2. Maintenance of past tense in storytelling
   3. Maintenance of present tense in storytelling
   4. Tense shifts based on introductory adverbial phrases
   5. Semantically appropriate use of clausal connectors
   6. Stating similarites and differences between two stimuli
   7. Sequential directions for use of a pay telephone
   8. Description of clothing and a person
   9. Explanation of the relationship between two items
   10. Barrier games
      a. Speaker in block arrangement
      b. Listener in block arrangement
      c. Speaker in barrier card game
   11. Twenty questions
   12. Creative storytelling
   13. Situational analysis (based on contextual demands)
   14. Expression and justification of an opinion

From Simon, C. S. (1984). *Evaluating communicative competence: A functional-pragmatic approach.* Copyright by Communication Skill Builders, Inc. Reprinted by permission.

based on that integration (Gallagher and Quandt, 1981; Lasky and Chapandy, 1976; Rees and Shulman, 1978), engage in verbal reasoning (Bereiter and Engelmann, 1966; Calfee and Sutter-Baldwin, 1982; Nelson, 1981), and evaluate the truthfulness and completeness of a message (Grice, 1975; Wiig and Semel, 1976).

2. Expressively, it should be determined if the student has sufficient skill to choose appropriate forms of language (Hannah, 1977; Loban, 1976), whether he or she can use these forms for varying speech acts (Bernstein, 1964; Glucksberg and Krauss, 1967; Halliday, 1973; Wells, 1973), and whether the student's communication style enhances or detracts from the listener's understanding of message content (Simon, 1979).

The procedure we use to collect this information is presented in Table 9–2. An introductory description of the procedure is given by Simon (1984a), and a detailed administration manual and materials are also available (Simon, 1984b). This procedure is meant to augment findings from standardized tests by providing opportunities for students to show their levels of skill in processing language and in using language in selected communicative contexts. It is not a test. It is a scenario that allows a clinician to systematically gather descriptive data on middle- and upper-school students as they are requested to assume listener and speaker roles.

EXAMPLES OF METHODS FOR SHARING DIAGNOSTIC INFORMATION

Notes for an IEP Staffing

At the multidisciplinary conference that precedes a student's entrance into a special education program, each team member has a limited amount of time to describe diagnostic findings and make recommendations. It is necessary to include, within this limited amount of time, the initial IEP objectives for the student.

It has been our experience that this meeting is one of the most crucial interactions we have with school staff and parents. During this conference, professional opinions from various disciplines are shared, parent frustrations and confusion surface, and decisions are made that profoundly affect the student's academic, personal, and social situation. The limited amount of time must be utilized effectively. To aid the clinician in presenting findings and recommendations, an outline is useful. The outline becomes a presentation plan that ensures that pertinent information is shared in a concise, organized manner. Our recommended outline consists of the following sections:

I. Self-Introduction
   A. Name and position
   B. Date student was seen
   C. Why student was seen (nature of referral)
II. Diagnostic Impressions
   A. Language processing
      1. Results from formal (standardized) tests
      2. Results from informal probes
      3. General impressions of language processing skills
   B. Expressive language
      1. Form and content (syntax and semantics)
         a. From formal measures
         b. From language sample
      2. Function
         a. Statement about language functions
         b. Examples of performance
      3. Style
         a. Verbal behavior
         b. Paralinguistic behavior
         c. Cognitive organization
      4. General impressions of expressive language skills
III. Recommendations
   A. General (special program placement)
   B. Specific (communication IEP objectives)

With this presentation plan and all data organized within it, the clinician will need approximately 7 to 12 minutes to summarize findings and recommendations. An example of this outline appears in Appendix 9–2 as it was used during an IEP staffing on an adolescent student at the junior high level. A detailed report such as presented in Appendix 9–2 takes 10 to 12 minutes. While the general outline can be used consistently, the degree of detail will vary from conference to conference.

Formal Diagnostic Report

The purpose of a formal report is to have in a student's cumulative file some description of his or her communication skills at various points in time. Following the initial evaluation, a formal report accompanies other paper work necessary to fulfill the guidelines of PL 94-142. When all requisite forms are completed, a student's name may be entered on the special education census for his or her district. At the end of each academic year, the student's placement in speech-language or other special education programs is reviewed. If the student continues in a special education program for three years or more, an updated evaluation and report are required.

Each school system usually has a recommended format for evaluation reports. The format is not as important as the content. Two different styles of formats are presented in Appendixes 9-3 and 9-4. The report presented in Appendix 9-3 has been reprinted from Simon (1980). The purpose of this report was to document the moderately severe expressive language skills of a child who was entering first grade. It was written by a consultant to the school system at the request of the child's parents. There has been an attempt to document the error patterns and their severity by showing the percentage of occurrence per obligatory context. Observations were made on the basis of a sentence imitation task and an unstructured language sample in which (1) the clinician and child talked and played, (2) the child interpreted sequential picture stories, and (3) the child transformed statements into questions that were addressed to a puppet.

As the reader will observe, the format and content of the report in Appendix 9-4 are quite different from the example shown in Appendix 9-3. The report in Table 9-4 was done by one of the authors, who is a speech-language pathologist within a public school system. The format reflects the guidelines presented by the district and PL 94-142, when the student is already enrolled in another special education program in the district and speech-language is a related service. In this case, the student was described as "learning disabled" and spent two periods per day in a resource room, but was mainstreamed for the remainder of his junior high school classes. He was originally seen as part of a screening procedure conducted for all special education students in his school. Although he passed the auditory and expressive portions of the screening tool, he evidenced obvious vocal pitch problems, and in conversation it was observed that he "talked around the topic" before actually getting to the point. A note was also made that he "lost sight of the task" on two sections of the screening procedure, indicating poor cognitive monitoring. When conversing with his language arts teacher a few days following the screening, she mentioned that this boy had difficulty expressing himself in classroom discussions, and his vocal style was frequently mocked by peers. On the basis of these informal observations, it was decided to request permission to evaluate his communication skills, despite his passing score on the screening test. His parents were relieved to receive the request, because they had difficulty in communicating with the boy and expressed frustration at his not remembering what he was told to do at home and at his frequently repeating the last few words of what they said when they gave him directives. They attributed their communication problems to "adolescence."

Regardless of a report's format, the clinician should provide a picture of why this individual appears to be an incompetent communicator and document the severity of the communication problems. This can be done by reporting standardized tests scores with an interpretation of the meaning of the scores and quantifying the results of the informal probes, whenever possible. Multiple examples of this type of reporting style are given in Appendixes 9–3 and 9–4.

Progress Reports

Progress reports can be written for parents or for cumulative files. The style will vary, depending upon the purpose. Usually, reports to parents are presented in a narrative format. The clinician frequently states the student's present objectives and indicates how much progress has been made on each objective. Although, some school systems send special education progress reports every nine weeks, along with academic progress reports, other systems provide a midyear semester report and an end-of-year report. It is suggested that on each progress report sent home, there be at least one positive comment! Parents of children in special education programs are bombarded with comments that describe their child's deficits; they need some "verbal strokes" periodically. A sample of a progress report sent to parents appears in Appendix 9–5.

Progress reports for cumulative files can be more data-oriented. An example of this type of format appears in Appendix 9–6. The purpose of this type of data organization is to have a compact display of baseline performance relative to subsequent levels of performance on tests as well as the improvement of form, function, or stylistic patterns evident in language samples. Simon (1979) developed this format as a means of establishing the merit of data obtained in a language sample. In other words, administrators are more easily convinced that a nonstandardized evaluation procedure is worthwhile if you can demonstrate that "the numbers game" can be played when discussing the result of intervention. This can be done by noting the decrease of error patterns and the increase of more productive cognitive-linguistic behaviors. These types of data are supplied next to standardized test scores.

An added advantage of the data from the Longitudinal Summary

Form (Appendix 9–6), can be a conversion of the data into a series of visual displays on a bar-graph that the student can view. Although test results might be stated in maturational ages on the Longitudinal Summary Form, all the clinician has to do is convert the data into *percentage correct* for the student's bar-graph. For example, a student may have received a maturational age of 10.9 on the Peabody Picture Vocabulary Test (PPVT). By looking at the ceiling (135) and the errors (24) you can calculate the percentage correct. In this case, the student responded accurately on 111 items. That yields a percentage correct score of 82%. This vocabulary notation can be placed on the same bar-graph as the declining percentage of ambiguous pronouns used in a sequential story. For example, +6/8 (75%) of the pronouns used had clear noun referents. A student can then view significant factors in his or her listener or speaker behavior and become more aware of how the various tasks in therapy have led to improvement of communication skills. This brings therapy to a "meta-pragmatic level" (Savich, 1983). It provides the perfect opportunity to have the student reflect upon the nature of communication and the advances that have been made in communication behaviors. The authors have found that students of elementary school age can understand and profit from such discussions about communication (even when they are unable to articulate the word). They develop an awareness of the factors involved in effective listening and speaking. This leads to better self-monitoring.

Transfer Report

There have been a great many changes in the knowledge base within speech-language pathology over the past decade. The operational model of one speech-language pathologist might be quite different from another. If a student moves from one school within a district to another, it is possible to interact informally with the new clinician who will be seeing the student. In addition, philosophies and methodologies are shared during district meetings, so that it is possible to become acquainted with the priorities and methodological preferences of one's colleagues. The type of smooth transition that results from this camaraderie is not possible when a student moves to another district or out of state.

The authors of this chapter developed the Communication Evaluation Summary Form (Appendix 9–7) as a replacement for an extensive narrative report. The purpose of this form is to provide the new clinician with an overview of the former clinician's conceptual model on which the student objectives have been based and provide an estimate of the student's current level of functioning on behaviors listed. At the end of the form, an average rating is given for each of the sections by adding all points within that section and dividing by the number of behaviors that been observed and rated. Appendix 9-7 provides an example of how this form can be utilized, and a blank copy of the form is given in Appendix 9-8.

Although the Communication Evaluation Summary Form was designed as a transfer report, it has since been used in additional ways. One of the authors has used this form as the basis of weekly interactions with team members in a private school that serves more severely impaired students. Team members have commented that the delineation of factors involved in the communication process has helped them better understand the complexity of a student's communication difficulties. Before using this form, which dissects the various facets of communication, they had conceptualized a student's problems within a receptive-expressive language dichotomy. It has aided them in understanding the pervasiveness of the student's cognitive-communication deficits, and it has become more apparent how these deficits have implications for the student's social, emotional, behavioral, and academic adjustment. These team members have responded favorably to the descriptive nature of information presented on the form as well as to notes placed under "comments," specific examples of behaviors provided, and the interpretation or implication of the findings.

Second, this same clinician has used the form during parent conferences. Like team members, parents are able to better grasp the current "state-of-the-art" in speech-language pathology and at the same time acquire a more comprehensive picture of how their child is progressing on specific skills.

The form, it appears, not only has value as a report on a particular student's communication skills, but it also acts as a "mini-in-service" on the nature of communication therapy.

In addition, both authors of this chapter have used the form as a checklist of behaviors that need to be evaluated. As the information on performance is gathered, it is dated. Follow-up observations can be compared with the baseline rating given to a specific skill.

OROFACIAL EXAMINATION CHECKLIST

There has been an emphasis on the presentation of diagnostic information on communication skills, particularly in the areas of pragmatics, language processing, and underlying cognitive organizational strategies. Appendix 9-9 is an Orofacial Examination Checklist. Just as the Communication Evaluation Summary Form can provide the clinician with a list of behaviors pertinent to processing and producing language, this checklist can provide some clinical guidelines on what should be observed about the structural integrity and functioning of facial areas as well as intraoral areas. For more detail on gathering observations listed on this form, see Mason and Simon (1977) and Mason (1980).

This form would be of particular use to clinicians working with more severely impaired students. The information that can be gathered systematically with the checklist can be transformed into a narrative summary that describes the nature of a student's oral-motor functioning and provides the basis for prognostic comments about the student's long-term possibilities for acquiring "normal speech."

SUMMARY

Evaluation reports should reflect the clinician's concern with auditory processing and with cognitive-linguistic, metalinguistic, and pragmatic behaviors observed. The types of notations that a clinician makes in a report not only describe a student's communication skills, but also comment on the clinician's operational theories and practices. In the field of speech-language pathology, research has expanded our knowledge about the communication process; this knowledge should be reflected in the types of evaluation performed and reports written. A report should signal to school staff who read it that the writer is a communication specialist, not just a speech correctionist. Such an observation has important implications for the quality of future referrals.

REFERENCES

Adler, S., and Birdsong, S. (1983). Reliability and validity of standardized testing tools used with poor children. *Topics in Language Disorders, 3*(3), 76–87.

American Psychological Association, (1982). *Learning and communication disorders: An abstracted bibliography, 1971–1980.* Washington, DC: Author.

Anastasiow, N. J., Hanes, M. L., and Hanes, M. L. (1982). *Language and reading strategies for poverty children.* Baltimore: University Park Press.

Bassett, R. E., Whittington, N., and Staton-Spicer, A. (1978). The basis in speaking and listening for high school: What should be assessed? *Communication Education, 27,* 293–303.

Beadle, K. R. (1979). Clinical interactions of verbal language, learning and behavior. *Journal of Clinical Child Psychology, 8*(3), 201–205.

Bereiter, C., and Engelman, S. (1966). *Teaching disadvantaged children in the preschool.* Englewood Cliffs, NJ: Prentice Hall.

Bernstein, B. (1964). Elaborated and restricted codes: Their social origins and some consequences. *American Anthropologist, 66,* 55–69.

Blank, M., Rose, S. A., and Berlin, L. J. (1978). *The language of learning: The preschool years.* New York: Grune and Stratton.

Bloom L., and Lahey, M. (1978). *Language development and language disorders.* New York: John Wiley and Sons.

Blue, C. M. (1975). The marginal communicator. *Language, Speech, and Hearing Services in Schools, 6*(1), 32–38.

Bottorf, L., and DePape, D. (1982). Initiating communication systems for severely-impaired persons. *Topics in Language Disorders, 2*(2), 55–71.

Boyce, N. L., and Larson, V. L. (1983). *Adolescents' communication: Development and disorders.* Eau Claire, WI: Thinking Ink Publications.

Brackett, D. (1982). Language assessment protocols for hearing impaired students. *Topics in Language Disorders, 2*(3), 46–54.

Bransford, J. A. (1979). *Human cognition: Learning, understanding and remembering.* Belmont, CA: Wadsworth.

Brown, K. L., Ecroyd, D., Hopper, R., and Naremore, R. (1976). A summary of communication competencies derived from the literature review. In R. R. Allen and K. L. Brown (Eds.), *Developing communication competence in children.* Lincolnwood, IL: National Textbook Company.

Bryen, D. N., and Gerber, A. (1981). Assessing language and its use. In A. Gerber and D. N. Bryen (Eds.), *Language and learning disabilities* (pp. 115–158). Baltimore: University Park Press.

Burns, W. J., and Burns, K. A. (1978). Checklist of perceptual-motor and language skills for developmentally handicapped preschoolers. *Perceptual and Motor Skills, 46*(3), 1211–1214.

Calfee, R., and Sutter-Baldwin, L. (1982). Oral language assessment through formal discussion. *Topics in Language Disorders, 2*(4), 45–55.

Chappell, G. E., and Johnson, G. A. (1976). Evaluation of cognitive behavior in the young child. *Language, Speech, and Hearing Services in Schools, 7*(1), 17–27.

Corsaro, W. A. (1981). The development of social cognition in preschool children: Implications for language learning. *Topics in Language Disorders, 2*(1), 77–95.

Culatta, B., Page, J. L., and Ellis, J. (1983). Story retelling as a communicative performance screening tool. *Language, Speech, and Hearing Services in Schools, 14*(2), 66–74.

Culbertson, J. L., Norlin, P. F., and Ferry, P. C. (1981). Communication disorders in childhood. *Journal of Pediatric Psychology, 6*(1), 69–84.

Dublinske, S. (1974). Planning for child change in language development/remediation programs carried out by teachers and parents. *Language, Speech, and Hearing Services in Schools, 5*(4), 225–237.

Dukes, P. J. (1981). Developing social prerequisites to oral communication. *Topics in Learning and Learning Disabilities, 1*(2), 47–58.

Flynn, P. T. (1978). Effective clinical interviewing. *Language, Speech, and Hearing Services in Schools, 9*(4), 265–271.

Fujiki, M., and Willbrand, M. L. (1982). A comparison of four informal methods of language evaluation. *Language, Speech, and Hearing Services in Schools, 13*(1), 42–52.

Gallagher, J. M., and Quandt, I. J. (1981). Piaget's theory of cognitive development and reading comprehension: A new look at questioning. *Topics in Learning and Learning Disabilities, 1*(1), 21–30.

Gardner, J. O. (1974). Identification of children for speech and language referral. *Journal of School Health, 44*(5), 255–256.

Geffner, D. S. (1981). Assessment of language disorder: Linguistic and cognitive functions. *Topics in Language Disorders, 1*(3), 1–9.

Gilbert, S. F. (1979). Early childhood education for the developmentally delayed: Diagnosis, intervention, evaluation. *Language, Speech, and Hearing Services in Schools, 10*(2), 81–92.

Glucksberg, S., and Krauss, R. M. (1967). What do people say after they have learned to talk? Studies of development of referential communication. *Merrill-Palmer Quarterly, 13,* 309–316.

Grice, H. P. (1975). Logic and conversation. In P. Cole and H. L. Morgan (Eds.), *Syntax and semantics* (Vol. 3: *Speech acts).* New York: Academic Press.

Gruenewald, L. J., and Pollack, S. A. (1973). The speech clinician's role in auditory learning and reading readiness. *Language, Speech, and Hearing Services in Schools, 4*(3), 120–126.

Halliday, M. A. K. (1973). *Explorations in the functions of language.* London: Edward Arnold Publishers.

Hannah, E. P. (1977). *Applied linguistic analysis* (Vol. II). Pacific Palisades, CA: Sen Com Associates.

Hasenstab, M. S., and Laughton, J. (1982). *Reading, writing and the exceptional child.* Rockville, MD: Aspen Systems.

Heyer, J. L., and Courtright, I. C. (1979). A communication profile for the developmentally disabled. *Language, Speech, and Hearing Services in Schools, 10*(4), 259–266.

Higginbotham, D. J., and Yoder D. E. (1982). Communication within natural conversational interaction: Implications for severe communicatively impaired persons. *Topics in Language Disorders, 2*(2), 1–19.

Hurvitz, J. A., Rilla, D. C., and Pickert, S. M. (1983). Measuring change in children with severe articulation disorders. *Language, Speech, and Hearing Services in Schools, 14*(3), 195–198.

Jackson, M. R. (1973). Methods and results of an every-child program for early identification of developmental deficits. *Psychology in the Schools, 10*(4), 421–426.

Jansky, J. J. (1975). The marginally ready child. *Bulletin of the Orton Society, 25,* 69–85.

Johnson, D. J. (1981). Factors to consider in programming for children with language disorders. *Topics in Learning and Learning Disabilities. 1*(2), 13–27.

Kagan, J. (1965). Impulsive and reflective children: Significance of cognitive tempo. In J. D. Krumboltz (Ed.), *Learning and the educational process.* Chicago: Rand-McNally.

Khan, L. M. L., and James, S. L. (1980). A method for assessing use of grammatical structures in language disordered children. *Language Speech and Hearing Services in Schools, 11*(3), 188–197.

Knight, H. S. (1973). Language referrals: A serviceable procedure. *Language, Speech, and Hearing Services in Schools, 4*(4), 196–198.

Kretschmer, R. R., and Kretschmer, L. W. (1978). *Language development and intervention with the hearing impaired.* Baltimore: University Park Press.

Lasky, E. Z., and Chapandy, A. M. (1976). Factors affecting language comprehension. *Language, Speech, and Hearing Services in Schools, 7*(3), 159–168.

Lee, L. L. (1974). *Developmental sentence analysis.* Evanston, IL: Northwestern University Press.

Leonard, L. B., Prutting, C., Perozzi, A., and Berkley, R. K. (1978). Nonstandardized approaches to assessment of language behaviors. *ASHA, 20*(5), 371–379.

Loban, W. (1976). *Language development: K–12.* Urbana, IL: National Council of Teachers of English.

Lucas, E. V. (1980). *Semantic and pragmatic language disorders.* Rockville, MD: Aspen Systems.

Lund, N. J., and Duchan, J. F. (1983). *Assessing children's language in naturalistic contexts.* Englewood Cliffs, NJ: Prentice-Hall.

Lynch, J. (1979). Use of a prescreening checklist to supplement speech, language and hearing screening. *Language, Speech, and Hearing Services in Schools, 10*(4), 258–299.

MacDonald, J. D. (1978). *Environmental language inventory.* Columbus, OH: Charles E. Merrill.

Mason, R. M. (1980). Principles and procedures of orofacial examination. *International Journal of Oral Myology, 6*(2), 3–20.

Mason, R. M., and Simon, C. S. (1977). An orofacial examination checklist. *Language, Speech, and Hearing Services in Schools, 8*(3), 155–163.

Mattes, L. J. (1982). The elicited language analysis procedure: A method for scoring sentence imitation tasks. *Language, Speech, and Hearing Services in Schools, 13*(1), 37–41.

McBride, J. E., and Levy, K. (1981). The early academic classroom for children with communication disorders. In A. Gerber and D. N. Bryen (Eds.), *Language and learning disabilities* (pp. 269–294). Baltimore: University Park Press.

McCabe, R. B., and Bradley, D. P. (1973). Pre- and postarticulation therapy assessment. *Language, Speech, and Hearing Services in Schools, 4*(1), 13–22.

McLean, J. E., and Synder-McLean, L. K. (1978). *A transactional approach to early language training.* Columbus, OH: Charles E. Merrill.

Menyuk, P., and Flood, J. (1981). Language development, reading, writing problems and remediation. *Orton Society Bulletin, 31,* 13–28.

Miller, J. F. (1981). *Assessing language production in children.* Baltimore: University Park Press.

Moore, D. M. (1971). Language research and preschool language training. In C. S. Lavetelli (Ed)., *Language training in early childhood education* (pp. 3–47). Urbana: University of Illinois Press.

Muma, J. R., (1978). *Language handbook: Concepts, assessment, intervention.* Englewood Cliffs, NJ: Prentice-Hall.

Musselwhite, C. R. , St. Louis, K. O., and Penick, P. B. (1980). A communicative interaction analysis system for language disordered children. *Journal of Communication Disorders, 13*(4), 315–323.

Nelson, N. W. (1981). An eclectic model of language intervention for disorders of listening, speaking, reading and writing. *Topics in Language Disorders, 1*(2), 1–24.

Nippold, M. A., and Fey, S. H. (1983). Metaphoric understanding in preadolescents having a history of language acquisition difficulties. *Language, Speech, and Hearing Services in Schools, 14*(3), 171–180.

Northcott, W. H. (1972). The learning impaired child: A speech clinician as an interdisciplinary team member. *Language, Speech, and Hearing Services in Schools, 3*(2), 7–19.

Pirozzolo, F. J. (1981). Language and brain: Neuropsychological aspects of developmental reading disability. *School Psychology Review, 10*(3), 350–355.

Potts, P. L., and Greenwood, J. (1983). Hearing aid monitoring: Are looking and listening enough? *Language, Speech, and Hearing Services in Schools, 14*(3), 157–163.

Prutting, C. A., and Kirchner, D. M. (1983). Applied pragmatics. In T. Gallagher and C. Prutting (Eds.), *Pragmatic assessment and intervention issues in language.* San Diego, CA: College-Hill Press.

Rees, N. S., and Shulman, M. (1978). I don't understand what you mean by "comprehension." *Journal of Speech and Hearing Disorders, 43*(2), 208–219.

Rupp, R. R., Smith, M., Briggs, P., Litvin, K., Banachowski, S., and Williams, R. (1977). A feasibility scale for language acquisition routines for young hearing impaired children. *Language, Speech, and Hearing Services in Schools, 8*(4), 222–233.

Savich, P. A. (1983). Improving communication competence: the role of metapragmatic awareness. *Topics in Language Disorders, 4*(1), 38–48.

Schwartz, E. R., and Solot, C. B. (1980). Response patterns characteristic of verbal expressive disorders. Language, Speech, and Hearing Services in Schools, 11(3), 139–144.

Siegel, G. M., and Broen, P. A. (1976). Language assessment. In L. L. Lloyd (Ed.), *Communication assessment and intervention Strategies.* Baltimore: University Park Press.

Simon, C. S. (1980). *Communicative competence: A functional-pragmatic program.* Tucson, AZ: Communication Skill Builders.

Simon, C. S. (1979). *Communicative competence: A functional-pragmatic approach to language therapy.* Tucson, AZ: Communication Skill Builders.

Simon, C. S. (1984a). Functional-pragmatic evaluation of communication skills in school-age children. *Language, Speech, and Hearing Services in Schools, 15*(2), 83–97.

Simon, C. S. (1984b). *Evaluating communicative competence: A functional-pragmatic approach.* Tucson, AZ: Communication Skill Builders.

Sonksen, P. M. (1977). The assessment needs of preschool children with handicaps of language development. *Child Care, Health, and Development, 3*(5), 319–323.

Sullivan, P. M., and McCay, V. (1979). Psychological assessment of hearing impaired children. *School Psychology Digest, 8*(3), 271–290.

Taylor, O. L., and Payne, K. T. (1983). Culturally valid testing: A proactive approach. *Topics in Language Disorders, 3*(3), 8–20.

Torgesen, J. K. (1982). The learning disabled child as an inactive learner: Educational implications. *Topics in Learning and Learning Disabilities, 2*(1), 45–52.

Tyack, D., and Gottsleben, R. (1974). *Language sampling, analysis and training.* Palo Alto, CA: Consulting Psychologists Press.

Vetter, D. K. (1982). Language disorders and schooling. *Topics in Language Disorders, 2*(4), 13–19.

Waller, M., Sollad, R., Sander, E., and Kunicki, E. (1983). Psychological assessment of speech and language disordered children. *Language, Speech, and Hearing Services in Schools, 14*(2), 92–98.

Wells, G. (1973). *Coding manual for the description of child speech.* Bristol, England: University of Bristol School of Education.

Westby, C. E. (1980). Assessment of cognitive and language abilities through play. *Language, Speech, and Hearing Services in Schools, 11*(3), 154–168.

Wiig, E. H., and Semel, E. M. (1980). *Language assessment and intervention for the learning disabled.* Columbus, OH: Charles E. Merrill.

Wiig, E. H., and Semel, E. M. (1976). *Language disabilities in children and adolescents.* Columbus, OH: Charles E. Merrill.

Wong, B. J. L. (1982). Understanding learning disabled students' reading problems: Contributions from cognitive psychology. *Topics in Learning and Learning Disabilities, 1*(4), 43–50.

Zink, G. D. (1973). Rehabilitative and educational audiology programming. *Language, Speech, and Hearing Services in Schools, 5*(1), 23–36.

APPENDIX 9-1

REVIEW OF SELECTED
EVALUATION PROCEDURES

I. CHECKLISTS AND QUESTIONNAIRES

Burns and Burns (1978)

Presents a checklist of perceptual-motor and language skills for developmentally handicapped preschoolers

Sonksen (1977)

Presents an outline of pediatric assessment needs of children with delayed or deviant language development

McBride and Levy (1981)

Presents a Student Evaluation Form that allows teachers to comment on the child's communication, classification, social-emotional readiness, and fine motor skills

Khan and James (1980)

Offers a checklist to help determine what structures a child might be expected to use consistently at different levels of language production, based on Brown's MLU stages; it is designed for children whose MLU falls between 2.0 and 5.0 morphemes

Heyer and Courtright (1979)

Permits clinicians to consider the total communication behaviors of profoundly to mildly retarded individuals and includes these categories: identification and background information, self-help skills, socialization skills, education, communication skills (attending, imitative, receptive, and expressive behaviors; semantic and cognitive skills; functional or interpersonal skills; articulation; voice and rhythm; oral-facial integrity; auditory skills)

Hasenstab and Laughton (1982)

Presents a list of high-risk expressive language behaviors that might indicate a child is more susceptible to later reading problems

Loban (1976)

Presents an Oral Language Scale on which teachers rate student performance in (1) skill in communication, (2) organization, purpose, and control of language, (3) wealth of ideas, (4) amount of language (regardless of quality), (5) vocabulary, (6) quality of listening, (7) quality of syntactic structure

Gruenewald and Pollak (1973)

Provides a list of components of reading readiness assessment and detailed outline of auditory activities that could be used as observational probes for attending behavior, listening skills, memory, and discrimination

Appendix 9-1 (continued).

Lynch (1979) — Questionnaire administered to teachers of preschool children to ascertain which students need preferential screening; it is based on the assumption that adults who have daily contact with a child in the school setting will be able to make valuable observations when asked the right questions, so that priority can be given to children who will probably need speech-language services

Blue (1975) — Presents a two-part checklist for focusing observation on an adolescent's communicative interactions in terms of those that are adult-initiated and those that are self-initiated

Potts and Greenwood (1983) — Provides a checklist for evaluating the functioning and effectiveness of a student's hearing aid

Flynn (1978) — Provides a questionnaire that can be used to provide information on a student prior to or as part of assessment

Knight (1973) — Provides a questionnaire to be given to the examining laryngologist for vocal abuse cases; by not requiring a narrative report from the physician, the rehabilitation program can be expedited and the form communicates to the physician the specific types of information needed by the speech-language clinician

II. RESEARCH QUESTIONS AND TASKS THAT CAN BE ADAPTED INTO CHECKLISTS AND ASSESSMENT PROBES

Brown, Ecroyd, Hopper, and Naremore (1976) — A review of developmental research on the communication behaviors of children from preschool through adolescence that can be used as a checklist for the following age groups: 3–5, 5–9, 9–12, and 12–18

Bassett, Whittington, and Staton-Spicer (1978) — A list of listening and speaking competencies that can and should be expected from students by the time they graduate from high school; can be used as the basis for a checklist of abilities to communicate effectively as citizens, in everyday interactions and on the job

Siegel and Broen (1976) — Guidelines are presented on the nature of assessment in the areas of (1) articulation, (2) understanding and use of grammatical structures, (3) understanding and use of vocabulary and concepts, and (4) the functional or interpersonal uses of language; guidelines are presented for evaluating the reliability, validity, and appropriateness of standardized measures for any one student being assessed

Corsaro (1981) — From a synthesis of research, pertinent questions are posed about the nature of communicative competence that can be applied to systematic observation of a child's skills

Moore (1971) — A synthesis of research implications on culturally different children and the types of skills they need by school entrance, such as elaborated syntax, use of a precise language of reference, superordinate class names, use of adjectives, adverbs, and logical connectors, social abilities, ability to use information to give appropriate answers to questions, sentence variety

Appendix 9–1 (continued).

O'Brien (1983)	A list of behaviors children should exhibit by the end of primary school in the areas of speaking facility, linguistic ability, vocabulary power, and reading-thinking abilities; can serve as a checklist
Bryen and Gerber (1981)	Presents descriptions of stimuli, administration procedures and methods for analyzing results of performance on language processing and language usage tasks
Wiig and Semel (1980)	Same as for Bryen and Gerber's list (1981)
Lucas (1980)	Presents a series of questions that clinicians can use as guidelines during the observation of a child's spontaneous language as well as a series of principles to guide in the selection of standardized tests
Johnson (1981)	Describes areas of assessment that a clinician should include in a testing format: sensory acuity, intelligence, nonverbal functions, attention, problem-solving or comprehension of the nature of a required task, strategy selection and usage, systems analysis (receptive and expressive language, including input-integration-output, and experience that involves perception, memory, symbolization and conceptualization), pragmatics, verbal mediation, and emotional factors
Dukes (1981)	A list of social prerequisites to oral communication
Jansky (1975)	Lists characteristics of the immature primary and elementary school child who has marginal language disabilities that need to be identified
Beadle (1979)	Presents guidelines for differential diagnostic evaluation of pertinent physiological, environmental, emotional, and language factors that may lead to learning and academic failures
Vetter (1982)	A series of questions (on language and thinking skills) is posed to serve as a guideline to teachers in determining where students are failing in formal communicative interactions in the classroom
Calfee and Sutter-Baldwin (1982)	Provides guidelines for analyzing the quality of a student's classroom discussion skills, including the ability to take both listener and speaker roles; retain, integrate and comment on information that has been shared; take turns informally; ask probing or clarification questions
Culbertson, Norlin, and Ferry (1981)	Describes interdisciplinary (medical-neurological, psychological, speech-language) collaboration methods to evaluate verbal and nonverbal cognitive abilities, perceptual and academic skills, and communication style; a profile of strengths and weaknesses is devised from the data
Pirozzolo (1981)	Neurological criteria for the differential diagnosis of visual-spatial and auditory-linguistic dyslexia are listed

Appendix 9-1 (continued).

Menyuk and Flood (1981)

Presents a paradigm for assessing syntactic-semantic metalinguistic awareness that could be used as part of an evaluation procedure with older students who are experiencing difficulty with reading and writing

Khan and James (1980)

Presents a model for grammatical assessment based upon a language sample taken in a "natural setting"

Anastasiow, Hanes, and Hanes (1982)

A sentence repetition task (on p. 61) systematically probes a student's ability to engage in the repetition of sentences that use increasingly complex "function words" (such as *while, either-or*)

Mattes (1982)

Presents a scoring procedure that can be used to obtain an in-depth descriptive analysis of responses produced on elicited imitation tasks

McCabe and Bradley (1973)

Presents an articulation testing protocol requiring 10 to 15 minutes of administration time (counting from 1 to 10, reciting letters of the alphabet, production of 40 words, spontaneous sentences, reading sentences, reading paragraphs, and conversation); a protocol data sheet is provided on which the clinician can record baseline and subsequent performances to analyze the percentage of accuracy

Hurvitz, Rilla, and Pickert (1983)

Presents a clinical articulation profile to measure baseline and progress

Culatta, Page, and Ellis (1983)

Provides stimulus stories and comprehension questions for use in a story-retelling task used as a communicative performance screening tool with elementary school children

MacDonald (1978)

The sampling procedure uses three production modes: imitation, conversation, and free play; the semantic-grammatical rules used or deleted are analyzed

Bloom and Lahey (1978)

Suggestions are presented for the analysis of a language sample by describing the context and behaviors of the other speakers, utterances of other speakers, child utterances (with attention to form, content and use), and child behaviors

Miller (1981)

Presents (1) a list of procedures for in-depth analysis of a child's free-speech sample, (2) procedures for analyzing syntactic and pragmatic behaviors, (3) elicited imitation procedures

McLean and Snyder-McLean (1978)

The Transactional Assessment Model is described and a communication assessment profile is presented, which summarizes findings on a child's expressive and receptive linguistic abilities and social and cognitive bases of performance; standardized tests that would be relevant to the evaluation of these areas are described

Appendix 9-1 (continued).

Gilbert (1979)
Provides a formal protocol (tests and subtests) and an informal protocol (observational) for diagnotic evaluation of communication behaviors of preschool children

Gruenewald and Pollak (1984)
Presents a protocol for Analysis of Language Interaction that analyzes the triad of language content or concepts, teacher-instructional language (written and oral), and student language; resulting mismatches in preparation and style are addressed in terms of accounting for academic difficulties

Brackett (1982)
Provides a list of skills that should be evaluated in hearing impaired students and recommends specific tests and analysis procedures

Kretschmer and Kretschmer (1978)
The Kretschmer Spontaneous Language Analysis Procedure is presented; this probes preverbal, syntactic, and pragmatic skills in hearing impaired students

Zink (1973)
Describes the Rehabilitative and Educational Audiology Profile (REAP) that quantitatively displays comprehensive evaluation results for auditory and visual channels, intelligence, language, articulation, motor development, social development, and educational performance for hearing impaired students

Sullivan and McCay (1979)
Specific tests are recommended for use with hearing impaired students in the areas of intellectual, behavioral and personality, academic achievement, neuropsychological, communication-language and vocational interest-aptitude assessment

Rupp, Smith, Briggs, Litvin, Banachowski, and Williams (1977)
An evaluation scale is presented for use in early habilitative planning for hearing impaired children; performance is subjected to a scoring of prognostic factors based upon evaluation of behaviors and circumstances that can positively or negatively affect programming efforts

APPENDIX 9–2
NOTES FOR AN IEP STAFFING

I. Self-Introduction
   A. Charlann Simon, Speech-Language Pathologist
   B. Seen October 3-4, 1983, for approximately 1½ hours total
   C. Referrals from three classroom teachers; "talks in circles," "runs words together," "talks too fast," "can't follow directions"
II. Diagnostic Impressions
   A. Language processing
      1. Formal tests
         a. PPVT-M: 12.3 ma (12.6 ca). Approximately age level on receptive vocabulary; slow response rate when selecting a picture
         b. Auditory Association (ITPA): +38/42. Easily comprehended how to complete comparative relationships in analogies; word-finding problems on six items
         c. Token Test for Children: Parts I–III = 100%; Part IV = 50%; Part V = 62%; auditory memory shows overload when he has to remember six critical elements (give example), and he is not picking up on subtle linguistic differences (example)
      2. Informal probes
         a. Detecting absurdities: Sentences +6/7; paragraphs +4/7 (examples of each); has difficulty remembering inconsistencies when several sentences have to be integrated
         b. Solving riddles: +8/9. He changed his mind on three items immediately after his initial response; some self-monitoring evident
         c. Memory for facts +12/21; errors were on items that appeared in paragraphs of three to four sentences; generally OK on one to two sentence presentations (examples)
         d. Paragraph comprehension: +4/5 on comprehension questions; got the gist of what he heard; disorganized answers to questions (example); if in a classroom situation, his comprehension of the material might not be evident due to his poor formulation of an answer to the comprehension question
         e. General impressions of language processing: Poor auditory memory and marginal auditory integration skills; emerging use of rehearsal and monitoring strategies
   B. Expressive language
      1. Form and content

Appendix 9-2 (continued).

    a. Formal

       Test of Language Development—Intermediate (TOLD–I)
       Sentence combining: 37th percentile

    b. Informal

       (1) MLU: 9.0 words per sentence when telling a sequential picture story; 93% of sentences were syntactically OK

       (2) Sentence complexity: Relied upon compound sentences 58% of the time and complex sentences 25% of the time

       (3) Metalinguistics: OK on shifting tense per adverbial cue (example); +2/9 on use of clausal connectors appropriately (example)

2. Function: Use of language for various purposes (description, explanation, stating an opinion, and so forth)

    a. Sequential storytelling: Comprehended the subtle cause-effect relationships; used only minimal sentences that labeled each story frame, only syntactic difficulty was maintenance of tense; semantically: ambiguous use of pronouns (example)

    b. Explanations (relationship between two objects): +1/4; minimal or inadequate specificity; poor organization (example)

    c. Directions (for use of a pay telephone): Only 50% of the segments could have helped a listener; egocentric

    d. Stating opinions: +0/4. Gave one-word responses with no justification (examples)

3. Style

    a. Verbal: three problem areas

       (1) Vocal fillers. During formulation he inserts multiple uses of "uh," "OK;" most repetitions are easy and cannot be described as "stuttering"

       (2) Irregular speech rate. Within a 26 word story, he made 13 significant pauses of between 1 and 4 seconds, which produces a "jerky" speech rate (play tape)

       (3) Unintelligible segments. 59% of his language sample sentences have unintelligible segments; a combination of sloppy speech habits and a self-imposed pressure to speak too rapidly (play tape)

    b. Paralinguistic: Nervous; poor eye contact

    c. Cognitive organization: Impulsive style that lacks a presentation plan (example)

4. General impressions of expressive language skills

    a. Form: Relies upon simple and compound sentences, probably because he is unsure of how to use clausal connectors; marginal comfort with English as a system as noted by his performance on

Appendix 9-2 (continued).

both formal and informal measures; syntactic errors were insignificant; profits from clinician modeling

b. Function: His difficulty with the manipulation of language for various purposes is characterized by incomplete and disorganized presentation of his thoughts

c. Style: Use of vocal fillers and prolongations of sounds might make it seem that he is stuttering; however, there is no tension and these fillers and prolongations seem to be compensations for formulation problems—stalling for time while he thinks about how he is going to say something; his speech rate is much too fast, which causes him to slur words together and not even take time to produce some sounds accurately; he is presently uncomfortable in communication tasks

III. Recommendations

A. General: Consider placement in the self-contained Communication Disorders Classroom with mainstreaming for mathematics, physical education, art or shop; build awareness of listener-speaker skills

B. Specific

1. J will be able to engage in self-evaluation of speech clarity when listening to taped samples of his performance and be in agreement with the clinician on performance adequacy 80% of the time by 6-1-84

2. J will be able to generate semantically appropriate sentences using 10 clausal connectors by 6-1-84

3. J will be able to provide sequential directions for the use of three household appliances by 6-1-84

4. J will be able to take notes on details he hears in news stories and use these notes to answer comprehension questions with 80% accuracy by 6-1-84

APPENDIX 9–3

FORMAL DIAGNOSTIC REPORT

Name: S. J.   Birthdate: 10-21-73   Present Age: 6.0
School: Burns Elementary   Teacher: J. F.   Date of Evaluation: 10-15-79
Evaluator: C. S. Simon

Phonology (production of speech sounds)

1. ɔ/r and w/r substitutions are inconsistent, but in error approximately 95% of the time; he was able to produce a good /r/ in the following contexts: Spiderman, forget, water-in, other-room, over-a.

2. ɔ/l and y/l and -/l errors in medial position of words approximately 80% of the time; most initial and final /l/ sounds were supplied.

3. s/ʃ substitutions approximately 90% of the time in all three word positions.

4. Consistent reduction of blends; for example, p/pl, t/st, b/bl, b/br, k and t/tr, g/dr, f/fl, g/gr, k/kr.

5. t/tʃ in medial word positions and k/tʃ in initial word positions consistently; final tʃ was not observed.

6. d/dʒ in initial word position; medial and final positions not tested.

Note: An articulation test was not given. All notations were derived from his taped language sample and responses on other tests.

Morphology (word endings that show tense, number and possession)

1. He has the plural -s in the /s/ and /z/ forms (as in books and chairs), but the -ez (as in boxes) is inconsistent.

2. He does not have the third person singular -s in its /s/, /z/ or /ez/ forms (as in jumps, pulls, pushes).

3. Adds -s inappropriately (Cats jumps or Boys plays).

4. Inconsistent use of -ed past tense marker -2/3 times, showing a 66% error rate.

5. He relies on -est for both comparative uses and superlative uses.

6. Test notations on Carrow Elicited Language Inventory (repetition of sentences) confirmed the following difficulties: first person singular -s and -ed past tense marker.

Syntax (grammatical sequencing of words in a sentence)

1. Inconsistent omission of auxiliary is/was -7/11 times, showing a 66% error rate.

Appendix 9–3 (continued).

2. Inconsistent omission of copular (linking) is/was -7/19 times, showing a 37% error rate.

3. Omission of copular *are/were* -3/3 times, showing a 100% error rate.

4. Omission of *do* in *What + do* questions (What do you want?/What does it say?) -6/6 times, showing a 100% error rate.

5. Inconsistent omission of auxiliary *will* -3/7 times, showing a 43% error rate.

6. Omission of infinitive *to* or substitution of a/to -5/6 times, showing an 83% error rate.

7. Inconsistent appropriate word order in wh-questions -4/8 times, showing a 50% error rate.

8. Confusion in use of definite/indefinite articles (a/the) -5/25 times, showing an error rate of 20%.

9. Inconsistent appropriate usage of irregular past tense verbs -9/20 times, showing an error rate of 45%.

10. Inconsistent omission of articles.

11. None of the spontaneous yes-no questions was correctly structured. His style was to use a statement uttered in a question inflectional pattern (You go to school?). However, when asked to transform a statement into a question on two occasions (such as "Ask the puppet if he goes to school"), he correctly structured the question (Do you go to school?).

12. Inconsistent difficulty using clausal connectors. The two sentences below are taken from his language sample. The first example shows his ability to embed and the second shows his difficulty in doing this:

I just need to put 'em in that room so I won't forget them.

When you found them we can see and that same other one.

13. Consistent use of *is* and *don't* with plural subject.

14. Test notations from Carrow Elicited Language Inventory (repetition of sentences) confirmed the following difficulties:

    a. Does not use *are* with a plural subject
    b. Inconsistent use of copular is/was
    c. Confusion in definite/indefinite article usage
    d. Does not use indirect object constructions
    e. Does not use compound and complex verb auxiliaries
    f. Substitutes *them* for *they*
    g. Doesn't seem to differentiate between *is, if, it;* they are used interchangeably during sentence repetitions

Appendix 9–3 (continued).

  h. Tendency to reduce sentence complexity, such as saying "Bill not coming" instead of "Bill isn't coming"
  i. Confuses subject/object roles during sentence repetitions
15. Of 134 sentences in the language sample, 80 showed one or more grammatical errors. In other words, 60% of his sentences were structurally inadequate.

Semantics (meaningfulness of words and combinations of words used)
  1. Labeling of colors was inconsistently accurate.
  2. Has difficulty explaining a complex idea 75% of the time. Examples include the following:
    a. This...you put some water in it and you look through here and water...it...water come out this little hole and lots come out.
    b. You turn 'em all over and you have one...and you found one...and you pick one and you need found another one and it need be the same.
    c. When it fall down here on side and here it won't fall down 'cause something am here.

GENERAL OBSERVATIONS

S. J. has a short attention span for a first grade student. He has considerable difficulty interpreting sequential picture stories and subordinating one idea to another, which are negative signs regarding reading readiness. He seems very receptive to linguistic stimulation and would probably welcome opportunities to learn how to code some of his more complex thoughts and observations linguistically. He has a keen sense of humor, but this frequently interferes with a cooperative attitude on tasks which he views as laborious.

Recommendations

  1. Periodic audiological examinations until at least age 10, to monitor possible intermittent middle ear infections.
  2. Enrollment in a language-development classroom for this academic year and reevaluation in June to consider his readiness for reading and other regular classroom activities the following September.
  3. Home language stimulation, done on an informal, clarification basis. For example, when he syntactically miscodes an idea or observation, parents should recode it and then proceed to interact with the child, such as:
      Child: What it is?
      Parent: What is it? It's a peacock.

Appendix 9–3 (continued).

4. Specific language goals in therapy or a language classroom would
   include:
   a. Develop the ability to tell a story from a series of sequential
   pictures.
   b. Develop the ability to explain events and describe observations
   clearly and coherently.
   c. Develop the ability to create a story that evidences a beginning,
   middle and conclusion.
   d. Clarify morphological and syntactic rules which are currently
   inconsistent or nonexistent.
   e. Develop articulation skills, beginning with those sounds that are
   being inconsistently produced correctly. Establish easy production
   of the sounds at the syllable level before progressing to words.

From Simon, C. S. (1984). *Evaluating communicative competence: A functional-pragmatic
approach.* Copyright by Communication Skill Builders, Inc. Reprinted by permission.

APPENDIX 9–4

COMMUNICATION EVALUATION

Name: D. C.   Birthdate: 7-15-70

School: Wright Jr. High   C. A. : 13.3

Grade: 7   Evaluation Date: 9-83

Parents: Mr. and Mrs. C.   Teacher: Ms. G.

Address: 2000 S. 2nd St.   Primary Language: English

        Tempe, Arizona   Speech-Language Pathologist:

                                        Charlann S. Simon

Phone: 839-3100

Student Number: 470117

Current Audiometric Screening   *Current Vision Screening*

   Date: 9-9-83 pass/fail   Date: 9-3-83 pass/fail

Reason for Referral

The Coordinator for Special Education asked me to screen all students
who were enrolled in special education programs at Wright Junior High
School. Although D. passed the screening test, he was asked to come in
for additional evaluation of observable vocal pitch problems. In addition,
his language arts teacher noted that he had difficulties expressing himself
coherently in discussions. During subsequent evaluation, auditory memory

problems and cognitive-linguistic difficulties became more apparent than they were on the screening test, which relied upon a series of brief responses.

Assessment of Functional Communication

D. is a prototypical "marginal communicator." He does not appear to have severe communication problems compared with other students in the caseload, nor do his problems really become evident until he is asked to express himself at higher cognitive levels; these higher levels (such as explanation or devising a set of sequential directions) necessitate organization of ideas before expressive formulation begins. In addition, it is necessary to know how to embed one related idea into another. What is immediately noticeable is that D. has not established a "vocal pitch identity." There are the natural breaks in pitch and lack of breath support that can be expected during puberty, but D. tends to lapse into a falsetto voice and sustains it when he is under stress. For example, when asked to give his opinion on four separate issues, he was very uncomfortable. The result was that on one occasion, 46% of his words were in falsetto and on another occasion, 33% of the words were in falsetto. On the remaining two trials, his voice was normal on all of 75 words used in stating the third opinion and on the three words used in his last statement of an opinion. The other task on which vocal abnormalities were observed was when he was asked to create a story about a picture. In addition, he kept forgetting the names he had given to the characters in his story. This made him very uncomfortable, which was reflected in his vocal pitch changes.

Types of Tests Administered and Results of Tests

Both formal (standardized) and informal procedures were used.

Formal

1. *Peabody Picture Vocabulary Test* (M): 11.3 MA. This measure indicated that he is approximately two years below his chronological age in receptive vocabulary. This would not have been predicted by his performance on the screening measure (STAL). Errors were scattered between the age 11–16 section of the test and included words such as plastering, triplet, tropical, fragment, parallel, precipitation, embracing, and judicial.

2. *The Token Test for Children* (DiSimoni). This measure of language processing revealed the following information:
On Part I (two critical elements—Touch the *red circle),* Part II (three critical elements—Touch the *large red circle),* and Part III (four critical elements—Touch the *yellow circle* and *red square),* he scored 100% accuracy. In each of the three parts, however, he engaged in verbal rehearsal three to four times and in self-correction of an initial choice on three to four trials per part of the test. Similar

Appendix 9-4 (continued).

compensatory behaviors were observed on Part IV (six critical elements—Touch the *small yellow circle* and the *large green square)*, but he was still able to score 90% accuracy. He commented after the test that the times when "all the chips were out" it was confusing. While this might have meant that his auditory memory was taxed or his visual distractibility was increased, his assessment was not completely accurate. When only the large chips were presented in Part V of the test, he scored 62% accuracy (+13/21 items). The manipulation of syntactic subtleties seemed to be the most confusing to him. For example, he responded exactly the same on these three directions: Touch—*with* the blue circle—the red square; Touch the blue circle *and* the red square; Pick up the blue circle *or* the red square. There were also three reversals such as in "Before touching the yellow circle, pick up the blue square," in which he manipulated the blue circle and the yellow square.

3. *Test of Language Development* (TOLD): Intermediate (I).
This measure includes five sub-sections. The test is normed for students up to age 12.11 years, but D. did not score above the 37th percentile on any one of the five sections. Specific findings were:

Percentile

a. Sentence combining   37
(asked to combine two+ simple sentences into a compact compound-complex sentence)

b. Characteristics   37
(asked to respond with a true-false to a series of statements stated in a factual manner)

c. Word ordering   1
(asked to unscramble and reorder a series of words in a grammatically correct sentence)

d. Generals   25
(asked to provide a classification name into which three items would fit)

e. Grammatic comprehension   37
(asked to listen to sentences and decide if they are grammatically correct)

Throughout this test, memory problems were evident. He even said at one point, "I keep forgetting these words!" These difficulties were most noticeable on word ordering and sentence combining. Not only did he have memory problems during word ordering, he

Appendix 9-4 (continued).

also lacked an intuitive grasp of language structure that would allow him to rearrange vocabulary and structural units in a grammatically correct manner.

Informal

Auditory Tasks

1. Identification of absurdities in
   a. sentences: +6/6
   b. paragraphs: +5/6

2. Integration of facts to solve a riddle: +6/7. There was a delay, however, of 3 to 10 seconds before he supplied the answer to each riddle, as he tried to review the information given.

3. Memory for facts: +13/21. He had particular difficulty remembering names. In addition, there is some evidence of sporadic attention problems. Six of the eight errors occurred in two of the stimulus items. It was as if he did not attend to these statements because he missed all of the associated comprehension questions.

4. Making inferences from presented material: +2/5. He was asked to listen to an eight-sentence paragraph and answer comprehension questions that necessitated his making logical inferences, because the answers were not directly stated. This was the most difficult of the auditory tasks for him. This task taxed memory and integration.

5. Comprehension of directions: +7/10. All of these were similar to Part V of The Token Test for Children. This was presented several days prior to the Token Test, so his later poor performance on Part V was predictable.

Metalinguistic Tasks

1. Tense shifts based on introductory adverbial phrases (such as "Last night.." whereupon he was to complete a sentence in the *past* tense): +3/8. He did not pick up on either the present or future tense phrases, but he performed better on past and present progressive.

2. Semantically appropriate use of clausal connectors (where he was given a clausal connector such as "because" and asked to formulate a sentence using it): +6/10. He was unable to use "until," "however," "so," "except for" in an appropriate manner.

Expressive Tasks

1. Sequential directions (for use of a pay telephone): +9/12. While he provided, in sequential order, most of the necessary

Appendix 9–4 (continued).

informational segments, much extraneous information was given and sometimes the content was quite rambling in nature. For example, "Usually you don't have to put in a quarter, but you put in a quarter or how much. It's usually up on top. It says a quarter."

2. Description of clothing (to someone on the telephone who could not see the items he was viewing): +0/4. He was asked to "paint a picture with words" for the listener, but his descriptions were both egocentric and extremely disorganized.

3. Explanations (about why two objects belonged together): +1/4. Once again, his lack of cognitive planning was evident. He tends to talk around the point before zeroing in on the point. For example, "You always have to have the shoe before you have the shoelace and then you have to have the lace before the shoe—but sometimes you don't and you don't have to tie it. It'd be better if you did because when you're running, it'd fly off. You take this shoe and you string the lace in through the shoe and then you tie it real nice and tight and it won't fall off."

4. Creative storytelling: +5/12. Only five of his story segments advanced the plot or provided a logical conclusion. He had extraordinary difficulty remembering the names he assigned to the various characters and as he was struggling with the names, he would forget where he was in the story-line. When the clinician said "And how does your story end?" he proceeded into an entirely new subplot. He could not devise a logical conclusion, perhaps because he could not remember what he had already related.

Assessment of Communication Problem

D. C. shows communication difficulties in the following areas:

1. Cognitive-linguistic organizational skills
2. Auditory memory or attention, or both
3. Vocal pitch consistency
4. Metalinguistic knowledge

Both his classroom language arts teacher and his resource teacher report similar observations. D. has difficulty focusing on the nature of a task and then remembering the task demands while engaged in it. He shows immature metalinguistic skills, as evidenced in his difficulty unscrambling sentences and formulating requested types of sentences. Auditorially he has difficulty with phonemic sequencing of sounds in 4+ syllable words and focusing on and remembering details and making inferences from information provided. When he engages in description or explanation, the product is rambling and disorganized. Vocal pitch problems are evident

Appendix 9–4 (continued).

when situations are stressful.

Recommendation of Goals and Instructional Objectives

It is recommended that D. be placed in communication therapy for improvement of auditory processing, expressive language, and voice problems. He should be scheduled for two to three times per week, and it could be anticipated that his programming will need to be continued upon high school entrance. Specific instructional objectives include the following:

D. Will be able to

1. listen to a tape recording of his performance during storytelling, explanations, or giving an opinion and decide whether or not his vocal pitch is normal or abnormal and correct performance as necessary

2. listen to the presentation of scrambled sentences of four to six words and reformulate a syntactically accurate sentence with 90% accuracy

3. provide a description of a stimulus picture 80% of the time that is
   a. clear to a listener in a barrier-game context
   b. syntactically well subordinated

4. focus on the nature of the task and cognitively organize
   a. explanations of why two objects go together on +3/4 trials
   b. his opinion or justification on at least three issues

5. listen to a tape recording that has three presentations of multisyllabic social studies vocabulary words on it and be able to correctly articulate at least 10 of these words

Charlann S. Simon, M.A. (CCC)
Speech-Language Pathologist

APPENDIX 9–5

SEMESTER PROGRESS REPORT

Date of Review   1-13-84

Child's Name   M. L.   Date of Birth   3-10-74

Program or Service   Speech-Language Therapy   Gr. Spec. Ed. -3

OBJECTIVES:

1. Accurate production of the /r/ sound in connected speech.
2. Use of self-cueing to facilitate word retrieval during confrontation naming of pictures.
3. Ability to process and follow four-element directions for the manipulation of objects in various spacial relationships.
4. Ability to provide an organized description for listener interpretation.

ASSESSMENT OF STATUS:

M. has made consistent progress during the first semester. He has achieved 80% to 100% accurate production of /r/ during oral reading and 60% during conversation. He attempts to use self-cueing (40% of obligatory context), but continues to rely on clinician cues. Limited comprehension of spacial concepts and attending deficits continue to interfere with his ability to follow directives. His ability to organize verbal descriptions has improved considerably. He has become more aware of listener needs.

RECOMMENDATIONS:

1. Continue with current speech-language therapy program: Once per week individually, two times per week in small group with one other child.
2. Continue classroom language group two times per week.
3. Ensure eye contact or attention before giving M. a direction.
4. Positively reinforce accurate /r/ production (e.g., verbal praise).

ADDITIONAL COMMENTS:

M. displays a positive, enthusiastic attitude in therapy. He is eager to please and is "self-rewarded" by his successful performance. He remains very sensitive to failure and will give up or refuse to participate if he views a new activity as too difficult, especially during group sessions. He seems highly motivated to improve his communication skills and puts forth a great deal of effort in both individual and group sessions when anxiety is reduced.

Date Sent to Parents   1-16-84   Person(s) Reviewing Placement:

Cynthia L. Holway

Speech-Language Pathologist

If you would like to discuss M's program in further detail or if you have any questions concerning the above information, please feel free to contact me at 988-2900.

APPENDIX 9-6

A LONGITUDINAL EVALUATION SUMMARY

NAME: D.M.   BD: 12-29-72   Entered Therapy: 10-7-82

S = spontaneous
D = Drill

dates of evaluations	PPVT	Auditory Association (ITPA)	Grammatical Closure (ITPA)	CELI	ACLC	Token	Goldman Fristo Test of Articulation	MLU (mean length of utterance)	Unsuccessful communication attempts S	Unsuccessful D	-ed regular past tense; story S	-ed past D	% Verbal Mazes S	% Verbal Mazes D	% Giant Words (slurred, rapid speed) S	% Giant Words D	Wh-question transformation S	Wh-question D	Semantic intent of pictured action (CCM Photos) S	Semantic intent D	Percentage of restricted sentences in sample
8-82 CA = 9.2	(A) 6.10	—	—	+2/7 28% 3.8% Total	2.90% 3.100% 4.40%	—	+78 96%	3.0 range 1-8	27%		40%		62%				0%		44%		87%
5-83 CA = 10.5	(A) 7.0	4.5	5.0	—	2.100% 3.90% 4.70%	—	—	3.9 range 2-10			60%	80%			61%		12%	30-68%	100%		58%
2-84 CA = 11.1 MA = 6.2	(M) 6.5	5.3	5.10	+15/30 50%	100%	100% 100% 80% 0% 21%		5.4 range 2-16	6%		71%	92%	40%		32%		60%	85%			40%

APPENDIX 9-7

COMMUNICATION SKILLS
EVALUATION REPORT

Date: 2-84

Student's Name: D. M.   Age: 11.1   Birthdate: 12-29-72   Clinician: C. Holway M.A. (CCC-S)

Background Information

(1) non-verbal until age 4½

(2) entered reporting therapist's caseload 10-17-82

(3) prior service: language-based classroom

(4) present service: 3× per week / 30 minute small group therapy with one other peer,
    2× per week / 30 minutes classroom language groups, language-based classroom

(5) progress: slow but steady with remarkable progress considering his developmental history

Formal Assessment (Test Scores) — see attached longitudinal summary

Informal Assessment Observations

Observations of performance on the following tasks have been noted to ascertain the quality of the student's skills in communication situations. Language concepts, language processing, the use of language for varying purposes and the articulation of speech sounds have been evaluated. Performance adequacy has been ranked on a 0-4 point scale: 0 = not present; 1 = present but inadequate (i.e., emerging skill or present but deviant); 2 = barely adequate (i.e., not consistent or generalized to a variety of contexts); 3 = adequate for MA (i.e., peformance is at an anticipated level considering IQ test scores); 4 = adequate for CA or quite good (i.e., a strong skill that is comparable or may even exceed performance of peers). When a particular skill has not been subjected to observation, the notation "NA" will be used to signify that information of that skill is not available.

I. Basic Language Concepts   Comments

  A. General fund of information
     1. in answering substantive questions   0 ①2 3 4   _____
     2. as reflected in word usage   0 1 2③4   at MA (6.5); word retrieval
        (vocabulary)   problems in conversation

  B. Comprehension and use of spatial concepts
     relative to
     1. moving self in space   0 1 2③4   _____
     2. moving objects in space   0①2 3 4   R/L;front/behind;on/above problems
     3. following directions for written work   0 1②3 4   _____
     4. classroom subject performance (e.g.,   0 1 2 3 4   NA
        geography)

  C. Comprehension and use of temporal concepts
     relative to
     1. orientation within time (e.g., aware-   ⓪1 2 3 4   relies on environmental structure
        ness of passing time; planning
        amount of time needed)
     2. vocabulary (before/after; while. . .)   0①2 3 4   variable
     3. classroom subject performance (e.g.,   0①2 3 4   _____
        history, narrative events in story/novel)

Appendix 9-7 (continued).

D. General Notations and Classroom Implications:

(1) difficulty with cognitive planning and organization of thoughts, but improvement evident
(2) needs lexical organization and associative categorization

II. Cognitive-Linguistic Organization

  A. Associative categorization   0 ① 2 3 4

    1. divergent (name 5 animals)   variable

    2. convergent (cat, dog, rabbit are all. . . ?)   0 1 2 ③ 4

  B. Semantic organization (i.e., advance cognitive planning of message content and sequencing of a series of related events so it is coherent)   0 ① 2 3 4   depends upon visual support available so sequence can be seen

  C. Syntactic skill

    1. ability to correctly code a series of scrambled words   0 1 ② 3 4   60% on 3-word

    2. form a structurally coherent sentence in adult grammar that maps intended meaning   0 ① 2 3 4   variable—depending upon contextual demands

  D. General Notations and Classroom Implications:

(1) difficulty with cognitive planning and organization of thoughts, but improvement evident
(2) needs lexical organization and associative categorization

III. Auditory Skills and Language Processing

  A. Auditory acuity (hearing level)   0 1 2 ③ 4

  B. Auditory perception

    1. sustained attention to auditory information   0 ① 2 3 4   up to 15 min. per task on good days

    2. discrimination between

      a. sounds (phonics)   0 1 ② 3 4

      b. similar words (except/accept)   0 1 ② 3 4   Wepman $x = +26/30, y = +9/10$

  C. Synthesis of sounds into words (blending)   0 1 ② 3 4

  D. Memory for information just heard   0 ① 2 ③ 4

  E. Separation of background noise from a message (message receives focus)   0 1 ② 3 4

  F. Linguistic processing

    1. comprehension of time, number, possession morphological markers   0 1 ② 3 4   80-100% drill; 50-70% conversation

    2. comprehension of syntactic nuances (i.e., is/has been; could/should)   ⓪ 1 2 3 4

    3. comprehension of semantic/syntactic relationships (i.e., understanding and remembering noun/modifiers; knowing what is big and what is little in "the big dog chased the little ball")   0 ① 2 3 4

  G. Cognitive/semantic processing

    1. comprehension of details

      a. within 1-3 sentences   0 1 2 ③ 4   when attending actively

Appendix 9-7 (continued).

b. within a paragraph   0 ① 2 3 4   attending and memory problems

2. integration of information segments
   a. getting the gist of a story   0 1 ② 3 4   _____
   b. combining 3 clues to solve a riddle   0 1 ② 3 4   _____
   c. providing a logical conclusion to   0 1 ② 3 4   likes this creative task
     a story

3. auditory evaluation
   a. absurdities (Noses are for hearing)   0 1 ② 3 4   100% sentence level; 0% paragraphs
   b. false statements/propaganda   0 1 2 3 4   NA
   c. incomplete directions for a task   0 1 2 ③ 4   excellent on therapy tasks

4. carrying out oral directions
   a. pointing to/manipulating objects   0 1 ② 3 4   _____
   b. paper and pencil tasks   0 1 2 ③ 4   _____

5. detection of nuances between synonyms (angry/enraged) and multiple meaning words (comb)   0 ① 2 3 4   _____

6. analysis of comparison and completion of analogies (grass is to green as sugar is to — white = color)   0 1 ② 3 4   Auditory Assoc. (ITPA) = 5.4 yrs.

7. understanding of figurative language (idioms, puns, proverbs)   ⓪ 1 2 3 4   only rote performance—not novel

8. detection of true or false factual statements from opinions   0 1 2 3 4   NA

H. General Notations and Classroom Implications:

(1) severe problems processing syntactic & semantic cues; limited concepts; memory & selective attention problems; frustration tolerence— low
(2) eye contact must be encouraged prior to receiving directions, use of rehearsal to improve retention of information and use of questioning for clarification

IV. Language Use
   Form (structure)
A. Degree to which (or percentage of time) sentence structure reflects adult grammar   0 ① 2 3 4   _____

B. Average number of words used in each sentence   - - - -   MLU = 5.4

C. Mastery of irregular forms (verbs - sing/sang; comparatives - good/better; plurals - tooth/teeth)   0 ① 2 3 4   verbs = 72% drill, nouns difficult

D. Use of semantically appropriate conjunctions (and/but) and clausal connectors (although/while/until. . .)   0 ① 2 3 4   _____

E. Maintenance of tense (a consistent time reference)
   1. conversation   0 ① 2 3 4   _____
   2. given an adverbial cue (Tell me what happened last year)   0 1 ② 3 4   minimal understanding of temporal domain
     a. sentence description of picture   0 ① 2 3 4   _____
     b. within a paragraph or story   0 1 ② 3 4   _____

Appendix 9-7 (continued).

F. Use of work endings (i.e., to show   0 1 ②3 4   considerable improvement
time, number and possession)

G. Sample of syntactic/morphological skills: (including the most and least syntactically
sophisticated performance)

(1) "Her putted clothes on to went to bed."
(2) "I am mad cuz Joe took my pen and din' ask!"

H. Sample of semantic appropriateness of words and word combinations:

"One more thing... Can I have one more thing?... uh... uhm... can (8 sec. pause)...
I done will be the last?"

(semantic intent: Can this be the last question so we'll be finished?; I want to stop!)

I. General Notations and Implications:

(1) behaviors observable during formulation difficulties: rolling eyes, blank stare, twisted
facial expression
(2) very responsive to: (a) modeling (syntax), (b) clinician cueing for cognitive-semantic organization
("stop and think—1, 2, 3, 4. . .")

Function (Use of language for varying purposes)

A. Instrumental ("I want. . .")
   1. make polite requests   0 1②3 4   capable but inconsistent use
   2. clear description of an object that   0 1②3 4   egocentric spontaneously but re-
      is wanted (by first analyzing how   sponds to cue "I can't read your mind."
      much information is needed for
      the listener to identify the
      desired object)

B. Regulatory ("Do as I tell you. . .)
   1. versatility in the use of direct,   0 1②3 4   better with adults than peers
      polite or indirect commands de-
      pending upon the participants
      and context
   2. give directions to a listener
      a. for arranging objects in a pattern   0 1 2③4   3-elements with blocks = 100%
         identical to the speaker's arrange-   6-element = 0-30%
         ment, when the listener and
         speaker cannot see each other
      b. for a sequential task (such as
         making a phone call)
      c. for participating in a game   0①2 3 4   egocentric; sequencing problems

C. Interactional ("Me and you. . .")
   1. interact with others socially in a   0 1②3 4   variable
      gracious manner
   2. general poise in using social rules   0 1②3 4
      (such as greeting, farewell, thank you)
   3. apologies and explanations of   0 1②③4   often apologizes
      behavior
   4. conversational skills
      a. initiation of a topic   0①2 3 4   variable function between a. and b.
      b. maintenance of a topic   0①2 3 4
      c. taking conversational turns   0①2 3 4

Appendix 9–7 (continued).

d. providing relevant answers to questions asked   0①2 3 4 _____

e. revision of a message that a listener indicates is unclear (rather than repeating the message verbatim)   0 1 2③4   consistently attempts but not always productive

f. respect for alternative points of view   0①2 3 4 _____

D. Personal ("Here I come. . .")

1. expression of a state of mind/health/attitude (I'm angry/My side hurts/It's the best I've felt in ages!)   0 1②3 4   a major advancement area

2. expression of feelings

a. one word statements ("mad")   0 1 2③4   correlates with behavioral improvement

b. explanation of feelings ("I'm really mad because my teacher said I wasn't listening, but I just didn't understand what I was expected to do.")   0①2 3 4 _____

3. tell an adult what is not understood in an accusation (I feel that I was right in hitting him because he hit me first)   0 1 2 3 4   NA

4. offer an opinion on an issue and supply a supportive statement for the opinion   0①2 3 4   "I like it because I like it"

5. supply basic identification and bio-graphical data (such as birthdate, address, full name, parents' occupations)   0 1②3 4   variable; information retrieval problems (aphasic-like)

E. Heuristic ("Tell me why. . .")

1. Asks adults questions

a. for clarification of incomplete in-formation they have received   0 1 2③4   uses spontaneously; unsure of his own processing skill

b. to systematically gather information (as in "20 Questions")   0①2 3 4 _____

2. curious inquiry (or interest in util-izing knowledgeable others to gain greater understanding of the world/issues   0 1 2③4   good!

F. Imaginative ("Let's pretend. . .")

1. engage in role-playing of various situations; pantomiming   0 1 2③4 _____

2. create a story that has a beginning, several logical intervening events and a reasonable conclusion   0①2 3 4   lack of narrative structure

G. Informative ("I've got something to tell you")

1. provide an organized description of a situation or object that features some details and subordinates others   0 1②3 4   beginning to use compound and complex sentences

2. interpret and relate content of a 4-6 frame sequential picture story

a. semantically appropriate mapping of content in each picture frame   0 1②③4   depends upon complexity of picture

Appendix 9–7 (continued).

   b. observation of cause/effect details   0 (1) 2 3 4   picks up on this in cued storytelling

   c. use of precise noun/pronoun referents   0 1 (2) 3 4   _____

   d. able to profit from or show im-   0 1 2 (3) 4   _____
   proved story quality after hearing a
   model story; paraphrasing the
   clinician

3. explanation of the realtionship   0 1 (2) 3 4   requires clinician cueing for full
   between two objects (vase/flower)   detail _____

4. compare and contrast attributes of
   a. 2 objects (needle/pin)   0 (1) 2 3 4   comprehends concept but poor syn-
   b. 2 vehicles (tricycle/bicycle) or   0 (1) 2 3 4   tactic skill interferes with explanation
   events (football/soccer)   _____

5. engage in evaluation of
   a. the appropriateness of one item in   0 1 2 3 4   NA _____
   contrast to another (thongs/boots
   for a hike)

   b. the quality of an event (such as   0 1 2 3 4   NA _____
   a movie) based upon a criteria of
   excellence

H. Sample of flexibility in language use: (4-frame picture story) "Sally was watchin t.v. an
eatin' tata chips. an an Then she was watchin t.v. The cookes spilt. . .an woke Spot up. An then
Sally went tu get. . .the kitchen an brought a dustpan an clean up the cook. . .chips. I'm done."

(Clarification) What's a "middle"? This is the middle?

I. General Notations and Classroom Implications:

1. upon enrollment in present program, D. only responded to direct questions; now, initiating and
maintaining conversation, questioning, descriptive information and comments, attempting to express
feelings and thoughts
2. syntactic limitations restrict complexity; organizational deficits

Style (individual characteristics that enhance or detract from one's communicative
effectiveness)

A. Supplies sufficient quantity of in-   0 (1) 2 (3) 4   depends upon word retrieval _____
   formation (doesn't expect listener
   to be a "mind reader")

B. Word finding (retrieval of needed   0 (1) 2 3 4   reduced frustration; self-cueing _____
   vocabulary and lack of empty   0 (1) 2 3 4
   words such as it, thing or stuff)

C. Organizes and coherently presents   0 (1) 2 3 4   _____
   ideas

D. Speaks fluently (without multiple   0 (1) (2) 3 4   revision of 40% of utterances _____
   revision of content) when express-
   ing thoughts

E. General sensitivity to the demands   0 1 2 (3) 4   _____
   of a communication situation
   (making appropriate modifications
   to consider the speaker, listener,
   message content, context)

Appendix 9–7 (continued).

F. Ability to interpret and use para-   0 1 2 ③ 4   strong skill _____
linguistic cues (body language,
intonation)

G. Effectiveness of voice
   1. natural pitch/intonation   0 1 ② 3 4   oral-motor problems interfere _____
   2. sufficient volume (depending upon   0 1 ② 3 4   can be excessive _____
   the proximity of the listener and
   context)

H. General intelligibility of speech   0 1 ② 3 4   improved, but still rapid and slurred
(clear production as contrasted to
slurred speech)

I. Sample of stylistic behaviors: "You need a pin. . .uh. . .uhh/ a needle a need to sewed it. . .
uhh. .uhh you have to need pin or it won' work. So you put the string. .uh. .uhh thread inside/ under
. .no. . .through to untie a you will knit. .NO! . . .fix your cloths."

J. General Notations and Classroom Implications:

(1) aphasic-style communication (retrieval-cognitive organization); sometimes abandons thoughts
or needs midway through expression
(2) classroom vocal volume may not be appropriate; if he has difficulty making semantic intent
clear, teacher questions and clarification attempts are useful

V. Speech
   A. Structural integrity of speech   0 1 2 ③ 4   _____
   mechanism
   B. Articulation of sounds (percentage   0 1 ② 3 4   _____
   of sounds correctly articulated in
   speech)
   C. Oral-motor skills
      1. volitional lip and tongue control   0 1 ② 3 4   variable, but improved _____
      2. diadochokinetic rate (rapid and con-   0 ① 2 3 4   _____
      sistent production of puh/tuh/kuh)
      3. articulation of 4-6 syllable words   0 1 ② 3 4   4 syllables = 50-100% _____
   D. Discrimination of correct/incorrect   0 1 2 3 4   NA _____
   production of speech sounds
   E. Stimulability of correct production   0 1 2 3 4   NA _____
   of error sounds
   F. Specific notations (such as number/type of errors):

(1) Goldman Fristo: d/e, b/v, s/z
(2) Conversational speech: multiple sound substitutions, omission of final consonant and
complete syllable, distortion of vowels

   G. General Notations and Classroom Implications:

(1) slurred, rapid, and sometimes unintelligible speech that has some neurological underpinnings
plus bad habits
(2) when asked to speak more slowly, intelligibilty is improved

VI. General Summary and Recommendations:
   A. Quantitative summary (average rating in each area)
      1. Language concepts   0 1 ② 3 4   (1.50) _____
      2. Cognitive-linguistic organization   0 1 ② 3 4   (1.60) _____
      3. Auditory skills and language   0 1 ② 3 4   (1.95) _____
      processing

Appendix 9-7 (continued).

    4. Language use
      a. form   0 ①2 3 4   (1.25) _____
      b. function   0 1②3 4   (2.06)
      c. style   0 1②3 4   (1.77) _____
    5. Speech   0 1②3 4   (2.20) _____

B. Narrative summary and recommendations:

   (1) SUMMARY: Although significant and consistent gains have been observed in language processing, expression, and intelligibility, deficits still characterize performance.
   (2) RECOMMENDATIONS:
      a. intensive and comprehensive therapeutic program with built-in generalization training
      b. continued attention to self-monitoring and use of questions to clarify what has been heard
      c. cognitive organization and intelligibility training

APPENDIX 9-8

COMMUNICATION SKILLS EVALUATION REPORT

Date:_____

Student's Name:_____ Age:_____ Birthdate:_____ Clinician:_____

Background Information

Formal Assessment (Test Scores) — see attached longitudinal summary

Informal Assessment Observations

Observations of performance on the following tasks have been noted to ascertain the quality of the student's skills in communication situations. Language concepts, language processing, the use of language for varying purposes and the articulation of speech sounds have been evaluated. Performance adequacy has been ranked on a 0-4 point scale: 0 = not present; 1 = present but inadequate (i.e., emerging skill or present but deviant); 2 = barely adequate (i.e., not consistent or generalized to a variety of contexts); 3 = adequate for MA (i.e., peformance is at an anticipated level considering IQ test scores); 4 = adequate for CA or quite good (i.e., a strong skill that is comparable or may even exceed performance of peers). When a particular skill has not been subjected to observation, the notation "NA" will be used to signify that information of that skill is not available.

I. Basic Language Concepts   Comments

  A. General fund of information

    1. in answering substantive questions   0 1 2 3 4   _____

    2. as reflected in word usage   0 1 2 3 4   _____
      (vocabulary)

  B. Comprehension and use of spatial concepts
    relative to

    1. moving self in space   0 1 2 3 4   _____

    2. moving objects in space   0 1 2 3 4   _____

    3. following directions for written work 0 1 2 3 4   _____

    4. classroom subject performance (e.g.,   0 1 2 3 4   _____
      geography)

  C. Comprehension and use of temporal concepts
    relative to

    1. orientation within time (e.g., aware- 0 1 2 3 4   _____
      ness of passing time; planning
      amount of time needed)

Appendix 9-8 (continued).

2. vocabulary (before/after; while. . .)   0 1 2 3 4   _____

3. classroom subject performance (e.g.,   0 1 2 3 4   _____
history, narrative events in story/novel)

D. General Notations and Classroom Implications:

II. Cognitive-Linguistic Organization

A. Associative categorization   0 1 2 3 4   _____
1. divergent (name 5 animals)

2. convergent (cat, dog, rabbit are   0 1 2 3 4   _____
all. . . ?)

B. Semantic organization (i.e., advance   0 1 2 3 4   _____
cognitive planning of message
content and sequencing of a series of
related events so it is coherent)

C. Syntactic skill

1. ability to correctly code a series of   0 1 2 3 4   _____
scrambled words

2. form a structurally coherent sen-   0 1 2 3 4   _____
tence in adult grammar that maps
intended meaning

D. General Notations and Classroom Implications:

III. Auditory Skills and Language Processing

A. Auditory acuity (hearing level)   0 1 2 3 4   _____

B. Auditory perception

1. sustained attention to auditory   0 1 2 3 4   _____
information

2. discrimination between

a. sounds (phonics)   0 1 2 3 4   _____

b. similar words (except/accept)   0 1 2 3 4   _____

C. Synthesis of sounds into words   0 1 2 3 4   _____
(blending)

D. Memory for information just heard   0 1 2 3 4   _____

E. Separation of background noise from   0 1 2 3 4   _____
a message (message receives focus)

F. Linguistic processing

1. comprehension of time, number,   0 1 2 3 4   _____
possession morphological markers

2. comprehension of syntactic nuances   0 1 2 3 4   _____
(i.e., is/has been; could/should)

3. comprehension of semantic/syntactic   0 1 2 3 4   _____
relationships (i.e., understanding and
remembering noun/modifiers; knowing what is big and what is little in
"the big dog chased the little ball")

From Simon, C. S. (1984). *Evaluating communicative competence: A functional pragmatic procedure.* Copyright 1984 by Communication Skill Builders, Inc. Reprinted by permission.

Appendix 9–8 (continued).

G. Cognitive/semantic processing
  1. comprehension of details
    a. within 1-3 sentences   0 1 2 3 4   _____
    b. within a paragraph   0 1 2 3 4   _____
  2. integration of information segments
    a. getting the gist of a story   0 1 2 3 4   _____
    b. combining 3 clues to solve a riddle   0 1 2 3 4   _____
    c. providing a logical conclusion to   0 1 2 3 4   _____
      a story
  3. auditory evaluation
    a. absurdities (Noses are for hearing)   0 1 2 3 4   _____
    b. false statements/propaganda   0 1 2 3 4   _____
    c. incomplete directions for a task   0 1 2 3 4   _____
  4. carrying out oral directions
    a. pointing to/manipulating objects   0 1 2 3 4   _____
    b. paper and pencil tasks   0 1 2 3 4   _____
  5. detection of nuances between syno-   0 1 2 3 4   _____
    nyms (angry/enraged) and multiple
    meaning words (comb)
  6. analysis of comparison and comple-   0 1 2 3 4   _____
    tion of analogies (grass is to green
    as sugar is to — white = color)
  7. understanding of figurative
    language   0 1 2 3 4   _____
    (idioms, puns, proverbs)
  8. detection of true or false factual   0 1 2 3 4   _____
    statements from opinions
H. General Notations and Classroom Implications:

IV. Language Use
  Form (Structure)
  A. Degree to which (or percentage of   0 1 2 3 4   _____
    time) sentence structure reflects
    adult grammar
  B. Average number of words used in   - - - - -   MLU = _____
    each sentence
  C. Mastery of irregular forms (verbs -   0 1 2 3 4   _____
    sing/sang; comparatives - good/
    better; plurals - tooth/teeth)
  D. Use of semantically appropriate con-   0 1 2 3 4   _____
    junctions (and/but) and clausal con-
    nectors (although/while/until. . .)
  E. Maintenance of tense (a consistent
    time reference)
    1. conversation   0 1 2 3 4   _____
    2. given an adverbial cue (Tell me what   0 1 2 3 4   _____
      happened last year)
      a. sentence description of picture   0 1 2 3 4   _____
      b. within a paragraph or story   0 1 2 3 4   _____

From Simon, C. S. (1984). *Evaluating communicative competence: A functional pragmatic procedure.* Copyright 1984 by Communication Skill Builders, Inc. Reprinted by permission.

Appendix 9-8 (continued).

F. Use of work endings (i.e., to show   0 1 2 3 4   _____
time, number and possession)

G. Sample of syntactic/morphological skills: (including the most and least syntactically
sophisticated performance)

H. Sample of semantic appropriateness of words and word combinations:

I. General Notations and Implications:

Function (Use of language for varying purposes)

A. Instrumental ("I want. . .")
1. make polite requests   0 1 2 3 4   _____
2. clear description of an object that   0 1 2 3 4   _____
is wanted (by first analyzing how
much information is needed for
the listener to identify the
desired object)

B. Regulatory ("Do as I tell you. . .")
1. versatility in the use of direct,   0 1 2 3 4   _____
polite or indirect commands de-
pending upon the participants
and context
2. give directions to a listener
a. for arranging objects in a pattern 0 1 2 3 4   _____
identical to the speaker's arrange-
ment, when the listener and
speaker cannot see each other
b. for a sequential task (such as
making a phone call)
c. for participating in a game   0 1 2 3 4   _____

C. Interactional ("Me and you. . .")
1. interact with others socially in a   0 1 2 3 4   _____
gracious manner
2. general poise in using social rules 0 1 2 3 4   _____
(such as greeting, farewell, thank you)
3. apologies and explanations of   0 1 2 3 4   _____
behavior
4. conversational skills
a. initiation of a topic   0 1 2 3 4   _____
b. maintenance of a topic   0 1 2 3 4   _____
c. taking conversational turns   0 1 2 3 4   _____

From Simon, C. S. (1984). *Evaluating communicative competence: A functional pragmatic
procedure.* Copyright 1984 by Communication Skill Builders, Inc. Reprinted by permission.

Appendix 9–8 (continued).

    d. providing relevant answers to   0 1 2 3 4   _____
       questions asked

    e. revision of a message that a listener 0 1 2 3 4   _____
       indicates is unclear (rather than
       repeating the message verbatim

    f. respect for alternative points of view 0 1 2 3 4   _____

D. Personal ("Here I come. . .")

   1. expression of a state of mind/   0 1 2 3 4   _____
     health/attitude (I'm angry/My side
     hurts/It's the best I've felt in ages!)

   2. expression of feelings

    a. one word statements ("mad")   0 1 2 3 4   _____

    b. explanation of feelings ("I'm really 0 1 2 3 4   _____
      mad because my teacher said I
      wasn't listening, but I just didn't
      understand what I was expected
      to do.")

   3. tell an adult what is not understood 0 1 2 3 4   _____
     in an accusation (I feel that I was
     right in hitting him because he hit
     me first)

   4. offer an opinion on an issue and   0 1 2 3 4   _____
     supply a supportive statement for
     the opinion

   5. supply basic identification and bio- 0 1 2 3 4   _____
     graphical data (such as birthdate,
     address, full name, parents'
     occupations)

E. Heuristic ("Tell me why. . .")

   1. Asks adults questions

    a. for clarification of incomplete in- 0 1 2 3 4   _____
      formation they have received

    b. to systematically gather information 0 1 2 3 4   _____
      (as in "20 Questions")

   2. curious inquiry (or interest in util- 0 1 2 3 4   _____
     izing knowledgeable others to gain
     greater understanding of the
     world/issues

F. Imaginative ("Let's pretend. . .")

   1. engage in role-playing of various   0 1 2 3 4   _____
     situations; pantomiming

   2. create a story that has a beginning, 0 1 2 3 4   _____
     several logical intervening events
     and a reasonable conclusion

G. Informative ("I've got something to tell you")

   1. provide an organized description of 0 1 2 3 4   _____
     a situation or object that features
     some details and subordinates
others

   2. interpret and relate content of a
     4-6 frame sequential picture story

Appendix 9–8 (continued).

a. semantically appropriate mapping   0 1 2 3 4   _____
   of content in each picture frame

b. observation of cause/effect details   0 1 2 3 4   _____

c. use of precise noun/pronoun referents   0 1 2 3 4   _____

d. able to profit from or show im-   0 1 2 3 4   _____
   proved story quality after hearing a
   model story; paraphrasing the
   clinician

3. explanation of the realtionship   0 1 2 3 4   _____
   between two objects (vase/flower)

4. compare and contrast attributes of
   a. 2 objects (needle/pin)   0 1 2 3 4   _____

   b. 2 vehicles (tricycle/bicycle) or   0 1 2 3 4   _____
      events (football/soccer)

5. engage in evaluation of
   a. the appropriateness of one item in   0 1 2 3 4   _____
      contrast to another (thongs/boots
      for a hike)

   b. the quality of an event (such as   0 1 2 3 4   _____
      a movie) based upon a criteria of
      excellence

H. Sample of flexibility in language use:

I. General Notations and Classroom Implications:

Style (individual characteristics that enhance or detract from one's communicative effectiveness)

A. Supplies sufficient quantity of in-   0 1 2 3 4   _____
   formation (doesn't expect listener
   to be a "mind reader")

B. Word finding (retrieval of needed   0 1 2 3 4   _____
   vocabulary and lack of empty   0 1 2 3 4   _____
   words such as it, thing or stuff)

C. Organizes and coherently presents   0 1 2 3 4   _____
   ideas

D. Speaks fluently (without multiple   0 1 2 3 4   _____
   revision of content) when express-
   ing thoughts

E. General sensitivity to the demands   0 1 2 3 4   _____
   of a communication situation
   (making appropriate modifications
   to consider the speaker, listener,
   message content, context)

Appendix 9–8 (continued).

F. Ability to interpret and use para- 0 1 2 3 4 _____
linguistic cues (body language,
intonation)

G. Effectiveness of voice
   1. natural pitch/intonation 0 1 2 3 4 _____
   2. sufficient volume (depending upon 0 1 2 3 4 _____
     the proximity of the listener and
     context)

H. General intelligibility of speech 0 1 2 3 4 _____
(clear production as contrasted to
slurred speech)

I. Sample of stylistic behaviors:

J. General Notations and Classroom Implications:

V. Speech

A. Structural integrity of speech 0 1 2 3 4 _____
mechanism

B. Articulation of sounds (percentage 0 1 2 3 4 _____
of sounds correctly articulated in
speech)

C. Oral-motor skills
   1. volitional lip and tongue control 0 1 2 3 4 _____
   2. diadochokinetic rate (rapid and con- 0 1 2 3 4 _____
     sistent production of puh/tuh/kuh)
   3. articulation of 4-6 syllable words 0 1 2 3 4 _____

D. Discrimination of correct/incorrect 0 1 2 3 4 _____
production of speech sounds

E. Stimulability of correct production 0 1 2 3 4 _____
of error sounds

F. Specific notations (such as number/type of errors):

G. General Notations and Classroom Implications:

Appendix 9–8 (continued).

VI. General Summary and Recommendations:
   A. Quantitative summary (average rating in each area)
      1. Language concepts   0 1 2 3 4   _____
      2. Cognitive-linguistic organization   0 1 2 3 4   _____
      3. Auditory skills and language   0 1 2 3 4   _____
         processing
      4. Language use
        a. form   0 1 2 3 4   _____
        b. function   0 1 2 3 4
        c. style   0 1 2 3 4   _____
      5. Speech   0 1 2 3 4   _____
   B. Narrative summary and recommendations:

APPENDIX 9–9
OROFACIAL EXAMINATION CHECKLIST

Robert M. Mason, Ph.D., D.M.D.,
Charlann S. Simon, M.A.

Patient name: _____ Age: _____ Date: _____
Examiner: _____

I. Facial Characteristics

 A. General appearance: normal color _____; normal symmetry _____;
  adenoid facies _____; other _____.

 B. Frontal view

  1. eye spacing: normal (one eye apart) _____;
   hypertelorism _____ ; other _____
   _____.

  2. zygomatic bones: normal _____; hypoplasia _____;
   other _____ .

  3. nasal area: septum (straight) _____;
   or deviated _____; nares _____;
   columella _____; septum/turbinate relationship _____,
   turbinate color _____; other notations _____
   _____.

  4. vertical facial dimensions:

   a. upper (40% of face) _____; other notations _____
    _____.

   b. lower (60% of face) _____; other notations _____
    _____.

  5. lips: cupid's bow present _____; muscular union _____;
   neuromotor functioning _____/i/ _____;
   /u/ _____; /p-p-p/ _____; other notations _____.

 C. Profile

  1. normal (straight or convex) linear relationship between bridge of nose, to base of
   nose, to chin _____;

   retrusion } maxilla _____;

        mandible _____;

   protrusion } maxilla _____;

        mandible _____;

Appendix 9–9 (continued).

    2. mandibular plane: normal_____; steep_____; flat_____.
  D. General notations:

II. Intraoral Characteristics
  A. Dentition
    1. general hygiene: good_____; needs improvement_____; caries_____;
    gingival hyperplasia or recession_____.
    2. occlusal relationships ("bite on your back teeth" and separate cheek from teeth
    with tongue depressor)
      a. first molar contacts:
        Class I—normal molar occlusion (mandibular molar is one-half tooth ahead
        of maxillary molar)_____;
        Class I malocclusion (normal molar relationship with variations in other areas
        of dentition)_____;
        Class II malocclusion (maxillary ahead of mandibular first molar)_____;

        Class III malocclusion (mandibular molar more than one-half tooth ahead of
        maxillary molar)_____.
      b. biting surfaces: normal vertical overlap (overbite)_____;
        excessive vertical overlap A_____/ P_____; normal horizontal
        overlap (overjet)_____; excessive horizontal overlap A_____/
        P_____; crossbite (mandibular tooth or teeth outside or wider than
        maxillary counterpart, or maxillary tooth or teeth inside mandibular counterpart)
        _____; notation of teeth involved_____; open bite
        (gap between biting surfaces) A_____/ P_____.
      c. sibilant production with teeth in occlusion: normal /s/_____;
      /z/ _____ ; /f/ _____ ; /v/ _____ .
  B. Hard palate ("extend your head backward")
    1. midline coloration: normal (pink and white)_____;
    abnormal (blue tint)_____.
    2. lateral coloration: normal_____; torus palatinus (blue tint surrounding a
    raised midline bony growth)_____.
    3. posterior border and nasal spine: normal_____; short_____.
    4. general bony framework: normal_____; submucous cleft_____;
    cleft_____; repaired cleft_____; other_____.
    5. palatal vault; normal relationship between maxillary arch/vault_____;
    narrow maxillary arch/high vault_____; wide maxillary arch/flat
    vault_____; other_____.
    6. general notations_____.
  C. Soft palate or velum (Examiner's eye level should be at patient's mouth level. Patient's
  head erect, mouth three-fourths open, and tongue not extended out of mouth.)
    1. midline muscle union (say "ah"): normal (whitish-pink tissue line)_____;
    submucous cleft (blue tint with A-type configuration during phonation_____;
    cleft_____; repaired cleft_____ __
    2. length: effective (closure of nasopharyngeal port possible during phonation)_____;
    ineffective (hypernasality noted)_____.
    3. velar dimple (where elevated soft palate buckles during phonation): normal 80%
    of total velar length (or 3-5 mm above tip of uvula)_____;
    other   notations_____.

Appendix 9–9 (continued).

    4. velar elevation: normal (up to plane of hard palate)_____;
reduced_____; other_____.

    5. range of velar excursion (up and back stretching during phonation):
excellent_____; moderate_____; minimal_____.

    6. presence of hypernasality during counting:
60s_____; 70s_____; 80s_____; 90s_____.

    7. general notations: regarding air loss on unphonated sounds (nasal emission) and nasal resonance on phonated sounds_____
_____ .

D. Uvula

    1. shape: normal_____; bifid_____; other_____.

    2. position: midline_____; lateral_____.

E. Fauces

    1. open isthmus_____; tonsillar obstruction of isthmus_____.

    2. tonsil coloration: normal (pinkish)_____; inflamed_____.

F. Pharynx

    1. depth between velar dimple and pharyngeal wall on "ah":
normal_____; deep_____; other_____.

    2. Passavant's pad: present during physiologic activity?_____

    3. adenoidal surgery (ask patient): intact_____; removed_____;
date of tonsil/adenoid removal_____

    4. gag response: positive_____; negative_____; weak_____

    5. general notations:_____

G. Tongue

    1. size: normal_____; macroglossia (rare)_____; microglossia_____

    2. diadochokinetic rate—an estimate of neuromotor maturation for speech (observe consistency and pattern of rapid movements during the 15-repetition sequence)
      a. normal movement patterns: tuh_____; luh_____; kuh_____;
puh-tuh-kuh_____; describe variations_____
_____ .

      b. mandibular assist; normal (until age seven and one-half)_____;
possible neuromotor delay for speech (after seven and one-half)_____

    3. lingual frenum: normal (tongue tip to alveolar ridge when mouth is one-half open)_____; short_____.

    4. general notations:_____

III. General Observations and Other Findings

From Mason, R. M., and Simon, C. S. (1977). An orofacial examination checklist. *Language, Speech, and Hearing Services in Schools, 8*(3), 155–163. Reprinted by permission.

TRANSITIONAL NOTE

Because of the available evidence that the quality of a student's communication skills has significant impact on classroom success, there has been an emphasis in earlier chapters on how to systematically observe communication skills. Chapter 10, by Sawyer, is an excellent transition from an emphasis on the observation of communication variables to the observation of specific classroom skills. It continues to be apparent how communication—speaking and listening—cannot be separated from reading and writing.

In Chapter 10, Sawyer shares her observations of the types of language problems she has observed in students referred to her clinic for their difficulties with reading. The nature of language processing is discussed in terms of its characteristics and how deficits in this area affect classroom performance, with particular reference to reading skill.

Berger (1978) has addressed the relationships between listening and reading comprehension in an article titled, "Why can't John read? Perhaps he's not a good listener." Her research, along with the findings from many other studies, suggests that poor readers generally have a reduced ability to *comprehend language* and "provides support for the conceptualization of reading comprehension as interrelated with language comprehension . . . .The interrelationship of listening and reading comprehension is further evidenced by a comparison of subject's scores on oral and written models of presentation for each task" (Berger, 1978, p. 637). These relationships are also discussed in the companion volume, *Communication Skills and Classroom Success: Therapy Methodologies for the Language-Learning Disabled.*

Berger, N. S. (1978). Why can't John read? Perhaps he's not a good listener. *Journal of Learning Disabilities, 11* (10). 633-638.

CHAPTER 10

Language Problems Observed in Poor Readers

D. J. Sawyer

Language processing refers to the perceptual and cognitive activity necessary to acquire, understand, and use language effectively. This activity takes place in the central nervous system and cannot be observed directly.

Problems related to language processing must thus be inferred from other, observable behaviors and, perhaps, developmental histories. Children with severe language problems typically receive their basic education in special settings for the language impaired. Children with all other degrees of expressive language and language processing problems may be found in regular classrooms.

Poor achievement in reading seems to be one significant observable characteristic of children with language problems. The purpose of this paper is to share information and insights concerning language processing and expressive language problems that have been gleaned from recent research findings and from personal work in the Syracuse University Reading Clinic. Increased awareness of observable deficits should lead to better in-classroom recognition of children with possible language problems so they can be referred for complete evaluation and so instruction for them can be based upon observable strengths and weaknesses.

WHAT IS A LANGUAGE PROCESSING PROBLEM?

A language processing problem is said to exist when, despite adequate auditory acuity and environmental stimulation, an individual has difficulty acquiring, understanding, or using language at a level that is considered appropriate for age and level of intelligence. Humans are genetically programmed to acquire language (Lenneberg, 1968). To do so we must hear, sort out, and organize the critical features of the specific language we hear and we must learn to produce the sounds and melody line. Critical features of spoken language include the phonemes or sound characteristics, syntax or word order, and semantics or meaning. Recognizing what are the critical features of language that must be attended to, classifying those features in such a way that they may be distinguished from each other, and developing a grammar or implicit rule system for decoding an utterance to meaning or encoding a thought into words all depend on adequate functioning of various cell networks within the central nervous system. Faulty processing of linguistic information might occur at the level of word order (syntax) and form (i.e., tense or inflection), at the level of interpreting meaning, or at the level of expressing meaning. Sometimes, language behavior suggests some degree of processing difficulties at all levels.

TYPES OF LANGUAGE PROCESSING PROBLEMS

Early in the study of learning problems, difficulties at the level of language reception received significant attention. Many children who seemed to have adequate auditory acuity still seemed to have problems receiving, understanding, and acting on messages. In time, researchers differentiated "hearing" ability into three distinct components—acuity, perception, and association. Acuity is defined as the clear reception of sound in the brain. Perception involves the ability to recognize differences between sounds, to store that information, and to recall that information at will. This is necessary to both decode speech (recognize that "pit" and "pat" are different words) and to produce speech (make the appropriate articulatory movements to produce minimally different sounds).

Association involves linking what is heard with the immediate circumstances surrounding the sound (i.e., recognizing that the word "cat" pronounced as a picture of a cat is held up is intended to be understood as a name label for the picture), as well as relating a current experience to previous experiences (i.e., relating this picture of a cat with other pictures of cats and with real cats). This aspect of hearing is commonly referred to as comprehension. Studies over the last 20 years have shown that each of these three abilities increases, among normal children, as a function of both maturity and experience. However, at a given age or grade, individual differences in these abilities are also linked to differences in levels of reading achievement. Current research suggests that language processing problems may be inferred when there are persistent difficulties in the following aspects:

1. Distinguishing significant characteristics of the speech signal despite adequate acuity.

2. Associating words heard with prior experience or relating them within the rules of syntax despite normal or above normal intelligence.

3. Producing language as a result of problems in retrieving words from memory or in coordinating their sequential ordering for the expression of ideas.

Although we do not yet know why these difficulties occur, recent research has given rise to a few plausible hypotheses that are currently being tested. An excellent discussion of the research to date, as well as the working hypotheses currently under investigation, may be found in Wyke's book (1978). Briefly, defects in the auditory processing of information within sound signals have been suggested as the cause of perceptually based language processing problems. Tallal and Piercy (1978) have proposed that differences at the perceptual level of language processing may be due to "defective processing of rapidly changing acoustic information and an associated, possibly consequential, reduced memory span for auditory sequence" (p. 82). "Rapidly changing acoustic information," in this situation, refers to differences in the speed of production associated with different single speech sounds. For example, /t/ ("tuh") is a rapidly produced sound in comparison to /1/ or /m/. The work of Tallal and Piercy (1978) suggests that some children cannot distinguish "rapid" sounds as easily as they can "slower" speech sounds. Language is made up of combinations of these fast and slow sounds, and difficulties in distinguishing them could explain why some children seem to take longer to learn language and why these same children evidence a poorer quality of speech, initially, as well as greater confusion in learning to understand and use language.

Beyond problems in perceiving the speech signal, Menyuk (1978) suggests that difficulties with the comprehension of speech might be due to impaired abilities to grasp and recall the specific relations between actors, actions, and objects. Sensitivity to these relationships requires that an individual develop awareness of the special distinguishing characteristics of nouns, verbs, determiners, and so forth, that constitute language. Menyuk suggests that difficulties in coming to recognize that words in each category are, somehow, different from those in other categories could interfere with a child's ability to acquire a range of grammatical structures. Such children would use only a small number of different types of grammatical forms and would become confused when faced with the problem of having to work out the meaning of more complex structures.

Characteristics of expressive language must reflect what has been received and how that has been organized, as well as the individual's ability to recall and produce. Problems involving memory and sequential order are common in the spontaneous productions of children with language processing problems as well as in their repetitions of words, sentences, or sets of numbers. However, the reasons for this behavior might be rooted in the receptive and associative processes involved in learning language as well as in the recall and production processes. What is clear is that quantitatively the language produced by these children is less and qualitatively, it is both less complex and less well formed than language produced by "normal" children of the same age (Morehead and Ingram, 1973; Vogel, 1975). Our own work with children exhibiting significant expressive language problems suggests that the degree of reading comprehension actually attained is likely to be significantly greater than the degree of comprehension the child can demonstrate verbally (Sawyer and Kosoff, 1981). When verbal expression is a significant problem, alternative methods for assessing comprehension must be employed.

LANGUAGE PROBLEMS AND SCHOOL ACHIEVEMENT

The most frequently cited evidence of success or failure in school is level of reading proficiency attained. Since about the 1950s, research focused on identifying why some children have difficulty acquiring reading skills has increasingly linked poor reading to deficits in various aspects of receptive and expressive language competence. Difficulties discriminating between similar speech sounds (e.g., *th*ine versus *v*ine) was perhaps the first aspect of language processing that was correlated with poor reading achievement (Wepman, 1960). In a very few years, however, researchers were noting that children with severe reading disabilities— dyslexia—demonstrated "imprecise articulation, difficulties in specific name finding and immature syntax" (Rabinovitch, 1968, p. 9). We were cautioned, however, that these same children generally were able to compensate sufficiently for these problems in daily conversation so that their communication efforts did not stand out as grossly aberrant. Time after time this fact is driven home with the cases we meet in the reading clinic. Parents may report that some unusual phrases pop out occasionally, "tee" for "Let's see" but attribute it to laziness—"He can say it if he wants to." Others note some immature use of grammar, "I gots" but attribute it to the poor grammar of playmates or "trying to get to us." Sometimes, parents and teachers note how quiet (nonverbal) a child is but attribute it to shyness. About 90% of the children we have worked with who show language processing problems have never been referred for a language evaluation, although many have received some speech therapy along the way to correct articulation problems. Failure to acquire basic reading skills prompts referral for a reading evaluation. Careful attention to the language patterns exhibited in the course of the reading evaluation, coupled with developmental histories and specific test behaviors, lead us to infer a language processing problem as the precursor to the reading problem.

Vellutino (1977) has proposed a verbal deficit hypothesis to account for severe difficulty in acquiring basic reading skills. His review of a range of research studies concerned with the performance of poor readers on various kinds of language processing tasks led him to conclude that deficits (perhaps best understood here to mean observable language behaviors that are less than adequate for the age group) in either semantic, syntactic or phonological processing of language, or deficits involving any combination of those language subsystems, probably account for the severe difficulties children who are considered to be dyslexic experience in acquiring reading skill. Numerous other researchers are continuing to examine the nature of language processing problems and to document the role of language processing abilities in reading acquisition. Increasingly more sophisticated and reliable techniques are being developed. The mounting evidence suggests that children with language processing difficulties at the phonological level are slower to learn language. Children having difficulties at the syntactic level generally use grammatically less complex sentences than their age mates. Children with difficulties at the semantic level as well as those having difficulties at the phonological or syntactic levels demonstrate confusion in understanding spoken language—presumably for different reasons. For all of these children, learning to read is a difficult and frustrating task.

RECOGNIZING CHILDREN WITH LANGUAGE PROBLEMS

Experienced researchers can generally infer the existence of language processing problems in experimental laboratory settings. Teachers and parents, however, need less formal, though reasonably reliable, means for inferring the likelihood that such a problem is affecting a particular child. Such information should have an impact on instructional planning. In this section the characteristics observed in personal experience with such students that, in combination, tend to suggest that language processing difficulties are at the heart of reading and learning problems will be described.

Limited Spontaneous Speech Flow. These children were not talkative, but when they did engage in conversation they used brief phrases or sentences and generally did not string these together. They made simple statements or asked brief questions. Their statements were generally concrete and tied to both personal experiences and the present. They engaged in far less description than others their age. For example, one 12 year old offered this on a Monday morning after having spent Sunday at an amusement park. "We went to the park yesterday. I rode on the rides. One went real fast. It was fun."

Word-Finding Difficulties. *Frequently* these children would, in conversation or in response to a question, indicate that they knew the word they wanted to say but just could not think of it. Sometimes they would substitute a related word or phrase (strawberry for raspberry or "the thing you push" for "pedal"), or sometimes they would simply smile and shrug and were reluctant to go on.

Occasional Production of Novel Words and Phrases. This might be related to the word finding problem cited earlier, but instances of these "odd" utterances were noted in about half the children in the reading clinic. One child, when told he was going to have his hearing tested replied, "My earsight is good." Another, when asked what his favorite ice cream treat was replied, "banana sundae split." In no instance did any child recognize that an error had been made. Such utterances were noted among children ranging in age from 8 to 16 years.

Use of "Immature for Age" Grammatical Forms. These children may use only the regular plural form (word plus "s"), such as gooses, sheeps, or foots, well into middle childhood and early adolescence. Difficulties with the appropriate form of the verb may also be apparent (I gots). However, a word of caution here is necessary. Sometimes children who are using inappropriate grammatical forms may only be reproducing the language forms used at home ("He come to see me"; "I done the dishes"). Teachers need to be sensitive to this possibility when trying to evaluate language behaviors.

Difficulty in Untangling the Relationships in More Complex Sentences. The following sentence, encountered as a question in a popular skill text, offers one example of this problem. "In what you just read did figured mean "thought" or did it mean "added and subtracted?" When asked this question following silent reading one student screwed up his face, scratched his head and asked "What did you say?" Repeating the question, however, was still not sufficient to help him organize a response. He could not sort out what the question was asking. The boy was 11 years old. When the examiner took the question apart for him, step by step, he was able to answer. For some children with language processing problems it may only be necessary to rephrase such a sentence. The examiner might rephrase as follows: "The word figured was used in this story. In figuring something out did the boy think or did he add and subtract?" Rephrasing of this sort helps the child to identify the focus of the question. The dependent clause that introduced the original question, coupled with the pronoun "it" to refer to something noted earlier, makes this a complex structure to work through for children with language processing problems.

Trouble Remembering Information and Repeating Information Presented Orally. Children with difficulties in this area are usually frustrating to live with and to work with. When sent to get more than one thing or told to do more than one task at a time, they forget. Several stage directions are difficult for them to follow; long sentences or questions are difficult for them to repeat. Teachers and parents often accuse them of not paying attention. Errors in repeating may involve leaving out information, mixing up the order of information, or simply being unable to figure out where to start. The illustrative sentence in item 5 above is one kind of sentence such children might have difficulty repeating. The structure is quite complex—more so than the sentences they spontaneously produce—and fairly long.

Subdued Personality. Children with language processing problems tend not to be as verbally expressive as their age mates, even with their peers. They seem unusually quiet, are generally timid, and tend to engage more in parallel or solitary play than in cooperative play. Most of the boys who have come to the clinic spent much time riding a bike. All of these children could name few if any friends. Most of them did not have close relationships with siblings. In school, these children generally were not harassed by other students; they tended to be ignored. Most academic subjects, and often even gym, art, and music, were sources of frustration and anxiety. Presumably, this was true because of their difficulty comprehending, remembering, and acting on oral directions.

Poor Spelling. This area, like reading, appears to pose a major problem for children with language processing problems. Their efforts tend to show overdependence on sound-symbol correspondence ("tha" for "the"; "thay" for "they"), letter omissions ("spe" for "strap"; "smk" for "smoke"), and letter sequence problems ("wiht" for "with") as well as confused application of spelling rules ("hade" for "had"). They seem to have trouble recognizing when a word does or does not fit the pattern or rule. Perhaps the problem stems from difficulty coordinating two interrelated facts (e.g., in had/hade [final e present] + [makes the vowel long]).

Poor Reading Comprehension. Many children with language processing problems have so much trouble with the recoding task of reading that they can devote little attention to comprehension. For example, Ray made many word recognition errors and he rarely stopped to reconsider the appropriateness of his productions—"devop" for "develop," "another" for "enough," "matching" for "machine," "fork" for "force," and so forth. He was not an unusually slow reader but he did frequently try to work out words using some partial cues and guessing. Self-correction of such errors was rare and comprehension was quite poor. However, some children may master the code at some functional level but still have difficulty with comprehension questions that require more than direct restatements of words or phrases from the text. For example, in a paragraph about sky divers, the author wrote that skydiving was almost like being in a dream. In the next sentence it described how divers feel when they leave the plane. The reader was expected to make the association between the feelings described (i.e., floating) and what one feels like in dreams. After Jon read this passage he was asked, "Why is skydiving like being in a dream?" He responded, "You're asleep." The problems often can be traced to failures in grasping relations in the text that are signaled by syntax, tense markers, and pronoun referents. Questions involving the sequence of events frequently pose problems.

Slow to No Progress in Reading. Usually the child shows persistent difficulties with the code despite *much* help. Universally, the records of these children show slow progress in reading coupled with very early comments concerning lack of readiness for reading instruction and much special attention by classroom teachers as well as special reading personnel. Teacher comments regarding reading progress typically include some of the following: "Can't seem to remember what we have worked on from one day to the next;" "Virtually no application of the skill lessons;" "Can't do the workbook pages independently."

While it is true that any child might exhibit *any* one of the above characteristics on occasion, children with language processing problems exhibit several if not most of these characteristics consistently. Combining personal observations of these behaviors with information from school records and previous interviews with teachers and parents will help the educator decide if there is sufficient evidence to warrant referral for professional language and learning evaluations.

REFERRING CHILDREN FOR PROFESSIONAL EVALUATIONS

When a teacher has reason to believe that a child may have a language processing problem, a referral for professional evaluations should be made.

Typically, such children should be evaluated by an audiologist, a speech-language pathologist, a psychologist, and a reading specialist. A summary of the teacher observations, descriptions of classroom behavior, and academic problems, as well as anecdotal information concerning the course of language acquisition—including examples of unusual language characteristics—should accompany any referral for a suspected language problem. Other professionals will use such information as a reference point in developing a focused evaluation in contrast, perhaps, to a general screening.

An audiologist will attempt to determine if hearing acuity is adequate for the development of language. Tone reception will be evaluated and, in some cases, the audiologist can also investigate the efficiency with which speech sounds and words are received and integrated. A speech-language pathologist will evaluate the quality (clarity and maturity) of speech production, language comprehension, and language production.

A psychologist will assess the child's general level of intelligence, based upon accumulated knowledge as well as reasoning or problem solving ability. Efficiency in using verbal versus nonverbal input-output modes for learning will also be assessed. A reading teacher will seek to assess the level of mastery attained on language-based prereading skills, such as blending and rhyming, as well as the level of achievement in specific reading skills—sound-symbol correspondences, comprehension of directions, work attack skills consistently applied, and listening comprehension versus reading comprehension performance. Taken together, such multidisciplinary evaluations will either support the teacher's intuitions concerning a language-based problem or reveal other possible explanations for the behaviors and academic progress that should be investigated or treated.

Evaluations by a range of nonclassroom professionals will take time, often several months. Even then they may not yield instructional recommendations that can be implemented immediately. Referrals should be made with a view toward obtaining additional support services for the child if warranted. Positive diagnoses of language problems might also help everyone concerned to better understand and accept the child and his or her special needs for emotional as well as academic support. In the final analysis, however, the classroom teacher must identify daily the possible strengths to build upon. He or she must test out hunches about possible instructional strategies that might make a difference. This is tedious and often frustrating work.

The three cases described on the following pages are exemplars of different types of language processing problems. They are offered in the hope that they will make the task of working with language-based learning problems a bit less mystifying.

INSTRUCTIONAL PLANNING FOR CHILDREN WITH EXPRESSIVE LANGUAGE AND LANGUAGE PROCESSING PROBLEMS

Jimmy

Jimmy was a second grader when he was referred to the Syracuse University (SU) reading clinic. He had received much special reading help in school in both first and second grades, but by March of second grade was still functioning as a beginning reader. Jimmy was shy, quiet, gentle, and likeable. He often seemed to "disappear" in the classroom.

Information from school records, previous testing results and examiner comments, and discussions with present and previous teachers, as well as observation of Jimmy in his classes and one morning of working with Jimmy informally on a one-to-one basis, provided the data base out of which conclusions and recommendations were drawn.

Records showed that Jimmy did not begin to talk until he was about two and a half years old. A test of hearing acuity administered at a medical center indicated normal hearing acuity. Jimmy had received special speech therapy since age three and by second grade his speech was quite clear. We interpreted the delayed onset of speech and poor speech production in early childhood as indicators that Jimmy had had difficulty making sense of the speech around him. If so, Jimmy had a language processing problem that involved perception, as contrasted to acuity.

An evaluation of the sound-symbol correspondences Jimmy had mastered by mid-second grade showed significant gaps. Jimmy had mastered the association between the sounds of consonants, consonant blends, and consonant digraphs when shown those letters and combinations in print. However, he had not mastered the operation in reverse—giving the name of the letter or letters that are associated with the sounds he heard at the beginning of a spoken word. For example, Jimmy could see "g" and say "guh," but when asked to name the letter that "gal" begins with he was unable to do so. It seemed possible that Jimmy might have learned to produce sound correspondences in isolation for segments of words he really could not distinguish when he heard the whole word. Jimmy did recognize about 40 words at sight on graded lists of words accompanying an individual reading inventory. Jimmy seemed to be using visual skills more than auditory skills to support his learning.

Teacher reports and informal testing indicated that Jimmy had difficulty holding information in short-term memory while trying to act on it, and he had trouble following directions when more than two separate actions were required. Additionally, he could not accurately repeat sentences of more than seven words. Jimmy also had great difficulty learning songs in music class, both in remembering the words and in keeping the details in sequence (as in "There was an old woman who swallowed a fly"). Further, Jimmy's spelling was "confused" when dealing with two or three letter words (e.g., "put" for "pot"; "tud" for "tub"), but it was incomprehensible for words of four or more letters. Jimmy would seem to "forget" the sounds in the middle and produce only letters that appeared (or might be heard) at the beginning and the end (ska for smoke; spe for strap). The problem for memory seemed greatest when verbatim recall, or action based on verbatim recall, was required. For example, Jimmy had much difficulty performing a task that required that he listen to directions and then mark pictured objects on a page in the order mentioned and with the symbols indicated in the spoken directions. Interestingly, Jimmy could listen to short passages—stories on an informal reading inventory—and answer questions about them. In fact, his listening comprehension for connected, elaborated ideas was adequate for his grade placement.

Other informal testing showed that Jimmy had difficulty isolating the component sounds in a word. Spelling (encoding) and decoding requires the ability to focus on separate sounds. Research on this ability—called auditory segmentation—indicates that it develops, at least in part, as a function of maturation of the central nervous system and is strongly related to success in beginning reading (Sawyer, 1981; Stanovich, 1982). Jimmy could separate either the initial or final consonant or blend from the rest of a word (i.e., lea-f; r-ough), but he could not hear the word "bite," for example, and show that it was composed of three distinct parts ("buh"- "i"- "tuh"). His performance on auditory segmenting was about on par with that of five or six year olds. It was not surprising that rhyming was also difficult for Jimmy when it is remembered that rhyming appears to be an early stage in segmenting. Rhyming requires the ability to focus on a part split off from a whole word and to then generate other words containing that same part in the same position. Jimmy at age eight years seemed to be just "getting the idea" of what rhyming was all about.

As an example of how segmenting difficulties complicated Jimmy's learning, consider his spelling of "jet," which was "jat." If you separate out the /j/ and say it in isolation you hear "juh." The sound "uh" is like "a" in "He saw a dog." Jimmy apparently heard "juh" at the beginning, wrote "ja" and then added the next sound he could clearly isolate and match to a letter "t" for "tuh." Jimmy might not have been aware that a middle sound was part of "jet." Or, in trying to note that he heard /j/ and /a/ at the beginning, he might have lost track of — forgotten—the middle sound. Probably both factors played a part, since his short-term memory was not strong.

Testing also showed Jimmy's comprehension skills to be weak. He was still unsure of such basic concepts as calendar time, seasons, or holidays of the year. He also had difficulty "reading" pictures to sequence them according to time (first, second, and so forth) or according to cause and effect. Such concepts and relational thinking techniques were needed if comprehension of written or spoken language, beyond direct recall, was to be advanced.

It was concluded that Jimmy's reading difficulties were related to slower than normal development of both the perception and comprehension aspects of language processing. Slow development was apparent in his acquisition of speech and in his mastery of language related concepts— auditory segmenting and rhyming—that support reading acquisition. At age eight years, it was difficult to say whether maturation would eventually overcome the processing difficulties Jimmy was experiencing or whether he would always need to compensate for them. In either case, reading instruction and the acquisition of general information had to be planned to maximize the abilities he did possess and to circumvent his difficulties.

It was recommended that decoding instruction should have a dual focus: (1) building a "whole word" recognition vocabulary of personally important or interesting words; (2) word analysis based upon phonograms or clusters that pair the vowel, which Jimmy did not yet isolate in spoken words, with a consonant (e.g., -ot, at, it). A developmental program such as the Merrill Linguistics (Rudolph, Wilson, Otto, and Smith, 1975), program or the SRA Basic Reading (Rasmussen and Goldberg, 1967) program was recommended. Furthermore, it was recommended that Jimmy's general education proceed despite his inability to read content area texts. Teachers were urged to capitalize on Jimmy's listening comprehension to help him grasp as much basic information as was possible in social studies and science. They were urged to eliminate demands for his completion of independent worksheets as well as for silent reading of texts. People working with Jimmy were encouraged to simplify directions so that statements were brief (five to six words) and staged according to the necessary parts of the task. For example, instead of saying, "Put an X on the picture in each box that does not belong," teachers were asked to say, "Find the one that doesn't belong" (while pointing to one set of boxes); then, "Put an X on it." "Now look in this box." The directions, "Find the one..." would be repeated. After two or three examples Jimmy could then be told "Look in each box. Mark the one that does not belong." Special help in the development of basic time, order, and relational concepts would have to be provided beyond reading or content area classes. All instructional personnel working with Jimmy—speech-language, reading, classroom—were urged to meet frequently and regularly to coordinate instructional goals, methods, and opportunities to apply new skills as they develop.

Different kinds of language processing problems require different kinds of instructional focus. The case of Jimmy illustrates problems probably stemming from the perception of language. Excerpts from two other cases are offered here to illustrate interpretation and planning in light of information that suggests problems stemming from associative difficulties and expressive difficulties. The management techniques initially suggested are also presented.

Jennifer

Jennifer was nine years old and was about to repeat third grade when she was seen at the SU reading clinic for an evaluation of her reading. Specifically, Jennifer was having difficulty comprehending classroom reading material. She had been referred to the school's reading teacher for extra help in phonics in first grade. This area had improved so no extra reading help was recommended during second grade. In third grade, Jennifer was again referred for special help in reading comprehension. Additional support was provided daily by the school reading teacher throughout the spring semester. Testing at the end of the third grade year showed Jennifer's reading achievement level to be at about the second half of the second grade.

On the day of testing at the reading clinic Jennifer's mother reported nothing unusual in Jennifer's developmental history. Intelligence testing showed Jennifer to be of average intelligence and, throughout the day, we found her to be pleasant and cooperative. However, she generally spoke only in response to questions and was generally described by the diagnostic team as "quiet."

Reading testing showed that Jennifer could accurately decode words at the third grade level. Her oral reading was fluent. However, when asked to either "retell" or to answer specific questions about what she had read, Jennifer had trouble. On second and third grade level passages she could only make single, broad statements about each (e.g., "It's about bears and honey"). She could not note details or even express an awareness of the specific situation around which a passage was organized. In response to specific questions about the passages she had read, Jennifer relied on personal experiences and general background information. Usually her responses were not clearly related to the question. When asked to read a first grade level passage we saw quite different behavior. At this level Jennifer was able to retell the story, including many of the details. She was also able to correctly answer nine to ten specific questions that were asked about what she had read.

An analysis of the sentence structures used in the three different passages revealed a significant difference in the length and complexity of the sentences. Jennifer had difficulty comprehending the material as the sentences became more complex. Subject-verb-object patterns were easy for Jennifer to understand. But when clauses were embedded to clarify or to add description (e.g., "It was the first time Bill went to camp," or "In fright I knocked on the windowpane"), Jennifer seemed to lose the details and retain only a sketchy impression of the paragraph. Her recalls consisted of mainly nouns (camp; trees; leaves). She could not distinguish these nouns according to topic versus detail.

Further exploration of Jennifer's comprehension difficulties using 2^2 level material (the second half of second grade) suggested that, at that level, sentences and single paragraphs were generally understood. She could both retell and answer specific questions. However, when information from two or more paragraphs had to be integrated before retelling or responding to questions, Jennifer was barely able to give a general statement about the material. She could not recall specific details nor integrate them.

Other testing suggested that Jennifer had difficulty both understanding directions and expressing relationships she apparently recognized. For example, it was frequently necessary to explain and rephrase directions for her before she could adequately proceed with a task. On a test designed to evaluate ability to read and follow directions, Jennifer read carefully and slowly and frequently reread a direction after once beginning to act on it. On several items she began incorrectly but reread, erased, and began again. Errors she did make seemed related to the fact that she did not isolate key words in the directions.

Throughout the day Jennifer spoke in short, simple sentences. She rarely elaborated on statements through use of specific details. Her definitions of words, when required, were usually global rather than precise. Although she appeared able to organize information appropriately, she was not always able to explain why she had organized as she did. For example, on a categorizing task Jennifer was able to select, from a group of eight words, the printed words "trapeze," "elephant," "lion," "clown," and "tent" as belonging together. However, she could not state that they were things in a circus.

Difficulties in interpreting the meaning of complex sentence structures, as well as some difficulty in expressing ideas she apparently had grasped, did appear to account for Jennifer's comprehension problem. This problem affected the interpretation of both spoken and written language.

Recommendations included providing developmental reading instruction for Jennifer at two levels—decoding and comprehension. Comprehension skills were to be developed using late first grade to early second grade level materials. Instruction would focus on teaching sentence interpretation as well as the integration of information across sentences and then across two paragraphs. Decoding skills could continue to be developed in the regular skill group settings provided for her classmates. Approaches to comprehension that highlighted the importance of thinking about meaning all along the way were recommended. These included the following: (1) Sentence completion—"Columbus sailed west because _____." (2) Cloze procedure—President _____ freed the slaves. (3) Context to anticipate upcoming events or details: "The day was dark and gloomy. Hurricane warnings were in effect and the winds were howling around the house. Suddenly, sheets of rain began to blow toward the beaches. Mary's father rushed in through the door and said, "_____ _____ _____ _____."

In addition, semantic maps or structured overviews were recommended to be used with Jennifer prior to reading as a graphic aid to focus her attention on the details related to what would be read as well as to help set a purpose for reading. For example, if a lesson on foods was to be taught in health, the teacher was urged to prepare the class for reading as follows:

1. Write title of unit on board—*Foods for Health.*
2. List different foods children name.
3. Have children group foods listed—foods that are alike.
4. Teacher gives the newly organized groups superordinate labels of the four basic food groups and "nonessential" foods (e.g., candy).
5. Teacher directs class—"Read the unit in your health books that tells what foods are needed to keep us healthy. As you read, think about these four basic food groups listed on the board. See what different foods the authors list in these groups that we didn't think of. Read, too, to learn why candy and cake are listed as "nonessential foods."

Opportunities for oral expression were also recommended. Among the strategies suggested were cooperative creation of an original story (one person starts, another picks up and adds, and so on), small group imitations of a newscast, dramatizing a favorite story, and creating an ending for a story being read to the class, then individually defending the ending chosen.

Unlike Jimmy, whose comprehension of oral language was a strength, Jennifer had difficulty grasping the meaning of even moderately complex language structures, whether spoken or written. Her oral language was limited to the use of simple sentences and, although she sometimes seemed to grasp word meanings and relationships at a level that was consistent with her grade placement, Jennifer often had difficulty expressing the knowledge she possessed. Whereas Jennifer reportedly had *some* difficulty learning the sound-symbol system in first grade, Jimmy's difficulties with the code were great and persisted throughout the primary grades. Both showed difficulties using language to express themselves, but in neither case was spoken language so different that they were referred for possible language therapy. Both received special educational attention primarily as a consequence of reading problems.

Michael

Michael was 11 years old and entering fifth grade when seen at the SU reading clinic for a reading evaluation. Michael had repeated first grade and had received extensive one-to-one reading help since first grade.

Michael's mother reported normal childhood development and described Michael as a friendly, sensitive boy who had recently expressed concern about his poor reading ability.

School records indicated that Michael had received regular instruction in Distar Reading (Engelmann and Bruner, 1974) during the fourth grade year, which was provided by the resource teacher. He had also received speech therapy that year to correct a moderate articulation problem. His teachers (classroom, reading, and resource room) reported that he had appeared to be making adequate progress in Distar during the period of September through February. However, in the early spring he seemed to regress. Teachers felt that he had lost many of the skills he had once had.

Testing indicated that Michael was a nonreader. He recognized only about 10 words at sight and used only initial consonants as aids in word attack. Once he had begun, Michael just kept "reading," often producing what seemed like gibberish. Furthermore, Michael demonstrated a limited ability to use language to communicate. He was asked to discuss a recent experience his Mother had told us about. We used this as a foundation to develop the following language experience story about sports.

Sports I Like

This summer I'm going to play football. In the fall I'm going to play basketball. In the winter I'm going to wrestle. In the spring I'm going to play baseball.

Michael's sentences were simple in structure and every sentence had the same format (time order prepositional phrase, subject-verb-object). His sentences lacked descriptive words and phrases. Michael was unable to read the story (four sentences) a few hours later. He did face the page and pretend to read. He recreated from memory a story similar to the first.

Tests of Michael's ability to understand spoken language—word meaning, sentence meaning, following directions—all showed above average ability when motor and recognition responses rather than verbal production responses were required. A test administered to compare sequential recall of digits when presentation was either auditory or visual, and when recall required either spoken or written responses, showed Michael to be performing at the level of an average seven to eight year old. His strongest performance occurred when he both saw and heard the digits and then wrote his recall of the sequence.

A series of other tests investigated Michael's ability to retell a story, to repeat multisyllable words, to repeat sentences and phrases, to use appropriate plural and past tense forms, and to spontaneously produce as many words as he could in one minute. On all of these tests, Michael's performance was well below average for his age. He confused order of both syllables in words and of words in phrases as well as the order of events in a story. He left out words in sentences he repeated, and his responses became unrelated groups of words. He showed limited awareness of regular plurals and past tense forms. Throughout the day Michael seemed to have difficulty selecting the exact words he needed to communicate and frequently came up with approximations of the words he wanted—"wagon ride" for "hay ride," berry shake for strawberry milkshake (both strawberry and raspberry flavors were available), "we go driving" for "we ride our bikes." Probes that could be answered with yes or no always helped examiners to clarify what Michael had intended to say.

Michael seemed to have a pervasive expressive language problem that affected both imitation and spontaneous production. It was concluded that Michael's reading difficulties probably stemmed from a more general language deficit. His inability to consistently produce word labels for thoughts and experiences appeared related to the difficulty he has had in correctly "labeling" individual sounds represented by letters as well as "labeling" words he met in print. His past reading instruction had emphasized letter-by-letter decoding. Labeling problems coupled with sequence problems probably accounted for his lack of progress despite intensive and careful instruction.

Recommendations were developed to focus on both reading instruction and approaches for general education. Since it appeared that Michael could take in and retain information when it was presented in specific ways, it was recommended that content area instruction use taped text materials, films, and other visual aids to expose him to basic information and concepts. In addition, checks on his acquisition of information and concepts would be most valid if they permitted *recognition* of correct answers (e.g., multiple-choice tests; locating places, features, and so forth, on a map) rather than demanding a creative, verbal formulation. A modified version of the language experience approach—whereby one-to-one discussion related to content area lessons are recorded in a notebook for cooperative reading and study later—was suggested as a substitute for notetaking, outlining, and supplementary reading experiences typically assigned at the middle school level and beyond.

Since Michael did recognize and use initial consonant sounds as clues to word attack, reading instruction that emphasized phonogram patterns in words was recommended. To promote opportunities for Michael to both learn and practice the techniques of initial consonant substitution as an aid to decoding, many and varied rhyming games, stories, and poems were recommended as well as a more formal instructional program such as the Merrill Linguistic Reading Program (Rudolph, Wilson, Otto, and Smith, 1975). Glass Analysis for Perceptual Conditioning (Glass, 1978) was also recommended as a later procedure to supplement the Merrill program and teach Michael how to attack multisyllabic words using the same "cluster" principle.

It appeared likely that the severity of Michael's language problems would continue to inhibit progress toward reading fluency. It was thus suggested that Michael also be helped to develop "survival" reading skills, such as the recognition of common signs, location of specific names in a phone book, gathering specific information from various kinds of newspaper ads, coping with different kinds of simple menus, and so forth.

The future did not look bright for Michael, whether for school success or for getting along in life. However, identifying the likely presence of a language processing problem was an important first step in attempting to reverse the history of school failure by refocusing instruction in ways that permitted Michael to use the abilities he does possess while circumventing those he does not have available to him. Language therapy and special academic support services will be necessary throughout Michael's educational career. Psychological support services might also be necessary at some point to help Michael accept himself and to help him learn how to live with his handicap.

SUMMARY

As teachers, we take for granted the fact that children come to a learning context in general and to school in particular with certain basic abilities that we can help them to build upon. Language competence is the ability we depend on most heavily; classrooms are language saturated. When children come to school unable to understand or use language effectively, they quickly learn to not participate, and teachers develop various theories or hunches to account for this limited participation. Until recently, so little was known about language processing problems that articulation differences had been about the only language related problem teachers had been prepared to consider. That problem explains why many of these children have been referred by classroom teachers and have received speech therapy, often for what was considered to be only minor problems. Research and experience now suggests that articulation problems in *some* children may signal more general language learning problems. These children need to be monitored as they begin to learn to read. Any difficulties they experience in acquiring reading should be noted and early referrals for reading, speech-language, or psychological evaluations should become routine.

REFERENCES

Englemann, S., and Bruner, E. C. (1974). *Distar reading.* Chicago: Science Research Associates.

Glass, G. G. (1978). *Glass analysis for perceptual conditioning.* Garden City, NY: Easier-to-Learn Materials.

Lenneberg, E. (1968). *Biological foundations of language.* New York: John Wiley and Sons.

Menyuk, P. (1978). Linguistic problems in children with developmental dysphasia. In M. A. Wyke (Ed.), *Developmental dysphasia.* London: Academic Press.

Morehead, D., and Ingram, D. (1973). The development of base syntax in normal and linguistically deviant children. *Journal of Speech and Hearing Research, 16,* 330–352.

Rabinovitch, R. D. (1968). Reading problems in children: Definitions and classification. In A. Keeney and N. Keeney (Eds.), *Dyslexia: Diagnosis and treatment of reading disorders.* St. Louis: C. V. Mosby.

Rasmussen, D., and Goldberg, L. (1967). *SRA basic reading program.* Chicago: Science Research Associates.

Rudolph, M. K., Wilson, R. G., Otto, W., and Smith, R. S. (1975). *Merrill linguistic reading program.* Columbus, OH: Charles E. Merrill.

Sawyer, D. J. (1981). The relationship between selected auditory abilities and beginning reading achievement. *Language, Speech, and Hearing Services in Schools, 12.* 95–99.

Sawyer, D. J., and Kosoff, T. O. (1981). Accommodating the learning needs of reading disabled adolescents: A language processing issue. *Learning Disability Quarterly, 4*(1), 61–67.

Stanovich, K. (1982). Individual differences in the cognitive processes of reading: I. Word decoding. *Journal of Learning Disabilities. 15*(8), 485–493.

Tallal, P., and Piercy, M. (1978). Defects of auditory perception in children with developmental dysphasia. In M. A. Wyke (Ed.), *Developmental dysphasia.* London: Academic Press.

Vellutino, F. R. (1977). Alternative conceptualizations of dyslexia: Evidence in support of a verbal-deficit hypothesis. *Harvard Educational Review, 47*(3), 334–354.

Vogel, S. A. (1975). *Syntactic abilities in normal and dyslexic children.* Baltimore: University Park Press.

Wepman, J. M. (1960). Auditory discrimination, speech and reading. *The Elementary School Journal, 9,* 325–333.

Wyke, M. A. (1978). *Developmental dysphasia.* London: Academic Press.

TRANSITIONAL NOTE

Through her case studies, Sawyer has given examples of the types of oral language deficits she has observed at the Syracuse University Reading Clinic. Reduced skill in the ability to express oneself may be one of the earliest indicators available to a teacher that a student has language-based classroom problems. Earlier chapters have provided additional examples of communication behaviors that have been observed in the high-risk population.

In Chapter 11, Hasenstab describes her approach to the evaluation of reading skills. The "psychosociolinguistic approach" she describes integrates various aspects of language—e.g., phonology, syntax, semantics, pragmatics and text cohension. As she has stated, both reading and spoken language tap into a *general language awareness.* This philosophical premise is evident in the conceptual model Hasenstab presents and the resulting evaluation procedures.

CHAPTER 11

Reading Evaluation: A Psychosociolinguistic Approach

M. Suzanne Hasenstab

Evaluation in reading is far from novel in concept or in practice. Procedures for determining reading ability in students have existed since instruction in reading began. The measurement of reading ability, mastery of so called "reading skills" and "documentation of reading problems," has been and remains a goal in both regular and special education programs. The central purpose of evaluation from a general theoretical perspective also applies to evaluation in reading—that is, to compile pertinent data that will assist in the composite illustration of abilities or deficits for a specified area. Salvia and Ysseldyke (1981) explain that the results of evaluation should provide professionals with information that will augment intervention for the fostering of strength areas and the remediation of those facets that show deficit. The issue of whether or not reading tests and other reading evaluation procedures accomplish this task is an area of current concern.

TESTS OF READING

Various measures are available that are designed to examine certain factors of reading. Tests that are considered "diagnostic" in purpose focus on the determination of problems or disabilities in the reading function of students. Achievement tests, on the other hand, attempt to specify areas of mastery or skill performance that indicate a level of operation. Content of such measures frequently overlaps, but the underlying testing purpose differs.

Within these broad purpose areas, reading evaluation may be formal (i.e., achievement testing by the school psychologist) or informal (i.e., teacher-made checklist of vocabulary comprehension). Procedures may entail the administration of standardized measures, criterion-referenced tests, or observational techniques. In addition, reading evaluation may take place in a group or individual context. Testing strategies of teachers and other professionals may actually entail a variety of tests with these different characteristic combinations in their attempt to secure applicable test results.

Diagnostic Reading Tests

The most common image of a diagnostic reading test is a formal, standardized, and individually administered examination. Many professionals include criterion-referenced tests. Observational information in the test battery, however, is still based on norm-referenced standardization. Diagnostic tests, as standardized instruments, attempt to compare a student's performance on test items with the performance of peers as represented by the normative population. How well the student fares in this comparison is expressed in scores that represent age or grade levels, percentile, ranks, or stanines. Many professionals still feel strongly that standardized instruments are the "best" measures of student ability and function. In reality, however, standardized tests in reading, as in other areas, vary extensively in technical adequacy, including limited samples, lack of reliability, and paucity of empirical evidence for validity (Salvia and Ysseldyke, 1981).

Technical quality of diagnostic tests is only one aspect that is of concern in reading evaluation. Another paramount issue relates to exactly what is being evaluated in diagnostic testing. Indeed, the question arises as to whether "reading" per se is measured at all. In theory, at least, diagnostic reading tests are developed in such a way as to tap reading ability through the presentation of items or tasks, subtests, or other components across a broad spectrum of reading and reading-related skills. Actual composition depends on the author's definition and perspective of reading, including what he or she determines as pertinent to the reading process (Hasenstab and Laughton, 1982a). In general, however, diagnostic reading tests most often include all or partial selections of the following areas:

- Oral reading
- Word analysis
- Word "attack" skills
- Word recognition
- Word meaning
- Reading rate
- Sentence or passage comprehension

We will consider the merits of each of these areas.

Oral Reading

The value of oral reading as a measure of reading ability is debatable, especially if comprehension of written material is the focus of testing. Yet mastery of oral reading has been a skill area traditionally deemed important to "reading development" in children, and it has been considered important to evaluate. Many teachers (and parents) still equate a child's ability to read and his or her ability to articulate fluently the printed words without error as a level of reading success or failure. Although this is one level of achievement, it is not "reading,"—that is, comprehension.

Diagnostic reading tests usually include oral reading subtests. Procedure requires the student to read aloud passges that are arranged in graduated order of difficulty. This order of difficulty coincides with a grade level or reading level mastery. Errors in oral reading are recorded by the examiner as well as associated reading activity behaviors, such as pointing to words, losing place, and so forth. Typical error classes are summarized by Salvia and Ysseldyke (1981) and are presented in Appendix 11–1. In addition to the attention to oral reading in diagnostic measures, there are reading tests that are categorized specifically as "tests of oral reading." Purpose and procedure are similar in both testing formats.

Oral reading poses an interesting dilemma for evaluation when reading is viewed as based in a "linguistic foundation" rather than a "skill mastery" perspective. Reading is part of written language. Written language is a visual form of communication. When a child sees words on a page, the input signal or stimulus is visual in nature. It is received and processed within the visual modality. Processing analyses of incoming data and subsequent comprehension require time. Once time demands are met, encoding of expressive behavior can occur (Hasenstab and Schoeny, 1982). In the case of reading, the coordinating expressive behavior or output avenue is also coded visually through writing (Fig. 11–1).

Written language and spoken language are both communication and linguistic forms; therefore, they share certain criteria. However, as Olson (1982) stresses, the forms are not identical or synonymous. He explains that "difficulties that children have in reading and learning to read may in part be traced to the particular structures and discrepancies...for...written text and those...[for] oral language" (p. 2). The linguistic process involves two operational directions: input or reception and output or expression. In spoken language, the primary input area is auditory, with supplemental data added by the other senses as sources of secondary verification. The complementary output avenue is motor-speech. As can be seen in Figure 11–1, there are parallels for written language.

In addition to sharing a psychosociolinguistic base, written and spoken language also share components that are the constructs of language. These

Figure 11–1. Model illustrating similarities and differences between spoken and written language.

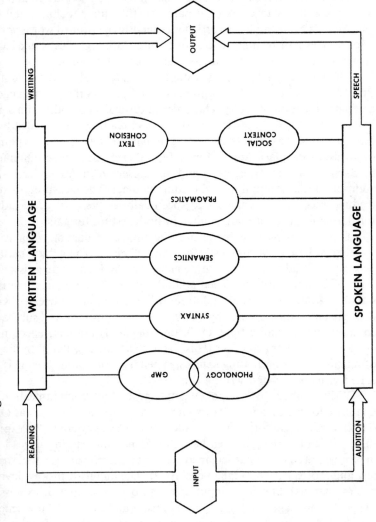

components have different representation and are coded by rules governing the modality. In spoken language, phonology represents the segmental and suprasegmental features of language, whereas in written language graphomorphophonemics (GMP) covers the parallel of letters, patterns, punctuation, and so forth. Syntax, semantics, and pragmatics are represented in both language forms but operate in either a visual or an auditory format (i.e., code requirements). In spoken communication, social and linguistic context modifies, enhances, constrains, and otherwise influences the interaction. Since a context of time and space is not usually shared in written language (except for passing notes in class), the component text cohesion is the governing contextual aspect. Because of the modality differences (visual versus auditory), codes, rules for coding and decoding, and application constraints for the components vary (Hasenstab and Laughton, 1982b).

In oral reading the reader is required to receive, process, and (it is hoped) comprehend a visual stimulus. However, he or she is then required to cross to the auditory-oral modality for expressive behavior via speech. This is frequently a difficult, or in some cases impossible, undertaking for beginning readers or children with acuity or processing modality deficits because oral reading uses both written and spoken communication avenues. Oral reading is actually a recoding (but not necessarily decoding) process of a visual code to an auditory code (Smith, 1973). The reader functions much as an interpreter taking the visual representation and coding it in the auditory-vocal form. Comprehension per se is not requisite; only a matching between the two codes. In fact, taking time to comprehend in the true sense of meaningful communication through written text actually slows down or otherwise interferes with precise oral reading. The process of oral reading can be influenced by two aspects: meaning and surface structure code. Adults and children who have proficiency with spoken and written language can balance these aspects, but children just beginning to develop written language or those with deficits cannot. Children who read orally and attend to meaning and interpretation based on their knowledge frequently fail to produce accuracy in oral reading, yet understand the passage content. Conversely, Bettelheim and Zelan (1981) point out that "error free, smooth reading aloud is unfortunately no proof that all is well" (p. 46). The reader may operate only in the arena of the code itself, merely exchanging grapheme representation for phonemic counterparts. There is no assimilation, relevance, meaning, or purpose ascribed to the printed text.

Mastery of oral reading as an aspect for evaluation is therefore deceiving. It is assumed that if a child can recode a word from printed to phonemic form he or she will understand the meaning of the word.

Therefore, if the child can read a passage efficiently he or she must also comprehend the content. However, children frequently become expert at recoding techniques. Hearing impaired children with strong phonetic emphasis in speech development therapy, for example, can become quite proficient in graphic-phonemic exchange. The following interaction was taped during a testing session of a bright, verbal hearing impaired ten year old child.

> Dr. H.: "Now, Jamie, read this paragraph out loud for me."
> Jamie reads the selected passage, quite appropriate for his developmental maturity, without error.
> Dr. H.: "That was fine. Now you tell me what the paragraph was about.
>   Tell me in your words what the author said in that paragraph."
> Jamie: "Uh - - - hmm. I dunno. Can I read it again?"

When asked to paraphrase a passage of equal difficulty after reading silently, Jamie was able to determine meaning and author intent without hesitation.

One additional consideration is important regarding oral reading. Proficient readers do not say each word to themselves as they read. Research has shown that reading rate and comprehension decrease when each word is recoded in the mind of the reader. In reality, words are grouped, received, and processed in meaningful units according to processing analyses and decisions. In oral reading we may instruct a child to "read in thought units," but the actual execution of that task may be entirely beyond children in early reading acquisition, those with language delays, and those with specific reading problems associated with the visual modality.

The use of oral reading as a vehicle for evaluation and as a measure of reading proficiency should be exercised with caution and awareness of what it does and what it does not represent. It is a skill of recoding. It does not guarantee that a child can *read*. Reading, because it is an input or receptive phase in the language-communication process, should result in comprehension of meaning and author intent. Oral reading elegance does not insure that. Oral reading can be of assistance to reading evaluation, however, when used as a foundation for miscue analysis (Goodman and Goodman, 1977), as discussed later in this chapter.

Word Analysis and Word Attack Skills

The emphasis on many aspects of word analysis and word attack techniques or skills emerges in part from the perspective that words are best understood if they can be recoded from their graphic form into their auditory representation. Word analysis actually entails much more than merely "sounding out" words or examining them in isolation. The result of word analysis should be comprehension, not just pronunciation. Diagnostic tests usually include subcomponents in these areas. Also, several tests are designed as diagnostic tests that specialize in evaluating word analysis mastery. Word analysis is the aspect associated with the ability to determine a word based on structural or contextual aspects. Such aspects relate to letter-sound representation (vowels and consonants), sequence of letter patterns (consonant or vowel clusters organization), syllable boundaries, syllabic emphasis or accent, and so forth.

Heilman (1968) summarizes word attack and word analysis domains across five main areas. The first is *phonetic or phonics analysis.* This aspect of word analysis is most often emphasized in diagnostic tests and is frequently interpreted to be at the summit of word attack strategies. In reality evaluation of a child's phonics skill determines how well he or she can recode from visual to auditory representation. The underlying skill principle is that of oral reading except that phonics subtests or components in diagnostic evaluation concentrate on letters, syllables, pseudowords, or actual words and the child's ability to pronounce them in accordance with visual to auditory exchange rules. Knowing "sounds" and blending them to articulate a word does not automatically ensure that the child comprehends the word. Yet comprehension is the ultimate purpose and goal in reading. A word may be a new to a child in both symbolic representations (auditory and visual forms), or so lacking in context, owing to isolation, that recoding value is lost if comprehension is the focus. Much can be said concerning the value or uselessness of phonics in the evaluation of reading, and the argument continues. Phonics and phonetic analysis should be seen for what they are: related skills but not an aspect of reading by themselves. They represent a low level entry (see Appendix 11-2) in the attempt to achieve comprehension of written text and are probably more useful to successful readers than those with language or reading deficits or children just beginning to use written language (Garrison and Heard, 1931; Heilman 1968; Robinson, 1971; Sexton and Herron, 1928; Smith 1973).

Another word analysis technique that does not guarantee comprehension relates to the *visual form* or *configuration* of the word. Words are visual stimuli that are characterized by a shape depending on the pattern of letters. Configuration cues are considered important from a "whole word" view. The form of the word represents its entirety rather than merely a sequence of isolated letters. Word configuration requires the ability to determine similarities and differences in visual stimuli with emphasis on form. In the strict sense, that is the first level of discrimination, with detailed determinations regarding individual elements (letters) at a second level of analysis. Form variation is an attribute of graphic format. However, it is a very rudimentary and general level of discrimination. Furthermore, in the actual reading process words are not treated as isolated forms. They are perceived in meaning units with other words. Form of a visual stimulus in reading is a feature of the total pattern but not a determination that can result completely in understanding of meaning.

Heilman's next category is *structural analysis* and concerns the student's comprehension of specific morphemes (prefixes and suffixes) and the manner in which they modulate meaning of a root or basic word. Structural analysis is a linguistic attempt to determine word meaning (but not necessarily word pronunciation); it represents growing sophistication in language mastery. Morphology is the last linguistic component to emerge in language development (Brown, 1973) and continues to refine and expand throughout the academic experience (Hasenstab, in press). A child's ability to determine the effect of morphological markers on total meaning of a phrase, sentence, or passage also contributes to semanticity (Kretschmer and Kretschmer, 1978) and syntactic expansion (deVilliers and deVilliers, 1978). Understanding of morphological alterations of words or variations of sentences therefore , contributes to meaning and subsequently comprehension and can allow entry at graphomorphophonemic (GMP), syntactic, and semantic levels (Fig. 11-2) (Hasenstab and Laughton, 1982a). Structural analysis of bound morphemes or root words does merit evaluation, but beyond the presentation of words with added prefixes or suffixes in isolation. Morphological additions should also be evaluated in the contextual meaning sense (category 4). In addition to prefix and suffix morphemes, other morphological features and their effects on phrase, sentence, or passage meaning merit evaluation. Such features might include negative markers, aspects of the auxiliary tense (be + present progressive [ing]; have + participle [en]; modals and quasi modals); adverbial and adjectival markers; and so forth. With younger children procedures such as those used by Berko (1958; Berko-Gleason, 1967) and also Brown (1973) might be helpful in determining awareness of morphological features. However, instead of using spoken items to accompany stimulus pictures, the task would require a written stimulus code of the morphological marker. This process could also be helpful in determining writing development by having the child write the correct feature application.

Use of *contextual clues* may be defined as the ability to determine a word, or more importantly its meaning and function, through the contextual relationship of the other words in the sentence or passage. This is a high level entry to comprehension and involves much more than examination techniques of a word in isolation. The ability to analyze words

Figure 11–2. The ladder effect of the PSL components in reading. From Hasenstab, M. S., and Laughton, J. (1982). *Reading, writing and exceptional children.* Reprinted with permission of Aspen Systems Corporation.

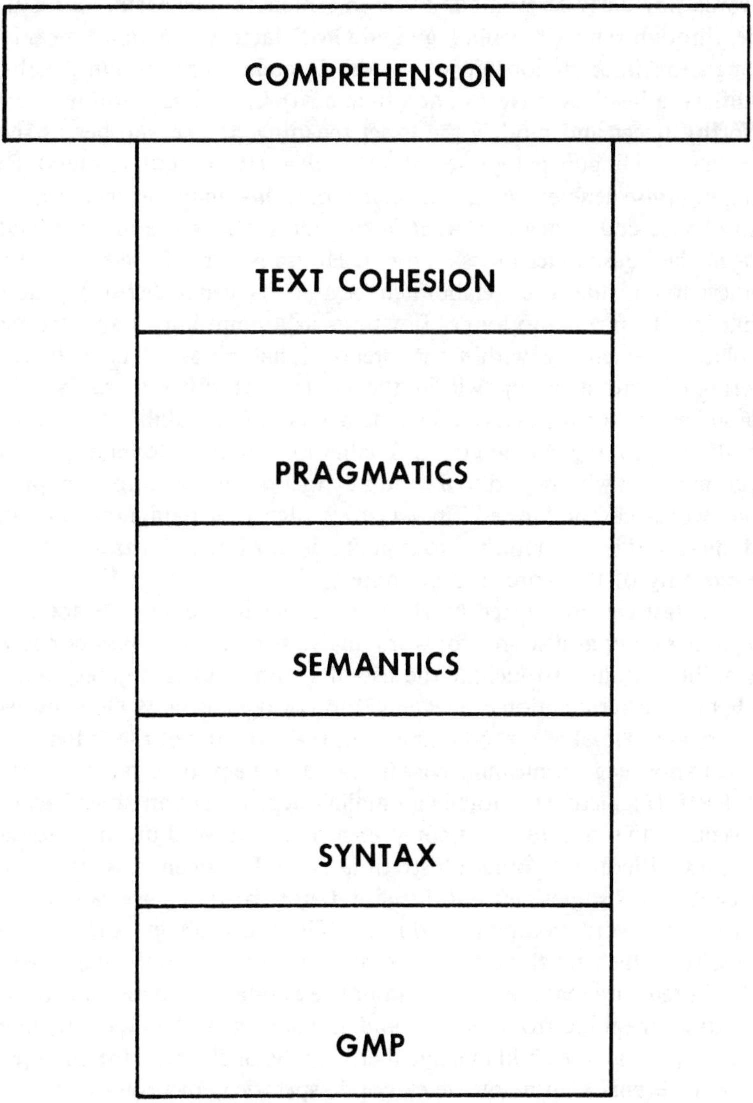

within context permits the determination of how the word functions meaningfully in a sentence, paragraph, or text. The value of contextual analysis is that the meaning of a word can be viewed in the perspective of its contribution to the total meaning that results from the interaction of all the words in the phrase, sentence, or passage. Meaning is not coded in words singularly or even additively in sentences. The surface structure code, through syntax morphology and GMP factors, facilitates meaning through the interrelationship of words. Content words (nouns, verbs), modifiers (adjectives, adverbs), and functors (prepositions, pronouns, and so forth) affect and modify the exact meaning of one another as they operate in the linguistic representation of ideas (Hasenstab, in press). For example, *house* denotes a certain meaning, *the house* indicates specification, *in the house* codes location, *went in the house* relays action, and *Paula went in the house* determines an event. House is part of the meaning of that event and has been elaborated beyond its usual dictionary noun definition. In fact, it no longer functions as a noun but as an adverbial of place interactively within the prepositional phrase. The ability to determine word meaning within the context of other words so that comprehension of a passage might be achieved is an ability that relates directly to reading as language. Evaluation in this domain presents important data with regard to a child's extraction of meaning from print. Target words can be "tested" in varying sentence or paragraph formats, and the reader is then required to explain, demonstrate, illustrate, or retell the meaning of the word in that context.

The last category listed by Heilman relates to the reader's ability to use *picture clues* as a source for word analysis. At a more elaborate level, this ability would also include the use of graphs, tables, figures, and so forth, in the determination of meaning. Employing illustrative clues involves an entry at the level of text cohesion (Fig. 11–2) and use of the individual's internal knowledge or meaning base in regard to the picture, graph, or other item itself. If a picture is a totally unfamiliar depiction of an object, action, or event, it does not augment comprehension of a word or, in a broader sense, text. Pictures or other illustrations should augment text. In reality, however, this is sometimes not the case. Before picture clues can be used to assist in word comprehension, a child must understand pictures themselves, which are also a form of symbolic representation. Young readers and children with reading deficits should be evaluated to determine if they can extract meaning from pictures and at what semantic-pragmatic level. For example, can the child merely label? Can he or she describe an object, action, or event? Can he or she elaborate specific depictions? Can he or she infer beyond what is seen? Older children should be evaluated on their ability to interpret graphs, tables, and similar material. This can be accomplished through written expression or verbal explanation.

The nature of words is actually characterized by several attributes or facets. Vellutino and Shub (1982) suggest five: graphic, orthographic, semantic, syntactic, and phonologic. An additional feature category would be contextual. Because words are multifaceted, word analysis strategies are actually used interactively by successful readers as they meet unfamiliar words in the text. Seldom do they merely "sound out" the target word. The evaluation of one form of word analysis (for example, phonetic analysis) gives only a partial view of a reader's facility in dealing with printed words and the meaning they represent. Therefore, diagnostic testing of word analysis strategies should result in data that illustrate (1) how a reader addresses words in the text, (2) the procedures he or she uses to determine their function and meaning, and (3) the effectiveness of his or her strategies. Word analysis strategies that permit entry into comprehension across several language component levels (structural analysis, context clues, picture clues) are more linguistically oriented then are those that merely tap analytic techniques at GMP level (phonetic analysis, configuration clues). Since reading is a language process, the goal in reading evaluation should be related to language as well.

Word Recognition

A subtest that is commonly included in diagnostic reading tests is one that is designed to determine a child's "sight vocabulary." Sight vocabulary includes words that are part of the reader's written language repertoire. Such words are recognized (and, it is hoped, understood) in their visual form. Usual testing procedure requires the reader to say words from lists or stimulus cards. The words are in isolation from other words and removed from a sentence frame. Word recognition, like the lower level strategies of word analyses, does not carry the guarantee of knowledge concerning what a word means or how it may be used. It often merely represents recoding skills and facility for blending sounds and marking syllables. Results of word recognition tests should be dealt with cautiously. It is not unusual for a reader to be able to identify a word in isolation yet be unable to successfully comprehend the meaning and function of a word in text.

The ability to know words "on sight," without having to resort to analysis strategies, is an important accomplishment in reading. Vellutino and Shub (1982) target word recognition or "whole word identification" as crucial in the development and mastery of written language. As an individual's sight vocabulary increases he or she can become more fluent in the reading process (provided of course, that his or her syntactic development is respected). Elaboration of a meaningful sight vocabulary permits a reader's written language repertoire to increase for both reading and writing, so that rate can be smooth and eventually flexible, and the ability to use contextual and linguistic data is enhanced. This all contributes to achieving comprehension.

The problem, however, is that word recognition tests fail to evaluate word recognition in that dimension. Such measures as exist do not ensure that the naming of a word is any more than an exercise in rapid use of phonetic analysis. Word identification implies more than attendance to the grapheme-phoneme exchanges between written and spoken language codes. True recognition of words in print concerns also the reader's recognition of that word's semantic, syntactic, morphological, and pragmatic aspects. He or she also needs to realize that words exist for the most part not in isolation from one another but in syntactic relationships with other words. Identification of words in a list or other stimulus format should be extended to evaluate word identification of those same words in sentences. These procedures can be combined with defining, demonstrating, or other tasks that illustrate the reader's identification of the target word as it operates in a particular text. In that way facets of meaning beyond the dictionary interpretation can be ascertained (affective, associative, connotative). Word identification can then provide more useful and informative testing data regarding ability in this area.

Reading Rate

The areas discussed to this point are quite familiar in the design of diagnostic reading tests. Reading rate measures, however, are less frequently included. The usual task associated with the determination of reading rate is concerned with the reader's ability to accurately and quickly read printed material that is conceptually familiar and structurally easy. The test is "how fast?" Reading rate, or more accurately, a person's ability to vary rate for different formats and purposes in reading is an area of reading mastery noted in successful readers. But it involves more than how quickly a reader can successfully complete a passage. Reading too quickly or too slowly can interfere equally with comprehension of the text.

Flexibility in reading rate is governed by three primary considerations. The first relates to the text itself. Aspects such as technical or elaborate vocabulary, complex syntactic structures, novel content, or involved conceptual presentation can singly or in combination require a reader to alter speed in reading to attain comprehension. Format of a particular text can also assist or interfere with reading rate. These factors would include print size and type, spacing of words or lines, page arrangement, and so forth. Some text formats are purposefully structured by author or printer to foster ease and rapid reading. Others appear formidable upon superficial examination.

The second consideration in rate flexibility is the reader himself. A reader selects and uses written material for his or her own purpose beyond which may have been intended by the writer. Regardless of text aspects the reader may choose a rate that suits his or her interest and purpose at that time. The important thing is that the choice is available—in other words, that the reader has sufficient ability to vary his or her reading rate as desired or as the text demands.

This choice availability leads to the third consideration, which is the match between the reader and the text. Age, experience, interest, linguistic and communicative sophistication, knowledge, and cognition of the reader must relate favorably to the text considerations. Even a fluent reader cannot hope to have choices in rate application with a passage that is unmatched to his or her particular reader composite. Beginning readers are quite limited in rate flexibility because they are new to the process as well as still in the acquisition phases of language in general. Experience in reading a variety of formats and learning the different purposes of reading will allow the development of rate flexibility. Determination of a reader's ability to vary reading rate rather than just the ability to read an easy passage quickly is an important evaluation component. Within diagnostic testing the question should be "Can the reader vary reading rate according to (a) text demands; (2) his or her own purpose?" This aspect of evaluation is not part of the standardized procedure of current diagnostic tests.

Reading Comprehension

Comprehension of printed material is not a skill or component or aspect of reading. It *is* reading. Whatever strategies, techniques, or procedures an individual uses to discern what printed form means must end in comprehension or a person is not reading. Diagnostic tests designed as reading comprehension instruments or those with comprehension subtests attempt to evaluate reading comprehension through administration of what are considered forms of comprehension, such as words, sentences, or passages. Passage comprehension is usually evaluated across three dimensions (Hasenstab and Laughton, 1982a). The first is *literal* comprehension and is directed toward how well the reader understands explicit information presented in the text. The second dimension is *inferential* comprehension and requires interpretation based on the text information. The third facet is *listening* comprehension, which requires recall after hearing a passage read aloud. The first two levels of comprehension address text as visually met by the reader and are aspects of comprehension of printed form. The third, listening comprehension, is not; this aspect lies in the domain of spoken language. What an individual comprehends of information presented in the spoken modality may not coincide with what he or she comprehends in the visual representation. Listening comprehension evaluation via recall procedures is a helpful and useful measure of language development and understanding, but in the spoken domain. An individual who reads a passage and then recalls it by retelling or writing information retains the visual input modality of reading. Procedures that combine and compare listening comprehension and visual comprehension by means of recall strategies can be very helpful in determining if a child has a reading or language deficit that is modality specific or one that emerges from the linguistic base itself.

Most often comprehension is tapped through the presentation of questions, although recall procedures may yield more accurate information regarding comprehension. In questioning, it is assumed that if the reader can answer a question correctly he or she has understood what he has been read. However, if the child does not respond correctly to a target question, it cannot by that fact be taken for granted that he or she does not understand the text. The child may not have understood the question. The ability to answer questions is a complex process that involves a level of sophistication regarding the pragmatic, semantic, syntactic, and morphological aspects of question forms themselves. Mastery of question form comprehension is part of language proficiency, not a reading skill. Frequently the stimulus question itself is more difficult for a language impaired child to comprehend than the content of the passage he or she has read. The ability to answer spoken and written questions should be evaluated from the broader perspective of language assessment rather than a measure of reading comprehension. The results cannot be interpreted without danger of misinformation. In most instances this condition of question comprehension is totally unaccounted for in diagnostic reading tests.

In addition to passage comprehension, diagnostic tests attempt to examine both sentence and word understanding. This may involve such tasks as drawing a line or circle or pointing to a picture or word that best depicts the meaning of a word, phrase, or sentence. A variation of this form of activity also displays a picture as the stimulus and provides a choice or words or sentences from which to determine a match. Definitions, explanations, synonyms, analogy completions, cloze procedures, demonstration, and action are also ways used in evaluating comprehension of words, phrases, and sentences (Hasenstab and Laughton, 1982a).

Comprehension at this level should not be generalized to a reader's ability to comprehend passages. Word understanding and even basic sentence meaning may be less proficient when placed in more complex structural formats of a passage.

Tests currently used for the evaluation of reading comprehension are generally unsatisfactory. Vellutino and Shub (1982) state that presently used tests have little theoretical basis, fail to reflect current linguistic research, and ignore aspects related to the cognitive and experiential requirements for comprehension. Tuinman (1973) poses the question of exactly what reading comprehension tests actually measure. From his in-depth evaluation of the five most frequently used tests, he concludes that the measures fail to ensure that errors that are found are due to reading miscomprehension. Format, content, procedure, and underlying perspectives of testing comprehension of printed language are definitely areas in need of updating and revamping. Standardized tests will have to be supplemented if an accurate view of a reader's comprehension is to be achieved.

Achievement Tests

Diagnostic procedures are used to determine the presence and extent of a reading or writing deficit. Achievement tests are aspects in determining a performance level or monitoring progress of a student. Achievement tests appear in a wider variety of forms than do diagnostic tests and may also have different purposes (i.e., screening versus class placement). In most instances achievement testing is concerned with skill mastery related to levels of accomplishment (age, grade, and so forth). Testing results supposedly indicate areas in which skills have been mastered and those in which they have not. Gaps in skill development are also frequently noted. Reading achievement tests are in the form of standardized tests (group and individual), informal commercially produced tests, or informal teacher-made measures. In some cases criterion-referenced tests are used, and for some programming decisions they are actually preferred.

Criterion-referenced tests offer some advantages over more traditional standardized approaches because they are not intended to compare a child with a normative population (which may be inappropriate). Performance is determined by whether or not a child can complete items designed to meet certain criteria deemed to be important. Theoretically, criterion-referenced tests can produce results that allow greater flexibility and individuality when applied to program design and objectives (Proger and Mann, 1973).

The most popular commercially produced achievement tests are of a battery designed with subtests that examine several different academic areas (Table 11-1). Reading components mostly relate to vocabulary (word recognition), general comprehension of words, sentences, or short passages, or phonetic analysis (or all of these). They do not attempt in-depth reading evaluation since overall academic functioning is the primary purpose of testing.

Reading achievement tests of all types suffer from the same problems as are evident in reading diagnostic instruments. Technical problems, absence of theoretical bases, questionable form, content, and procedure, and ignorance of linguistic, cognitive, and learning principles all contribute to the questionable data that result. Karlin (1971) suggests that achievement tests are useful as screening devices in that they can target children in need of more in-depth evaluation. As far as reading is concerned, great caution must be exercised in placing trust in either global reading scores or skill area scores defined by grade or age level equivalents. A child may perform specified tasks according to a correlation with a said normed sample—for example, naming words in a list—but that information does not specify how or how well he or she deals with written language.

Summary of a Critique of Current Reading Evaluation Procedures

Reading evaluation emerges from a laudable assumption that is also at least theoretically sound. That is, if we can evaluate reading ability in an individual so as to determine how well he or she uses the process, we can then go about the business of augmenting deficits and developing further proficiency. The practice of reading evaluation, however, does not sufficiently accomplish this end. Serious criticism has been leveled against reading evaluation and with just cause (Goldberg and Schiffman, 1972; King, 1977; Salvia and Ysseldlyke, 1981; Smith, 1973). Evidence of problems across many dimensions has been aptly illustrated. That is not to say that strides are not being made in an attempt to develop accurate and appropriate systems for evaluation. A vast body of knowledge has emerged in recent years that addresses the nature of reading as language rather than as an academic area or skill in itself. We have also learned a great deal regarding language and communication and the relationship that exists with cognition, social considerations, and learning in general. Yet little if any of this knowledge is reflected in the methods used to evaluate reading even at the most basic levels of testing. For example, it is accepted that words vary in meaning based on context of other words and the intent

Table 11-1. Achievement Tests with Reading Subjects

Test	Areas Evaluated
Comprehensive Test of Basic Skills (CTBS). E. Tiegs and W. Clarke. Monterey, CA: McGraw-Hill (1968, revised 1970).	Reading vocabulary Reading comprehension
Metropolitan Achievement Test (MAT). B. Balow, H. Bixler, W. Durost, G. Prescott, and J. Wrightstone. New York: Harcourt, Brace, Jovanovich (1970).	Reading vocabulary Word analysis Reading comprehension
Peabody Individual Achievement Test (PIAT). L. Dunn and F. Markwardt. Circle Pines, MN: American Guidance Service (1970).	Reading vocabulary
Wide Range Achievement Test (WRAT). J. Jastak, S. Kijou, and S. Jastak. Wilmington, DE: Guidance Associates of Delaware (1973, revised 1975).	Reading vocabulary
SRA Achievement Series. R. A. Naslund, L. P. Thorpe, and D. W. Lefever. Chicago: Science Research Associates (1954, revised 1958, 1963, 1978).	Word-picture association Reading vocabulary Reading comprehension
Woodcock-Johnson Psychoeducational Battery: Tests of Achievement. R. Woodcock and M. Johnson. Hingham, Maine: Teaching Resources Corp. (1977).	Reading vocabulary Reading comprehension Word analysis

From Hasenstab, M. S., and Laughton, J. (1982). *Reading, writing and exceptional children.* Rockville, MD: Aspen Systems. Reprinted with permission of Aspen Systems Corporation.

of an author. Yet we persist in targeting words in isolation as the measure of word identification. Worse yet, the criterion for task success is saying the words with no attention to comprehension—an aspect that is assumed. Changes are difficult but crucial in light of new learning. In the meantime children, however, are still failing to gain facility for written language under the traditional approaches to reading evaluation and subsequent instruction based on testing results. They may eventually master the skills targeted on the test, but they still cannot read.

Awareness of the inability of certain individuals to use written language effectively has been noted in professional literature since the 1870s (Kussmaul, 1877; Morgan, 1896). Individuals were described as having normal visual acuity, intelligence, and speech but were unable to comprehend or write any printed information except for a few simple words. The condition was originally termed *word blindness* but was later labeled *dyslexia.*

Attempts were made to classify the characteristics of those who were unable to read or write (Orton, 1937), and speculation was made as to possible causes (Robinson, 1946). Characteristics and causes have continued to be sources of research and discussion (Wallace and Larsen, 1978), with good reason. The greatest source of academic failure is reading disability (Strang, 1969). Amid this great concern professionals have also devised a wealth of nomenclature and a variety of definitions. Research and study has continued to advance our knowledge of reading and writing that is currently accepted as linguistic and communicative in nature. New data are directly applicable to investigations concerning disabilities of written language as well. Olson (1982) states that "the central problem in reading and writing...is linguistic" (p. 1). The central deficit of reading disability is the inability to comprehend language in the written or visual code (Smith, 1971; Spiro, Bruce, and Brewer, 1980; Sticht, 1977). Deficits in reading emerge from deficits in the language components and they may affect both spoken and written language to a greater or lesser degree—or in some cases may be modality specific. Language deficits are best viewed along a continuum of severity with mild problems at one end, such as a delay in articulation development, to a total inability to code or represent any internal knowledge linguistically at the other end. The language deficit may interfere predominantly with one component of language—for example, a pragmatic deficit. However, because of the interactive nature of the linguistic components, some effect is frequently evident across all aspects.

In view of current information available and the altered definitions of reading, writing, and written language deficits as they pertain to language, it would seem logical that language would be the legitimate basis for reading evaluation as well.

LANGUAGE AS THE BASIS FOR READING EVALUATION

Gradually more and more professionals are moving toward the acceptance of written language as a form of communication. Much of this acceptance is evident only in selected literature, professional presentations, and academic course offerings. The filtering from theory and discussion to actual use and application is still too often the exception rather than the rule of practice. There are several basic evaluation strategies presently in use that are linguistically oriented. They can be carefully structured to accent the evaluation of reading so that it pertains to written language function.

A Model to Begin With

Hasenstab and Laughton (1982a) present a fundamental model based on the psychosociolinguistic components of language as related to reading and writing. The elaborated term of *psychosociolinguistic* (PSL) is applied to the components because of the inherent relationship of language to cognition and social factors. The model is governed by several underlying assumptions:

- Reading is a linguistic process.
- Reading is therefore governed by the PSL components.
- The rules generated by the PSL components for reading are specific to written language. (Reading is not spoken language written down.)
- The PSL components are mutally interactive in the reading process.
- Simultaneous use of the PSL components is the best assurance of comprehension.
- Comprehension represents the verification of hypothesis generated through the PSL components.

Aspects and Structure of the Model

The model is based on the nature of written language and is structured about the PSL components as manifested in that form. The five aspects are: text cohesion, pragmatics, semantics, syntax, and graphomorphophonemics. The model is concerned with how printed format represents these components and the linguistic knowledge of the individual reader of the rules, roles, and application strategies related to these components for comprehension and production in written language. In this sense reading and writing are seen as the ability to code and decode knowledge via written symbolic representation.

Text Cohesion. Halliday and Hasan (1976) describe text as being of three facets: (a) a semantic unit, (b) a unit of language in use, and (c) passage. These facets produce a unified whole. Text cohesion is a tie that allows ideas represented in written form to hold together. It is that PSL component that governs the relatedness between sentences, as in cataphoric and anaphoric reference, paragraph structure, use of conjunctive forms, and so forth. Cohesion is coded via vocabulary (semantics) and structure (syntax and graphomorphophonemics). Text cohesion also concerns physical aspects (titles, pictures, and so forth), structure of information (paragraphing, dialogue, and so forth), and attributes that differ one written form from another (story format, essay format, and so forth).

Text cohesion is usually ignored in discussions of reading and writing even in current literature, yet it is extremely important as a component in written language. The statement that reading and writing are parallel but not identical to listening and speaking is frequently made. One aspect, beyond the differences depicted in Figure 11-1, is the absence of spoken and social context in written language (Olson, 1982). Spoken language, by virtue of a shared time and space and the ability of the speaker to monitor the listener as to the comprehension of his or her intent and meaning, accounts for cohesion. Written language, on the other hand, is dependent upon aspects of text cohesion interrelated with the other PSL components to accomplish the communication of information from author to reader.

Pragmatics. The area of pragmatics is presently entertaining a vast amount of attention and popularity. Much of this attention is directed toward the role of pragmatics in spoken language, but the issues also relate to written language. Underlying intent (Clark and Clark, 1977; Dale, 1980; Dore, 1973; Searle, 1969, 1975), discourse rules (Chapman, 1981; Kretschmer, 1980; Snow, 1977), presupposition and awareness of audience (Foppa and Kaserman, 1979; Greenfield, 1978; Halliday and Hasan, 1976), and cuing of old and new information (Clark and Haviland, 1977; Haviland and Clark, 1974) are all governed by pragmatics and are operational in written language. The domain of pragmatics relates closely to text cohesion and concerns function, purpose, style, and register of written language. Pragmatics is cued through the surface structure components of syntax and graphomorphophonemics. Like text cohesion, it is frequently ignored or merely alluded to even in current literature that addresses application in written language.

Semantics. The component of semantics is perhaps the most elusive and esoteric aspect of language (Hasenstab, in press). It is extremely difficult to study and is usually underdefined in its nature and role in language. Semantics governs meaning but beyond the usual interpretation of vocabulary. Reading evaluation and consequent intervention have been concerned with word and superficial sentence meaning but only cursory attention has been directed to semantics in relation to paragraph or text. Comprehension of sentences, paragraphs, and text is dependent on context provided by the text and previous and current knowledge of the world (and language) possessed by the reader. Semantic propositions that underlie sentences are coded via syntax and graphomorphophonemics and contribute to the attaining of comprehension.

Schema theory, emerging from research on memory, comprehension, and learning (Bartlett, 1932; Kintsch, 1974; Kintsch and Green, 1978; Piaget, 1952), offers a workable foundation for understanding the relationship between meaning in the broader perspective of language, cognition and similar aspects, and cognitive processes of organization, memory, and the coding of meaning in the form of written language.

Syntax. The contribution of syntax to the process of reading has been well defined (Smith and Goodman, 1971; Smith, 1973) and continues to hold focus in current literature. The primary role of syntax is to code, via structural aspects, the pragmatic and semantic PSL components. Syntax is also one vehicle of text cohesion, although in itself it is considered a low level entry to comprehension. Since syntax continues to be refined and expanded throughout the elementary school years (Chomsky, 1969), development is frequently evident in both spoken and written language. Awareness of what aspects of syntax a child understands and uses in spoken language (Klee and Paul, 1981) is a legitimate basis for determination of syntactic mastery in written language.

Graphomorphophonemics (GMP). The GMP component (Kretschmer, 1979) pertains to the rules that govern how words are written, modification cues for meaning changes, and aspects of punctuation. It concerns a sense of letters, spelling patterns, and grapheme-phoneme exchanges. GMP is to written language as phonology is to spoken form. Like syntax, GMP codes the other PSL components and assists in determining meaning and intent. GMP in itself does not yield comprehension. It may allow recoding of a word from an unfamiliar written representation to a familiar spoken symbol, but it is inefficient for connected written language.

The Ladder Effect

The PSL components in written language may be viewed as a ladder, with each stem operating as an access or entry level at which to hypothesize in order to attain comprehension (Fig. 11–2). The entry levels relate and tap into the existing cognitive and linguistic knowledge of the reader for that level. For example, the individual may begin to "attack" a written passage at GMP level, but this only allows a word by word (or less efficiently a letter by letter) hypothesis formulation and a long and circuitous route to the goal of comprehension. Each level is dependent on other levels for the most efficient progress in reading. Therefore, hypotheses must be made at all levels, but because the domains of the PSL components govern different aspects of language (and therefore reading), some levels will provide more direct links to comprehension than others (text cohesion, pragmatics, semantics versus syntax or GMP). Successful readers actually use all levels simultaneously or enter at whatever point is deemed necessary to determine precise aspects of meanings. In order to use all levels effectively, experience and learning must be directed toward awareness of all the PSL components. Unfortunately, such has not been the practice.

Evaluation of Reading Based on the Model

The model presented here and forming the basis for the Hasenstab and Laughton textbook on written language (1982a) can serve as a starting point in reading evaluation. Table 11-2 summarizes model components that are represented in selected standardized tests. However, in order to evaluate systematically across all of the PSL components, supplementary testing is vital. It is the contention of Hasenstab and Laughton (1982a) that unless systematic examination of the reader's operation in relation to all of the PSL components is undertaken, a complete language perspective is being ignored. Strategies of evaluation that are helpful are paraphrase and recall, miscue analysis, analysis of written language samples, and task observation.

Text Cohesion and Pragmatics. The PSL components of text cohesion and pragmatics can be evaluated through analyses of written language samples or by task observation and structured discussion with a reader. Evaluation based on written language samples should be composed of a collection of examples rather than a single one. The student's ability to apply PSL components may be noted using the following questions as guidelines (Hasenstab and Laughton, 1982a, p. 75).

- Is there a title?
- Does the title relate to the context of the passage?
- Do the introductory sentences cue text format (story, essay, and so forth)?
- What is the format of the passage (story, essay, letter, poem, and so forth)?
- Does the sample collection contain variations in format types?
- What format variations are represented?
- What format variation is used most frequently?
- Are format requirements carried throughout the passage (story grammar, essay development, letter form, and so forth)?
- Is paragraphing used (unless a poem)?
- Are paragraphs marked, and if so, how?
- Do paragraphs relate to the passage's central theme?
- Do sentences within each paragraph tie together?
- How are sentences tied together (tense, conjunctions, repetition of information, and so forth)?
- How is old and new information coded (articles, pronominalization, cataphoric or anaphoric reference, relativization, and so forth)?

- Is information prioritized and in what way?
- Is intent clear?

Younger children and children with severe delays in language acquisition who are not yet using written expression may be evaluated by observation and questioning or directives from the examiner. Recommended questions and directives are presented below. These can also be used in addition to written language sample analyses. Specific questions must, of course, relate to a particular child's age and estimated experiences.

Questions relating to purpose of books and reading:
- What is a book?
- Why do you (or does anyone) read?
- What can books tell us?
- What is the author telling you (select a passage for reading)?
- What is the topic? (What is this book or passage about?)

Questions relating to format:
- Show me _____ (parts of a book, cover, page, title, author, letter, word, sentence, paragraph, beginning, end, table of contents, index, and so forth)
- What does a _____ (title, table of contents, glossary, and so forth) tell you?
- What kind of book is this (books or passages representing various formats: animal story, fairy tale, poem, and so forth)?

Questions relating to contextual clues:
- What can you tell me about the picture (or other graphic illustration) in this book or passage?
- Does the picture (or graphic illustration) relate to the text?

Semantics. For a true perspective regarding a reader's grasp of meaning, semantics should be evaluated at word, sentence, and passage levels. Word meaning may be accomplished through subtests on various standardized tests, as can some precursory measure of sentence comprehension. In addition, miscue analysis has been used quite extensively by several researchers as a strategy for evaluation in reading (Bettelheim and Zelan, 1981; Burke and Goodman, 1970; Carlson, 1975; DeLawter, 1975; K. Goodman, 1967, 1969; Y. Goodman, 1970; Lipton, 1972; Nurss, 1969; Wardbaugh, 1969; Weaver, 1980; Zintz, 1980; Zutell, 1977). Miscue analysis allows insight into the strategies and processes that a reader uses in his or her approach to written language. It also provides information concerning background experiences, vocabulary preferences, general knowledge, and, in some cases, attitudes toward a topic or reading in general. The advantage of miscue analysis is that it examines words in context rather than in isolation. Two helpful sources for miscue analysis are the Reading Miscue Inventory (RMI) developed by Y. Goodman and

Table 11-2. Application of the Model Through Existing Diagnostic Reading Tests

GMP	Syntax	Semantics	Pragmatics	Test Cohesion
Consonant, vowel, letters, etc.: Botel (1978) Spache (1972) Gates-McKillop (1962) Roswell-Chall (1959) Durrell (1955) Stanford Diagnostic (1977) Woodcock Reading Mastery (1973) Blends: Spache (1972) Syllabication: Botel (1978) Spache (1972) Gates-McKillop (1962) Roswell-Chall (1959) Silent Reading Test (1970)	Test of Syntactic Abilities (1978)	Word recognition (in context): Silent Reading Test (1970) Stanford Diagnostic (1977) Word opposites: Botel (1978) Word definitions: Gates-McKillop (1962) Nelson-Denny (1973) Stanford Diagnostic (1977) Phrase meaning: Gates-McKillop (1962) Woodcock Reading Mastery (1973) Sentence comprehension: Stanford Diagnostic (1977)		

Table 11-2 (continued).

GMP	Syntax	Semantics	Pragmatics	Test Cohesion

Rhyming words:
  Botel (1978)
 	
Nonsense words:
  Botel (1978)
  Gates-McKillop (1962)
 	
Spelling:
  Durrell (1955)
  Gates-McKillop (1962)
 	
Word recognition (out of context):
  Botel (1978)
  Spache (1972)
  Gates-McKillop (1962)
  Silent Reading Test (1970)
  Sipay (1974)
  Stanford Diagnostic (1977)
  Woodcock Reading Mastery (1973)
		Passage comprehension:
		  Spache (1972)
		  Durrell (1955)
		  Gilmore (1968)
		  Nelson-Denny (1973)
		  Stanford Diagnostic (1977)
		  Woodcock Reading Mastery (1973)		

From Hasenstab, M. S., and Laughton, J. (1982). *Reading, writing and exceptional children.* Rockville, MD: Aspen Systems. Reprinted with permission of Aspen Systems Corporation.

Burke (1972) and Weaver's (1980) discussion of miscue interpretation. Bettelheim and Zelan (1981) provide a perspective of psychological explanation of miscues and the preoccupation of young readers with applying meaning to text.

With regard to sentence comprehension, Kamm (1979) stresses analysis of specific information and detail and synthesis of underlying meaning through sentence paraphrase or restatement with form variation. In paraphrase or restatement, the meaning remains intact but the surface structure is altered (therefore this is also a measure of syntactic flexibility), or words may be changed. For example, the following sentences change in surface structure or vocabulary but retain the underlying proposition.

Mommy made cookies.

Mommy baked cookies.

Mother made cookies.

The cookies were baked by Mommy.

To evaluate semantics from the broader perspective of passage meaning, paraphrase and passage retelling or rewriting is of benefit. Attention should be directed toward the balance or imbalance of noting detail and the ability to comprehend the underlying meaning of the passage. If questioning is used, the considerations discussed previously should be carefully entertained. In addition, correct answers to questions that are analytical and directed toward detail (What is the boy's name? Where did he go?) are no guarantee of comprehension of the passage. Guidelines for evaluating passage comprehension are as follows (Hasenstab and Laughton, 1982a, p. 76):

• Can the child ascertain the underlying meaning?

• Can the child infer information that is not explicitly stated in the text?

• Can the child draw implications beyond the text?

• How does the child treat new vocabulary or concepts?

• Does the child impose his or her own meaning on the text?

Schema theory application is also very useful, as mentioned earlier. Determination of reader comprehension according to factors of schema selection, availability, and maintenance will contribute to the reader composite. It is suggested that the explanation of schema theory by Pearson and Spiro (1980) be consulted.

Syntax. The area of syntax can be evaluated through analysis of a collection of written language samples. The Test of Syntactic Abilities (TSA) (Quigley, Steinkamp, Power, and Jones, 1978) is a commercial measure that is helpful in a general examination of syntax and structures represented in a child's language repertoire. The examiner who is evaluating syntax should be familiar with syntactic development and the aspects of syntax (base structure and transformations). Complexity of sentences varies according to the nature of the transformations used. Frequently testing procedures are inappropriate because the evaluator does not sufficiently understand the nature and role of syntax in written language. An evaluation of syntax through a spoken language sample is also helpful in determining the overall level of syntactic development of a child. This should be compared to the written sample to determine continuity across language modes. In addition, observation of syntactic forms that are understood by the child in spontaneous interaction and in reading should be noted. Performing designated tasks and paraphrasing are helpful techniques.

These general quidelines should be addressed:

• What sentence forms does the child understand and use in (a) spoken language; (b) written language?

• Does the child use a variety of sentence forms in speaking and in writing?

• Does the child understand a variety of sentence forms in listening and in reading?

• Does the child effectively code his or her meaning and intent via syntax in written and spoken modes?

Table 11-3 describes "high risk language behaviors" that a student with potential reading problems might show.

Graphomorphophonemics (GMP). Of all the PSL components, this area has received the greatest attention (Table 11-2), at least at the phoneme-grapheme level. It is suggested that attention also be directed toward the morphological features and how they alter meaning and the linguistic functions of punctuation, capitalization, spacing, and so forth, for the coding of text cohesion, pragmatics, and semantics.

Reading and Writing

One further issue should be brought into focus in the discussion of evaluation in reading. It concerns the relationship of reading and writing. The fact that they are both part of the written language process has permeated this chapter. Indeed, literature increasingly indicates that reading and writing are not just related but are mutually supportive in development. Acquisition in reading is reflected in expansion and refinement in writing, and vice versa (Applebee, 1977; Morris, 1981). Therefore, they should both be addressed in evaluation of written language. Even very young children can be evaluated along the lines of purpose and function of reading and writing (Is this a word? Show me a letter. Make a letter, and so forth) and in the areas of text cohesion and pragmatics. Traditionally reading has been

Table 11–3. Possible Reading High-Risk Indicators Related to Spoken Language

I. Phonology

Developmental delay in articulation acquisition
Multiple omissions, substitutions, and distortions in speech sound
    production
Poor intelligibility of speech
Disruption in prosody
Difficulty in sound orientation
Problems in selective auditory attention
Problems in sustained auditory attention
Inability to determine nature of sound (human versus
    environmental)

II. Syntax

Use of restricted forms in sentences
Use of ungrammatical forms
Overuse of short basic sentences
Limited application of transformations
Lack of appropriate pronoun use
Limited variety of sentence forms
Misapplication of articles, deictic forms
Inability to sequence information (auditory)

III. Semantics

Limited vocabulary
Narrow use of semantic cases
Failure to understand verbal directions
Failure to understand discourse
Limited concept development
Underdeveloped schema
Inability to synthesize auditory information

IV. Pragmatics

Failure to communicate intent
Inability to follow turntaking routines
Failure to cue the listener to the topic of discussion
Failure to use clarification strategies when misunderstood
Overdependence on performatives
Inability to comprehend and communicate old and new
    information

an academic area of its own, and writing has been addressed in the realm of language arts or English. In reality, however, they are the input and output aspects of the same system. Reading and writing, like their counterparts in spoken language, are also best learned and therefore best evaluated with regard to their existence for communication (Harste, Burke, and Woodward, 1981; Holt and Vacca, 1981). Isolated skills do not allow fluency in the use of written language, nor do they tell that an individual has mastered the process. Stotsky (1982) stresses that written expression allows for the exercise of the form particular to written language. Therefore, activities of recall, paraphrase, inferencing, and so forth, require the internalization and use of written language rules. Writing demands active involvement in reading. Kroll's (1977) much-quoted comment applies: "writers write reading" (p. 7).

SUMMARY

The evaluation of reading is a concern of professionals and parents alike. The mastery of reading is considered a mark of success in our society, and in many cases it is actually a requirement for survival. Yet many children fail to acquire literacy. An understanding that reading is language, that reading *and* writing constitute the process of written language, and that written language is not spoken language written down is emerging and receiving acceptance. Integration of this knowledge must now be made into the areas of evaluation and subsequent intervention. Written language mastery is more than mastery of skills—it is the acquisition of a communication system and should be addressed as such.

REFERENCES

Anderson, R., and Ortony, A. (1975). On putting apples into bottles: A problem of polysemy. *Cognitive Psychology, 7,* 167–180.

Applebee, A. (1977). Writing and reading. *Journal of Reading, 20,* 534–537.

Barclay, J. (1973). The role of comprehension in remembering sentences. *Cognitive Psychology, 4,* 229–254.

Bartlett, F. (1932). *Remembering.* Cambridge, MA: Harvard University Press.

Bettelheim, B., and Zelan, K. (1981). *On learning to read.* New York: Alfred A. Knopf.

Berko, J. (1958). The child's learning of English morphology. *Word, 14,* 150–177.

Berko-Gleason, J. (1967). Do children imitate? In *Proceedings of the International Conference on Oral Education of the Deaf.* Washington, DC: A. G. Bell Association for the Deaf.

Brown, R. (1973). *A first language.* Cambridge, MA: Harvard University Press.

Burke, C., and Goodman, K. (1970). When a child reads: A psycholinguistic analysis. *Elementary English, 47,* 121-129.

Carlson, K. (1975). A different look at reading in the content areas. In W. Page (Ed.), *Help for reading teachers.* Urbana IL: National Conference for Reading Teachers. ERIC Clearinghouse on Reading and Communication Skills.

Carpenter, P., and Just, M. (1975). Sentence comprehension: A psycholinguistic processing model of verification. *Psychological Review, 82,* 45-73.

Chapman, R. (1981). Exploring children's communicative intents. In J. F. Miller, *Assessing language production in children.* Baltimore: University Park Press.

Chomsky, C. (1969). *The acquisition of syntax in children from 5 to 10.* Cambridge, MA: MIT Press.

Clark, H., and Clark, E. (1977). *Psychology and language.* New York: Harcourt Brace Jovanovich.

Clark, H., and Haviland, G. (1977). Comprehension and the given-new contract. In R. Freedle (Ed.), *Discourse production and comprehension.* Norwood, NJ: Ablex.

Dale, P. (1980). Is early pragmatic development measurable? *Journal of Child Language, 7,* 1-12.

DeLawter, J. (1975). The relationships of beginning reading instruction and miscue patterns. In W. Page (Ed.), *Help for reading teachers.* Urbana, IL: National Conference on Research in English, ERIC Clearinghouse on Reading and Communication Skills.

Dore, J. (1973). *The development of speech acts.* Unpublished doctoral dissertation, New York: City University of New York.

Foppa, K., and Kaserman, M. (1979). *Some determinants of modifications in child language.* Nijmegen, The Netherlands: Max Planck Institute of Psycholinguistics.

Garrison, S., and Heard, M. (1931). An experimental study of the value of phonetics. *Peabody Journal of Education, 9,* 9-14.

Goldberg, H., and Schiffman, G. (1972). *Dyslexia—problems of reading disabilities.* New York: Grune & Stratton.

Goodman, K. (1967). Reading: A psycholinguistic guessing game. *Journal of the Reading Specialist, 6,* 126-135.

Goodman, K. (1969). Oral reading miscues: Applied psycholinguistics. *Reading Research Quarterly, 5,* 9-30.

Goodman, K., and Goodman, Y. (1977). Learning about psycholinguistic processes by analyzing oral reading. *Harvard Educational Review* (Special issue) *47,* 317-333.

Goodman, Y., (1970). Using children's reading miscues for new teaching strategies. Reading Teacher, *23,* 455-459.

Goodman, Y., and Burke, C. (1972). *Reading miscue inventory: Manual procedure for diagnosis and remediation.* New York: Macmillan.

Greenfield, P. (1978). Informativeness, presupposition, and semantic choice in single word utterances. In N. Waterson and C. Snow (Eds.), *The development of communication.* New York: John Wiley.

Halliday, M., and Hasan, R. (1976). *Cohesion in English.* London: Longman.

Harste, J., Burke, C. and Woodward, V. (1981). Children's language and world: Initial encounters in print. In J. Langer and M. Smith-Burke (Eds.), *Bridging the gap: Author meets reader.* Newark, DE: International Reading Association.

Hasenstab, M. S. (in press). Refinement and expansion in language acquisition. In J. Laughton and M. S. Hasenstab (Eds.), *Acquisition of communication.* Rockville, MD: Aspen Systems.

Hasenstab, M. S., and Laughton, J. (1982a). *Reading, writing and exceptional children.* Rockville, MD: Aspen Systems.

Hasenstab, M. S., and Laughton, J. (1982b). Two faces of language. *Journal of the Speech and Hearing Association of Virginia, 23,* 57–63.

Hasenstab, M. S., and Schoeny, Z. (1982). Auditory processing. In M. S. Hasenstab and J. Horner (Eds.), *Comprehensive intervention with hearing impaired infants and preschool children.* Rockville, MD: Aspen Systems.

Haviland, S., and Clark, H. (1974). What's new? Acquiring new information as a process in comprehension. *Journal of Verbal Learning and Verbal Behavior, 13,* 512–521.

Heilman, A. (1968). *Phonics in proper perspective.* Columbus, OH: Charles E. Merrill.

Holt, S., and Vacca, J. (1981). Reading with a sense of writer: Writing with a sense of reader. *Language Arts, 58:* 937–941.

Kamm, J. (1979). Focusing reading comprehension instruction: Sentence meaning skills. In O. Pennock (Ed.), *Reading comprehension at four linguistic levels.* Newark, DE: International Reading Association.

Karlin, R. (1971). *Teaching elementary reading: Principles and strategies.* New York: Harcourt Brace Jovanovich.

King, M. (1977). Evaluating reading. *Theory Into Practice, 16,* 407–418.

Kintsch, W. (1974). *The representation of meaning in memory.* New York: John Wiley.

Kintsch, W., and Greene, E. (1978). The role of culture-specific schemata in the comprehension and recall of stories. *Discourse Processes, 1,* 1–13.

Klee, T., and Paul, R. (1981). A comparison of six structural procedures. In J. F. Miller (Ed.), *Assessing language production in children—Experimental procedures.* Baltimore: University Park Press.

Kretschmer, R. (1979). *Language development in the hearing impaired: Assessment and educational planning needs.* Paper presented at Atlanta Area School for the Deaf, Atlanta, GA.

Kretschmer, R., and Kretschmer, L. (1978). *Language development and intervention with the hearing impaired.* Baltimore, MD: University Park Press.

Kroll, B. (1977). *Writer and reader as complementary roles.* Paper presented at North Central Reading Association, Champaign, IL.

Kussmaul, A. (1877). Disturbance of speech. *Cyclopedia of Practical Medicine. 14,* 581–875.

Lipton, A. (1972). Miscalling while reading aloud: A point of view. *Reading Teacher, 25,* 759–762.

Morgan, W. (1896). A case of congenital word blindness. *British Medical Journal, 2,* 1376–1379.

Morris, D. (1981). Concept of word: A developmental phenomenon in the beginning reading and writing process. *Language Arts, 58,* 659–667.

Nurss, J. (1969). Oral reading errors and reading comprehension. *Reading Teacher, 22,* 523–527.

Olson, D. (1982). The language of schooling. *Topics in Language Disorders, 2*(4), 1–12.

Orton, S. (1937). *Reading, writing and speech problems in children.* New York: W. W. Norton and Co.

Pearson, P., and Spiro, R. (1980). Toward a theory of reading comprehension instruction. *Topics in Language Disorders, 1,* 71–88.

Piaget, J. (1952). *The child's conception of number.* New York: W. W. Norton and Co.

Proger, B., and Mann, L. (1973). Criterion-referenced measurement: The world of gray versus black and white. *Journal of Learning Disabilities, 6,* 72–84.

Quigley, S., Steinkamp, M., Power, D., and Jones, B. (1978). *The test of syntactic abilities (TSA).* Beaverton, OR: Dormac.

Robinson, H. (1946). *Why children fail in reading.* Chicago: University of Chicago Press.

Robinson, H. (1971). *Phonics instruction—when, what, for whom? Teaching word recognition skills.* Newark, DE: International Reading Association.

Salvia, J., and Ysseldyke, J. (1981). *Assessment in special and remedial education* (2nd ed.). Boston: Houghton-Mifflin.

Searle, J. (1969). *Speech acts.* London: Cambridge University Press.

Searle, J. (1975). Indirect speech acts. In M. Cole and J. Morgan (Eds.), *Syntax and semantics,* (vol. 3). New York: Academic Press, pp. 59–82.

Sexton, E., and Herron, J. (1928). The Newark phonics experiment. *Elementary School Journal, 28,* 691–701.

Smith, F. (1973). *Psycholinguistics and reading.* New York: Holt, Rinehart and Winston.

Smith, F. (1977). *Understanding reading: A psycho-linguistic analysis of reading and learning to read.* New York: Holt, Rinehart and Winston.

Smith, F., and Goodman, K. (1971). On the psycholinguistic method of teaching reading. *Elementary School Journal, 71,* 177–181.

Snow, C. (1977). The development of conversation between mothers and babies. *Child Language, 4,* 1–22.

Spiro, R., Bruce, B., and Brewer, W. (1980). *Theoretical issues in reading comprehension.* Hillsdale, NJ: Erlbaum.

Strang, R. (1969). *Diagnostic teaching of reading.* New York: McGraw-Hill.

Sticht, T. (1977). Comprehending reading at work. In M. Just and P. Carpenter (Eds.), *Cognitive processes in comprehension.* Hillsdale, NJ: Erlbaum.

Stotsky, S. (1982). The role of writing in developmental reading. *Journal of Reading, 25,* 330–340.

Tuinman, J. (1973). Determining the passage dependency of comprehension questions in five major texts. *Reading Research Quarterly, 9,* 206–224.

Vellutino, F., and Shub, M. J. (1982). Assessment of disorders in formal school language: disorders in reading. *Topics in Language Disorders, 2*(4): 20–33.

Wallace, G., and Larsen, S. (1978). *Educational assessment of learning problems.* Boston: Allyn and Bacon.

Wardbaugh, R. (1969). *Reading: A linguistic perspective.* New York: Harcourt, Brace and World.

Weaver, C. (1980). *Psycholinguistics and reading: From process to practice.* Cambridge, MA: Winthrop Publishers.

Zintz, M. (1980). *The reading process: The teacher and the learner.* Dubuque, IA: William C. Brown.

Zutell, J. (1977). Teacher informed response to reader miscue. *Theory into Practice, 16*(5), 384–391.

APPENDIX 11-1

TYPES OF ORAL READING ERRORS ADDRESSED IN DIAGNOSTIC TESTING

1. Aid. The examiner is required to pronounce the word for the reader. Error is recorded by an underlined bracket.

2. Gross mispronunciation. Pronunciation that varies greatly from the actual word presented. Error is recorded by phonetically writing above the word.

3. Omission. A word or group of words is skipped by the reader. Error is recorded by circling omitted words.

4. Insertion. Words are added to a reading passage. Error is designated by a caret (∧) and words recorded.

5. Repetition. Words or groups of words are repeated. The repeated words are underlined with a wavy line.

6. Substitution. Words or groups of words are replaced. Errors are recorded by underlining and writing in the substituted words.

7. Inversion. Changes are made in sentence word order. Errors are indicated, as in "boy tall."

8. Partial mispronunciation. Only a part of a word is mispronounced. Errors are recorded phonetically.

9. Disregard of punctuation. Failure to observe punctuation by pause or intonation pattern as required. Error is recorded by circling the punctuation mark.

10. Hesitation. A pause of 2 seconds or more before a word is pronounced. Error is indicated by a check mark (✓) over the word.

From Salvia, J., and Ysseldyke, J. *Assessment in special and remedial education* (2nd ed.). Boston: Houghton-Mifflin. Reprinted with permission.

APPENDIX 11–2

Barlow, B., Bixler, H., Durost, W., Prescott, G. and Wrightstone, J. (1970). *Metropolitan achievement test (MAT)*. New York: Harcourt Brace Jovanovich.

Bond, J., Balow, B., and Hoyt, C. *Silent reading diagnostic tests*. Ardmore, PA: Meredith Corporation.

Botel, M. (1978). *Botel reading inventory*. Chicago: Follett.

Dunn, L., and Markwardt, F. (1970). *Peabody individual achievement test (PIAT)*. Circle Pines, MN: American Guidance.

Durrell, D. (1955). *Durrell analysis of reading difficulty*. New York: Harcourt Brace Jovanovich.

Gates, A., and McKillop, A. (1962). *Gates-McKillop reading diagnostic tests*. New York: Teacher's College Press.

Gilmore, J., and Gilmore, E. (1968). *Gilmore oral reading test*. New York: Harcourt Brace Jovanovich.

Jastak, J., Kijou, S., and Jastak, S. (1973, 1975). *Wide range achievement test (WRAT)*. Wilmington, DE: Guidance Associates of Delaware.

Karlsen, B., Madden R., and Gardener, E. (1977). *Stanford diagnostic reading test*. New York: Harcourt Brace Jovanovich.

Naslund, R., Thorpe, L., and Lefever, D. (1978) *The SRA achievement tests*. Chicago: Science Research Associates.

Nelson, M., and Denny, E. (1973). *The Nelson-Denny reading test*. Boston: Houghton-Mifflin.

Quigley, S., Power, D., Steinkamp, M., and Jones, B. (1978). *The test of syntactic abilities (TSA)*. Beaverton, OR: Dormac.

Roswell, G., and Chall, S. (1959). *Roswell-Chall diagnostic reading test of word analysis skills*. New York: Essay Press.

Sipay, E. (1974). *Sipay word analysis tests*. New York: Educators Publishing Service.

Spache, G. (1972). *Diagnostic reading scales*. Monterey: California Testing Bureau.

Tiegs, E., and Clark, W. (1970). *California reading test*. Monterey: California Test Bureau.

Woodcock, R. (1973). *Woodcock reading mastery tests*. Circle Pines, MN: American Guidance Service.

Woodcock, R., and Johnson, M. (1977). *Woodcock-Johnson psychoeducational test battery: Tests of achievement*. Hingham, ME: Teaching Resources Corporation.

TRANSITIONAL NOTE

Evaluation results should yield, as Hasenstab has pointed out, information about a student's strengths and weaknesses in communication and classroom skills. Sometimes it is impossible to gather this information through the sole use of standardized tests. Informal probes can provide observational refinements that lead directly to relevant programming.

The use of informal evaluation measures has been addressed in earlier chapters and elsewhere in the literature (Leonard, Prutting, Perozzi, and Berkeley, 1978; Muma, 1978; Siegel and Broen, 1976). Although federal guidelines for compliance with PL 94-142 note the need for standardized scores on students placed in special education programs, that does not mean that teachers are restricted from using informal observational procedures or are required to administer numerous standardized tests. The goal of evaluation is description; this means that the educator and clinician need to apply the principles of their operational (conceptual) model of "student competence" to the development of evaluation procedures that permit observation and analysis of student skills.

In Chapter 11, Hasenstab has described procedures for evaluating the student's reading process. It is a comprehensive procedure aimed at collecting data on various aspects of related skills. In Chapter 12, Sawyer, Dougherty, Shelly, and Spaanenberg focus on one component skill in the reading process—auditory segmenting. Being able to segment words in sentences and sounds in words is a basic assumption of phonics programs. If a child cannot perform these metalinguistic tasks required by a phonics program, the educator should be aware of this as soon as possible. Sawyer and co-authors discuss the nature of segmentation and provide specific suggestions on how teachers can observe a student's skill in coping with segmentation demands.

Muma, J. R. (1978). *Language handbook: Concepts, assessment, intervention.* Englewood Cliffs, NJ: Prentice-Hall.

Leonard, L. B., Prutting, C., Perozzi, J. A., and Berkeley, R. K. (1978). Non-standardized approaches to the assessment of language behaviors. *ASHA, 20,* 371–379.

Siegel, G. M., and Broen, P. A. (1976). Language assessment, in L. L. Lloyd (Ed.), *Communication assessment and intervention strategies.* Baltimore: University Park Press.

CHAPTER 12

Auditory Segmenting Performance and Reading Acquisition

D. J. Sawyer, C. Dougherty, M. Shelly, and L. Spaanenburg

Since the 1930s reading researchers have been attempting to identify factors that might be related to reading acquisition. Inquiry has focused on intelligence, perceptual processing skills, cognitive (thinking or reasoning) skills, and linguistic knowledge. Quite recently, researchers have explored the possibility that learning to read is affected by an individual's explicit awareness of the component elements of the speech stream. This ability to think about language as a signal system, apart from the messages conveyed by the system, requires that children think about language they hear in ways that typically are not essential for using spoken language to communicate.

Spoken language is produced in a continuous stream; there are no physical breaks between words. Our ability to identify separate words within a phrase or sentence, or to separate a single word into its component sounds, is a mental process we learn to impose on what we hear. Spoken words, and ultimately sounds, thus become psychologically "separate" units. When a child encounters written language, the spaces between words show them to be separate units, while the focus of beginning reading instruction serves to demonstrate the separation of sounds. If children have not yet acquired the awareness of words and sounds as psychologically separate units, can they profit from instruction that requires them to match (or "map") visual units (words and letters) onto splinters of the speech stream that the teacher models but which they (the children) cannot yet achieve independently? This chapter will (1) present a discussion of the relationship between children's conscious awareness of the component elements of the speech stream and their ability to achieve mastery over the written code, (2) review and summarize early research on this topic as well as current research being conducted at Syracuse University, and (3) provide educators with suggestions for applying the research findings as they seek to promote greater success among beginning readers.

RELEVANT RESEARCH

Reading has long been acknowledged as a language art—an activity that is related to and dependent on knowledge of language and ability to use language for communication. Mattingly (1972) noted that listening and speaking are primary language activities, whereas reading is a secondary, language-based activity. As such, reading requires a conscious awareness of the primary language activities. Various researchers have shown that this conscious or explicit awareness may be observed when children demonstrate their ability to isolate words and word parts when presented orally. Savin (1972) noted that children who have not acquired this explicit awareness of the elements of spoken language often are able to memorize some pieces of beginning reading instruction but are then unable to reason about how these pieces fit together in the process. For example, these children might memorize the members of the "at" family that the teacher has presented repeatedly, but they will be unable to figure out (or understand from the teacher's instruction) what those words have in common. Thus, they will be unable to decide if "bicycle" is or is not a member of the "at" family (p. 323).

Research on language awareness has examined children's awareness of word units and their awareness of word parts—syllables and sounds. Overall, ability to isolate the component elements of speech (to auditorially segment the speech stream) appears to develop between the ages of three and seven years. However, Rosner and Simon (1971) found that not every child had acquired the ability by sixth grade, and Dougherty (1981) discovered that developmentally disabled adults show significant variations in their abilities to isolate segments of spoken language.

The development of awareness of words as elements of the speech stream appears to involve distinguishing between word and nonword auditory stimuli as well as differentiating meaningfulness (semantic units) from order (syntactic function) units. Downing (1970) found that five year olds had difficulty distinguishing a spoken word when taped stimuli were presented and they simply had to indicate whether each item they heard was "a word" or was not. The items presented included a nonverbal sound, a single meaningless vowel sound, a single word, a phrase, and a sentence. Downing noted that no child's understanding (or recognition) of a word was equal to the concept of a word that teachers have in mind.

Karpova (1955) found that Russian children between the ages of three and a half and seven demonstrated stages in the development of word awareness. The children were asked to identify the first word, second word, and so forth. She noted a slow development of word consciousness beginning with semantically salient units and culminating in words that perform syntactic relational functions but lack much independent semantic identity. Thus, the words in "John ran home" will be isolated at an earlier age, because each word carries a clear semantic message, whereas the words in "John ran to the car" will not be easily isolated until a later age. "To the" will be linked to "car" by younger children who have not yet discerned the syntactic functions of these words and thus their importance or separateness in the speech stream.

Various other studies have examined word awareness among children four to seven years old with approximately the same results: (1) awareness of words in spoken language develops over time; and (2) five and six year old children often lack a clear understanding of words as units at the very time when reading instruction requires that they focus on these and smaller units in order to learn to decode (Holden and MacGinitie, 1972; Huttenlacher, 1964; Reid, 1966). One explanation for the gradual development of word awareness, as well as for the ages at which word awareness becomes a dependable ability, relates word awareness to cognitive development as described by Piaget. Papandropoulou and Sinclair (1974) found that children are not able to consistently conceive of words as objects of study in their own right (cannot demonstrate word segmenting) until they reach the concrete level of cognitive functioning as described by Piaget. Templeton and Spivey (1980) pursued the matter further and found that preoperational children were unable to talk about language abstractly (had little understanding of "word"). Children in the transitional stage between the preoperational and concrete operational stages demonstrated a better understanding of "word." However, only children who could be judged as functioning at the concrete level were able to demonstrate a fairly clear understanding of "word." They noted that level of cognitive development (according to Piaget) is often a better indicator of word awareness than is chronological age. This may be precisely why other studies have found some students, ages 10 to 60, who still do not have a well-formed, dependable concept of "word" upon which to base their learning to read efforts.

Children's awareness of syllables and sounds in words has also been investigated and here, too, it is important to understand that the isolation of one sound from others in a spoken word or syllable is a mental but not a physical possibility. Research on speech production and perception using a device that is capable of producing a visual image of speech (a spectrograph) has demonstrated that speech is not made up of strings of individually produced phonemes. Rather, in normal speech, the smallest unit of sound produced is approximately equivalent to a syllable (Liberman, Cooper, Shankweiler, and Studdert-Kennedy, 1967). That is, the smallest bit of the speech signal that humans receive and respond to usually contains information about two or three phonemes. If they are to respond to reading instruction that attempts to pair a written letter with a sound, children must learn to ignore what they actually hear and begin to think about spoken language *as if* it were composed of strings of phonemes. For example, teachers teach children that the letter "d" has the sound "duh" and encourage them to use that sound for "d" whenever it appears. However, MacGinitie (1975) points out that since it is not possible to isolate a stop consonant such as "d" from the accompanying vowel, the sound of "d" in "dog" is actually quite different from the sound of "d" in "dead." As you read this, stop to say each of these two words separately. Note the slight but identifiable difference in the position of your tongue and lips as you produce the beginning part of each word. The different vowel in each word "colors" your production of the "d" in each.

Studies of the development of sound awareness in children, as well as the relationship of this awareness to success in beginning reading, have shown that syllables are easier to isolate than phonemes or sounds and that the ability to isolate phonemes is related to success in the decoding aspect of reading. Liberman, Shankweiler, Fischer, and Carter (1974) examined preschoolers, kindergartners, and first graders. They found that syllables could be isolated by 46% of the preschoolers, 48% of the kindergartners, and 90% of the first graders. However, although none of the preschoolers could isolate phonemes, and only 17% of the kindergartners could do so, 70% of the first graders were successful at the task. The findings of several other studies support the progression toward mastery of sound awareness as well as the fact that not all children have achieved these levels of language awareness at the time that reading instruction is begun.

Liberman (1973) compared the ability of first graders to segment words into phonemes with their performance on a word recognition test. She found that among those who fell in the lowest third of the reading test, one half had failed the phoneme segmentation task. However, among those in the upper third on the reading test, none had failed the segmenting task. Sawyer (1975) examined the relationship between first graders' abilities (in December) to segment sentences into words as well as words into sounds and their end-of-year achievement on the Stanford Achievement Test, (Madden, Gardner, Rudman, Karlsen, and Merwin, 1973). Statistically significant correlations were noted for phoneme segmenting ability and achievement on the subtests of paragraph reading, word study skills, and spelling (.61, .48, and .46, respectively). Furthermore, there was a significant correlation between the ability to segment sentences into words and performance on the word reading subtest (.58). When overall achievement on the achievement test was considered, 76% of the children who had not reached criterion on the phoneme segmentation task (8 of 10 items correct) scored below the fifth stanine in reading performance. Only 12% of the children who achieved criterion on the segmenting task scored below the fifth stanine.

Several other studies have reported findings that confirm the relationship between segmenting ability, as an index of language awareness, and success in beginning reading. However, there has been some concern that relationships, in and of themselves, cannot explain whether awareness of words and word parts is an essential prerequisite for learning to read or if it develops as a consequence of reading instruction. In his review of the research on cognitive processes and word decoding, Stanovich (1982) noted that there is some evidence on both sides of the issue. It appears likely that phonemic segmenting, particularly, facilitates learning to decode and that learning to decode extends and enhances children's phonemic segmenting performance.

The research on auditory segmenting ability and beginning reading has been primarily correlational. As such, it has demonstrated that a relationship exists but has offered little information of practical value to teachers. How can teachers use this information to promote success in beginning reading? Is segmenting performance useful in making decisions about how to instruct? Should segmenting be taught before, or along with, beginning reading? A few studies have addressed these issues, but they have essentially involved small numbers of children or special populations. The remainder of this chapter will discuss a series of studies on auditory segmentation that have been conducted from the Syracuse University Reading and Language Arts Center. Collectively, the findings of these studies provide some concrete suggestions for pupil evaluation and instructional planning for the teaching of reading in light of the developmental phenomenon referred to as language awareness.

THE PROGRAM OF RESEARCH AT SYRACUSE UNIVERSITY

Interest in auditory segmentation at the Syracuse University Reading Clinic was piqued by various chapters in the book by Kavanagh and Mattingly (1972) that examined the relationships between speech and learning to read. The first study (Sawyer, 1975) spawned a program of research that continues to the present time. We are learning that a child's ability to segment the speech stream auditorially may have powerful implications for understanding and responding to individual variation in readiness for beginning reading instruction.

How Important is Auditory Segmenting Ability to Success in Beginning Reading?

To examine this issue, a test of auditory segmentation was developed. It tapped four levels of awareness—words in sentences, component words in compound words, syllables in words, and sounds (phonemes) in words. All 87 boys enrolled in first grade classes in a suburban elementary school were administered (1) individual tests of vocabulary comprehension—Peabody Picture Vocabulary Test (PPVT, Form B; Dunn, 1965); (2) group measures of auditory discrimination and auditory blending—subtests of the Gates-MacGinitie Readiness Skills Test (GMRST) (Gates and MacGinitie, 1966); and (3) the individual test of auditory segmentation. In June, Stanford Achievement Test reading scores were obtained and relationships between and among the various variables were examined. The finding of this exploratory study yielded the seed out of which new questions and subsequent studies have grown. In summary, this study demonstrated the following results:

1. Twenty-one boys failed to achieve criterion on the phoneme task. For them, phonemic segmentation ability appeared to be only one of a complex of auditory abilities, necessary for the processing of spoken language, that contribute to success in beginning reading. Statistical tests (multiple correlation and regression source of variance) applied to permit inferences concerning the relative strengths of each of the auditory abilities measured (discrimination, blending, and phoneme segmentation) showed that none, by itself, could adequately predict end-of-year reading achievement. Neither was vocabulary comprehension, by itself, an adequate predictor. When considered in combination, however, the four factors accounted for about 42% of the variance observed in end-of-year reading achievement among the inadequate segmenters (Sawyer, 1981).

2. Auditory segmenting ability is associated with measured achievement in reading. When all 87 boys were considered, the ability to segment words in sentences was significantly correlated with word reading (.58), whereas ability to segment phonemes in words was significantly correlated with paragraph reading, word study, and spelling.

3. Vocabulary comprehension was significantly correlated with the total segmenting scores (.58) among those 21 who did not achieve criterion on the phoneme level subtest, but was negatively related to segmenting performance when all 87 boys were considered.

4. Competence in phoneme blending is associated with phoneme segmenting ability (a significant correlation of .41 was obtained) and appears to develop earlier than phoneme segmenting. Subsequent studies supported this conclusion.

5. Among boys who were not yet proficient phoneme segmenters, a progression in the awareness of distinct phonemes was apparent. Awareness of the elements of spoken language appeared to progress from the level at which children fail to consistently recognize words as units to consistent awareness of words as units; and from isolation of a syllable size unit within a word to isolation of one or more phonemes in a word (Sawyer, 1983).

Can Auditory Segmenting Be Taught?

The second study in our series examined the effects of training in phonemic analysis on both auditory segmenting performance and word recognition performance. Spaanenburg (1982) tied this study to the previously identified relationship between the Piagetian level of conceptual development a child has attained and performance on segmenting tasks. Working with all children enrolled in first grade in a suburban elementary schoool in September, she individually assessed level of ability to conserve number, mass, and volume and rated each child as having high, medium, or low ability as a conserver on the basis of the sum of their scores obtained for all three kinds of tasks combined. The 69 children were then randomly assigned to either an experimental or a control group. The experimental group was given six weeks of daily small group instruction in the manipulation of words in strings and sounds in words using the Auditory Motor Program in Perceptual Skills Curriculum (Rosner, 1973). The control group was read stories, in small groups, twice each week. At the end of treatment, three levels of auditory segmentation ability were assessed (word, syllables, sounds) as well as recognition of words taught within the ongoing reading program in the classrooms. Ten weeks later these tests were readministered.

Spaanenburg found that the level of concept attainment children demonstrated on the conservation tasks was significantly related to performance on only the syllable level of auditory segmentation. That is, high conservers generally had high scores on syllable segmentation but did not, as a group, also have higher sentence or phoneme segmentation scores than children who were medium or low conservers. Furthermore, the treatment group did not differ significantly from the control group in ability to perform any of the segmenting tasks or the word recognition tasks either immediately after training or ten weeks later. Level of conceptual development within the treatment group did not affect performance on the segmenting or word recognition tasks. Finally, children in both the experimental and control groups made significant gains in their performance on both the segmenting tasks and the word recognition tasks between the first (November) and second (January) test periods.

We interpreted these findings to suggest that while attainment of concrete operations may be necessary for children to be able to examine language as a system apart from the meaning conveyed through utterances, the application of logic to an understanding of the perceptual world, in and of itself, does not appear to provide a clear advantage for either learning to segment language or for learning (remembering) words taught. Second, despite some evidence to the contrary in the literature on auditory segmenting training, we interpreted this carefully executed study to suggest that training in word and word-part analysis *that is not tied to the daily reading activities* children encounter has little potential for enhancing either segmenting or word recognition performance.

Might Beginning Reading Instruction Be More Effective if it is Tied to the Level of Segmenting Competencies Children Possess?

Time after time studies have reported a relationship between segmenting performance and reading achievement. In light of Spaanenburg's findings (1982) regarding the impact of direct teaching of segmenting tasks on reading achievement, our next series of studies examined the possible implications for teaching reading that knowledge about individuals' segmenting performance might permit.

Dougherty (1981), working with a population of developmentally disabled adults, administered a diagnostic battery designed to aid in the initial grouping for reading instruction—an elective course offered by a state-funded College for Living program. The results of this battery yielded profiles of current reading status as well as information that was used to infer potential for reading success. Following up on the findings of our original study, potential for success was determined by combining the results of a receptive vocabulary test, the Peabody Picture Vocabulary Test (Form B) (Dunn, 1965); a measure of ability to blend sounds into real words, the Roswell-Chall Auditory Blending Test (Roswell and Chall, 1963); a listening comprehension measure using passages from the Classroom Reading Inventory (Silvaroli, 1976); and a measure of auditory segmentation, the Sawyer Test of Auditory Segmentation (STAS) (preliminary version of Level II) (Sawyer, 1983). Two different kinds of auditory segmenting tasks were presented via the STAS. First, a child listened as the examiner said a sentence (e.g., Tom runs). The child was to draw one block from a pile on the desk, place it before him or her, and give the block the name of one of the words in the sentence the examiner had given (i.e., Tom). The process was repeated until one block for each word in the sentence was lined up before the child. The sentences ranged from two to ten words. The second task required that a child listen to a word the examiner pronounced, think about the separate sounds that make up the word and draw one block from the pile for each separate sound in the word. For example, for "tea" the child would draw one block and name it "tuh." He or she would then draw a second block and name it "ē." Eighteen words were presented containing from two to four separate sounds.

Analysis of the 23 individual profiles led to the formation of three distinct instructional groups. The approach to reading instruction in Group I emphasized sight recognition of whole words. Students in this group generally recognized no more than 10 to 15 words, were unable to read sentences at a preprimer level, had generally poor blending and segmenting skills, but did demonstrate vocabulary knowledge (PPVT) and listening comprehension sufficient to suggest that they might be able to extend their levels of reading performance.

Instruction for Group II focused on students' transition from a sight approach to a code emphasis approach for word recognition. In general, these students were able to recognize about 100 words at sight and were able to comprehend material written at about the first to second grade level. Their auditory blending and segmenting skills were stronger than those of the students in Group I but were not yet approaching mastery. Listening comprehension and word knowledge (PPVT) suggested potential to read at levels greater than they currently demonstrated.

Group III instruction adhered to a code emphasis approach. Students in this group were able to decode passages written at about the third grade level but often had difficulty with comprehension. Their auditory blending and segmenting skills approached mastery level. Generally, they guessed at words based on context and configuration. They did not apply phonics skills for decoding even though they possessed some knowledge of phonic elements.

Following two semesters of instruction each adult was again tested. Twenty-one of the 23 demonstrated significant growth in reading but no significant differences were found between the preliminary and later measures of auditory segmenting. Correlations for the raw scores on the

STAS and the San Diego Quick Assessment Test (LaPray and Ross, 1972) were .74 at the beginning of the program and .84 at the end. We concluded that this increase in the relationship between segmenting ability and decoding success occurred because decoding instruction for each was geared toward application of the level of segmenting ability available. Those who were primarily aware of words as units of language received a whole word approach to decoding, whereas those who were aware of some parts in words were taught both whole words and significant phonic elements, such as phonogram patterns, initial consonants, and blends as aids to decoding. Those who had nearly mastered phonemic segmentation were immersed in phonic-based instruction. It appeared that knowledge of segmenting ability might be used to make decisions about the kind of beginning reading instruction from which individuals might benefit most.

In light of our experience with developmentally disabled adults, we began to wonder about the power auditory segmenting ability might have to predict beginning reading achievement. We were particularly interested to learn if performance on the STAS might enhance the power of established measures of reading readiness to predict reading achievement at several time points during the first grade year.

In cooperation with a suburban school district, a study (Dougherty, 1982) was implemented to investigate the following questions:

1. Is performance in auditory segmenting in January of first grade predictive of end-of-year reading performance?

2. How will the predictive power of the STAS compare with that of other readiness measures already in use?

3. Since learning to decode requires both analysis of spoken and written words and synthesis of parts of words, will instruction using analysis techniques to supplement a primarily synthetic approach (Distar) yield higher levels of reading performance at the end of first grade than instruction using the synthetic approach alone?

In this district, children who did not score at the 46th percentile on the GMRST in either October or January of kindergarten were considered "at risk" for success in the standard basal reading series (Durr, Pescosolido, and Hayward, 1978). These children were placed in Distar reading (Englemann and Bruner, 1974) for the first year or two of their reading experiences. However, in one of the three primary buildings, all children were placed in Distar reading for the first grade year.

All children in Distar reading in the first grade classes in the district were included in the study ($N = 93$). The study was explained to teachers and training was provided in the supplementary analysis techniques to be used. These included auditory and visual analysis of words in context using mainly sentences and stories dictated by children, and auditory and visual analysis of words in isolation, using activities based upon Rosner's Auditory Motor Program (1973) but joining visual presentations of words to be analyzed auditorially.

In January, 12 Distar groups were in progress in seven classrooms. Following preliminary testing for reading skill, intelligence, and auditory segmenting, treatments were randomly assigned (Distar only or Distar plus analysis) to matched pairs of instructional groups. For eight weeks the regular classroom teachers provided ten minutes of additional instruction each day in the Distar program for those groups assigned to Distar only, and ten minutes of experiences using the analysis tasks they were trained to provide for the Distar plus analysis groups. The children were individually tested at the end of eight weeks and end-of-year reading performance on the Iowa Test of Basic Skills (ITBS) (Hieronymus and Lindquist, 1978) was also collected.

April testing, immediately following the treatment, showed that all children in the Distar plus analysis groups, regardless of level of segmenting ability at the start of the study, made greater gains in word recognition than children who had been in the Distar only groups. Experience in the auditory and visual analysis of words, provided as part of the reading experience each day, seemed to support reading acquisition. It appears that such experiences demonstrated, for children, how to apply to the decoding process the awareness of language elements that they already possessed. It is important to note, however, that method of instruction did not affect growth in segmenting ability. Neither treatment group was superior to the other in the April measure of segmenting performance. If auditory segmenting ability develops, in part, as a consequence of reading instruction, it appears that experiences in blending sounds may be equally effective in helping children to refine their awareness of language elements as experiences in both blending and segmenting.

The superiority of the "plus" groups was evident on the end-of-year performance on the ITBS but the difference was no longer statistically significant. This was perhaps due to differences in the intent of the post-test measures of reading used in April and the performance on the ITBS. For purposes of the study, reading achievement was equated with number of words recognized in lists and in passages. The ITBS scores, of course, reflect comprehension of text, listening comprehension, and language usage skills as well as word analysis and vocabulary. No independent measure of word recognition was taken in June, so the opportunity to examine this phenomenon was not available.

In order to address questions 1 and 2 of this study—questions concerning the ability of STAS performance to predict first grade reading achievement—a series of statistical procedures was applied. First, correlations were calculated for performance on each of the "predictor" variables (readiness measures) with January word recognition scores, April word recognition scores, and May ITBS total reading scores. Table 12-1 shows the degree of association noted for each index of reading readiness gathered with each of the measures of reading achievement.

Two significant observations should be made concerning the relationships noted in Table 12-1. First, the degree of association between performance on the STAS and measures of reading performance at each time point are high and similar, regardless of the specific measure of reading achievement used—word recognition or a more comprehensive battery of reading and related skills. Second, both the measure of vocabulary comprehension and performance on the reading readiness battery demonstrated stronger correlations with a global index of reading achievement (ITBS) than with specific word recognition scores at different time points. Further, the correlations with word recognition performance were considerably smaller than those noted for the STAS. This suggests that the STAS may be a better proxy for those reader abilities that support beginning reading, whether narrowly or broadly defined. However, the PPVT and the GMRST appear to be better predictors of reading achievement later in the acquisition process, when word recognition competency is established at some level, and may begin to be *applied* for various purposes.

Finally, the data obtained for this study were statistically tested to ascertain whether the STAS contributed to the power of other variables to predict beginning reading success. Multiple regression analyses were performed. The first showed that performance on the STAS in January of first grade was a powerful and significant predictor of achievement on the May ITBS. Additional regression analysis showed that even after accounting for the strong ability of age, vocabulary comprehension (PPVT), and reading readiness (GMRST) to predict reading achievement, the STAS added significantly to the prediction equation. Segmenting ability appeared to be a significant factor in understanding the variables associated with the reading acquisition process and proved to be a powerful index of later reading achievement.

How Does Auditory Segmenting Ability Relate to Reading Acquistion over Time?

The suburban school district that had participated in the Dougherty (1982) study agreed to participate in a longitudinal study that involved first grade and kindergarten children. This study was designed to address three questions:

Table 12-1. Correlation Coefficients for the Predictors of First Grade Reading Achievement with Measures of First Grade Reading Achievement at Different Time Points

Predictors	Reading Achievement Measures		
	January—WR	April—WR	May—ITBS
PPVT (January of first grade)	.24*	.14	.42†
GMRST (January of kindergarten)	.42†	.39†	.71‡
STAS (January of first grade)	.69‡	.58‡	.64‡

PPVT, Peabody Picture Vocabulary Test; GMRST, Gates-MacGinitie Readiness Skills Test; STAS, Sawyer Test of Auditory Segmentation; WR, word recognition; ITBS, Iowa Test of Basic Skills.
*Significant at the .05 level.
†Significant at the .001 level.
‡Significant at the .0001 level.

1. What is the power of the Sawyer Test of Auditory Segmentation (STAS) to predict reading achievement beyond grade one? (2) Can performance on the STAS be diagnostically interpreted so that appropriate recommendations for supplemental language awareness experiences might be made? (3) Will supplemental language experiences affect the acquisition of reading?

In October of 1982, the STAS and a measure of word recognition was administered to 265 first graders. In addition, PPVT scores were available for 185 students who had participated in prekindergarten screening, and GMRST percentile scores (GMPCT) were available from kindergarten testing for the 84 children in one of the three primary schools involved in the project. In June of 1983, measures of segmenting and word recognition were again administered. In addition, scores on the ITBS were collected for all 265 students and reading group placement was noted for everyone. We believed that reading group assignment reflected teacher perceptions of students' relative success in the actual instructional program being used. As such, reading group was, perhaps, a more valid index of reading achievement than are results of standardized tests. ITBS scores were collected again at the end of second grade. Correlations were calculated.

Table 12–2. Correlation Coefficients for Selected Predictors of First Grade and Second Grade Reading Achievement with Various Measures of Reading Achievement

	Reading Achievement Measures							
	Grade One						Grade Two	
	Fall		Spring				Spring	
Predictors	Reading Group	Word Recognition	Reading Group	Word Recognition	ITBS Word Analysis	ITBS Reading	ITBS Word Analysis	ITBS Reading
Segmenting (October 1, N = 265)	.59	.55	.54	.62	.51	.56	.57	.58
PPVT (Kindergarten, N = 185)	.42	.44	.37	.39	.37	.46	.21	.38
GMRST (Kindergarten, N = 84)	.74	.64	.51	.55	.55	.54	.38	.55

PPVT, Peabody Picture Vocabulary Test; GMRST, Gates-MacGinitie Readiness Skills Test; ITBS, Iowa Test of Basic Skills.

Table 12–2 shows the correlations obtained for the October of first grade administration of the STAS with the various measures of reading achievement. A consistent and continuous relationship between segmenting performance and subsequent reading performance through second grade is apparent. Table 12–2 also shows correlations obtained for the PPVT and the GMRST with the measures of reading achievement.

Regression analyses applied to data available at the end of the first grade year supported our earlier findings (Dougherty, 1982). The STAS again was a significant element when combined with scores from the PPVT and the GMRST in predicting end of first grade reading achievement. The STAS accounted for significantly more of the variance in reading performance on the first grade ITBS than could either of the other two predictors do separately. Although similar analyses have not yet been conducted using the end of second grade data, the size of the correlations noted in Table 12–2 suggests that similar relationships among the variables are likely to be found for that time point as well.

Implications of the Research Observations for Classroom Practices

In our opinion, there are sufficient data to argue that educators should use information regarding children's abilities to segment spoken language as a building block for planning beginning reading experiences. It cannot be assumed that every child has these requisite skills. Appendix 12–1 lists diagnostic probes that a teacher may use to assess children's ability to segment at the word and phoneme level. These probes may be initiated with a small group of four or five. Children who do not seem to perform appropriately should be taken separately to evaluate further. The same probes may be used in either a group or individual setting.

Experimental Programs to Develop Segmenting and Reading

Since our data continued to demonstrate the power of performance on the STAS to predict reading achievement at several subsequent time points, we next examined the possibility that specific instructional experiences could be implemented within kindergarten and first grade classrooms to foster growth in segmenting and reading. A program of such experiences was developed. It was rooted in a few logical assumptions concerning the relationship between segmenting and beginning reading.

The effectiveness of the program is still being examined, but findings to date are interesting and even promising.

The instructional program that was designed and implemented assumed the following: (1) Explicit awareness of words and sounds in spoken language contributes to or supports the acquisition of reading competencies, (2) growth in awareness of language units proceeds in a predictable order, (3) those children who demonstrate even rudimentary awareness of individual sounds as units within the speech stream at the time when reading instruction begins prove to be the better readers at subsequent time points. In keeping with these assumptions, experiences were designed to help children become aware of increasingly smaller elements of the spoken language in an attempt to promote achievement in reading.

Entry into our instructional sequence, dubbed the "Supplemental Language Program," is determined by the level of explicit language awareness a child demonstrates on the STAS (separate forms are now administered to all kindergartners and all first graders in the participating school district each autumn). Children who show little or limited awareness of words in sentences and no awareness of parts in words are placed in *word awareness* groups within their classrooms. Those who show firm awareness of words but little or no awareness of parts in words are placed in *syllable and sound awareness* groups within their classrooms.

The word awareness groups are engaged in supplemental (to the ongoing readiness or beginning reading instruction) activities for five to ten minutes daily. These activities are conducted by the classroom teachers and focus attention on isolated words within familiar phrases or dictated sentences and stories. These activities include marching and clapping to beats, pointing to different words in a familiar phrase the teacher had written on the board and had read aloud (e.g., "Someone's been eating my porridge!"), building sentences and stories using a "slotting" or replacement technique (e.g., "My doll is _____," with children taking turns supplying a word that makes sense in the slot). First grade word awareness groups also dictate stories. Teachers cut apart the separate sentences and have the children cut apart the separate words in a sentence, reconstruct a given sentence using the cut out words, and then reconstruct the story. Duplicates of the stories are also made and children circle "long" words, words with tall letters, and so forth. These activities help children to recognize that spaces signal boundaries between written words and serve to focus attention on some of the internal characteristics of individual words (length, shape, multiples of a single letter) that will aid discrimination between words at a later time when actual recognition of specific words begins to be stressed.

Syllables and sound awareness experiences, for those who demonstrated basic awareness of words, include clapping or hopping for each syllable in a spoken word, rhyming and seeing where rhymed words are the same and different, hearing and seeing sentences such as "I can run," and noting that when "can" is changed to "am" ("I am run"), "run" sounds odd or "funny." The children are encouraged to suggest the necessary change of "run" to "running." Children also learn to listen for other inflectional endings (e.g., -s, -ed) and to see that words with such endings are longer than the original word. Again, these metalinguistic activities supplement the ongoing readiness and reading experiences for about five to ten minutes each day; they are designed to help children become explicitly aware of some of the elements of spoken language. Later in kindergarten and throughout first grade, the Auditory Motor Program (Rosner, 1973) is also used. This program provides teachers with carefully sequenced lessons for syllable and sound awareness and provides appropriate lists of words for each lesson, thus easing the burden of preparation for teachers.

During the first year of these supplementary language experiences, teachers were enthusiastic about the effect of the prescribed experiences on student achievement. First grade "at risk" children were showing greater interest in reading and more success than they (or similar groups in previous years) had been able to achieve earlier. Kindergarten teachers generally reported success for the children who were moving from word awareness to awareness of word parts. However, they did not see much progress among those children who were in the basic word awareness groups. Again, the probable relationship between Piagetian levels of concept development and word segmenting was suggested. Perhaps those children did not have sufficiently developed cognitive abilities to permit them to recognize or internalize the goal of phrase and sentence segmenting activities during their kindergarten year.

The Effect of Supplementary Language Experiences

Comparisons of selected measures of first grade achievement for two successive classes suggest that a full year of supplementary language awareness experiences in kindergarten may have an important impact on first grade reading achievement. Table 12-3 shows mean scores and standard deviations for segmenting, word recognition, and selected ITBS scores. The 1981–82 class had the language awareness supplement for five months in first grade; the 1982–83 class had a full year of supplement in kindergarten but virtually no supplement in first grade. Comparisons of their reading

Table 12-3. Selected Means and Standard Deviations for the Achievement of Two First Grade Classes

1981-82 First Grade*			1982-83 First Grade†		
	X	SD		X	SD
Fall–segmenting	22.8	8.4	Fall—segmenting	26.4	6.6
June—segmenting	30.1	4.5	June—segmenting	31.5	3.6
June—word recognition	50.5	22.4	June—word recognition	57.7	20.9
ITBS—word analysis	65.5	19.0	ITBS—word analysis		
ITBS—reading	63.2	16.8	ITBS—reading	75.5	19.8

ITBS, Iowa Test of Basic Skills.
*Five months of supplementary activities in first grade.
†Ten months of supplementary activities in kindergarten.

readiness scores and PPVT results at kindergarten entrance showed the two classes to be quite similar (mean differences of one or two points on the different measures were not statistically significant). It might be concluded that first grade performance differences may be due to the timing and duration of the supplementary language awareness experiences provided.

Current and Future Research

During the 1982–83 school year, a second longitudinal study was launched, which is still in progress. We gathered a variety of descriptive data for 179 kindergartners. These data include demographics, achievement measures, and indices of development. We plan to follow the progress of this class through the end of their third grade year. Our objective is to investigate the relationship between and among auditory segmenting and other recognized indices of readiness for reading. Information accumulated through previous studies suggests the possibility of a continuum in the emergence of readiness factors that link oral language competence to the acquisition of reading competence. The hypothesized continuum of auditory-cognitive skills, leading from language to reading, pegs auditory blending as the first skill to emerge, followed by discrimination, segmenting, analysis of printed words, and comprehension of written language.

Complex statistical procedures are being employed to test the validity of this hypothesized continuum.

A second question of interest involves the relationship between physical and mental development during the kindergarten-primary years and subsequent reading achievement. Over the years, numerous variables have been found to correlate significantly with subsequent measures of reading achievement. Since so many and diverse abilities have been identified as predictors of later achievement in reading, we are interested to learn if it is possible to identify specific spans of time, during the kindergarten to third grade years, during which particular abilities might be most potent in their power to predict subsequent reading performance. Discovery of such "critical periods of prediction" (Shelly, in preparation) might serve to clarify the educator's task regarding reading readiness factors—what to test for, when, and what to do about the results. Information gleaned concerning a possible continuum in the emergence of readiness factors, as well as possible "critical periods" in the relationship between measures of learner competence and indices of reading achievement, should contribute to greater efficiency and effectiveness in educational testing and instructional planning practices.

SUMMARY AND CONCLUSIONS

Children's ability to separate the stream of speech into words, syllables, and sounds has been linked to both development and reading (decoding) acquisition for at least 20 years. Yet, the fact of that relationship has had little impact on educational practices. A program of research at the Syracuse University Reading and Language Arts Center first developed a valid and reliable test to assess auditory segmenting abilities and then designed a series of studies to address questions of segmentation in relation to development, training, and reading acquisition.

At this time, our findings suggest that auditory segmenting ability is an essential foundation upon which reading acquisition pivots. Furthermore, it appears that this ability is subject to refinement in kindergarten and first grade as a consequence of experiences designed to highlight increasingly smaller units of the speech stream while relating these to the structure of written words. Finally, we have some evidence to suggest that, among developmentally disabled adults, attaining mastery over the code during the initial stages of reading acquisition is more efficient and effective when the size of the unit addressed during decoding instruction (whole word, phonogram, or phoneme) is matched to the size unit (whole word, syllable, phoneme) an individual was able to consistently isolate within spoken sentences or words. When we combine this finding with the growth noted among two first grade classes in our longitudinal study (Table 12-3), we conclude that explicit awareness of words and sounds in spoken language is a significant factor to consider in designing and delivering beginning reading instruction to any age learner.

Material is presented in Appendix 12-1 (at the end of this chapter) to provide suggestions for assessing children's explicit awareness of words and sounds in spoken language. Implications of their performance for beginning reading instruction are also noted. Teachers wishing to implement a readiness and beginning reading program that capitalizes on information about children's explicit language awareness may refer to the section of this chapter that describes, in detail, the experimental program that we have been piloting.

REFERENCES

Cazden C. (1974). Play with language and metalinguistic awareness. *International Journal of Early Childhood, 6,* 12-24.

Dougherty, C. (1982). *First graders' segmenting ability, method of instruction, and beginning reading performance: A readiness perspective.* Syracuse, NY: unpublished doctoral dissertation, Syracuse University.

Dougherty, C. (1982). *First graders' segmenting ability, method of instruction, and beginning reading performance: A readiness perspective.* Unpublished doctoral dissertation, Syracuse University, Syracuse, NY..

Downing, J. (1970). Children's concepts of language in learning to read. *Educational Research, 12,* 106-112.

Dunn, L. (1965). *Peabody Picture Vocabulary Test.* Circle Pines, MN: American Guidance Service.

Durr, W. K., Pescosolido, J., Hayward, G. A. (1978). *The Houghton Mifflin Basal Reading Series.* Boston: Houghton Mifflin.

Gates, A., and MacGinitie, W. (1966). *Gates-MacGinitie reading tests—readiness skills.* New York: Teacher's College Press and Boston: Houghton-Mifflin Co.

Englemann, S., and Bruner, E. C. (1974). *Distar reading.* Chicago: Science Research Associates.

Hieronymus, A. N., and Lindquist, E. F. (1978). *Iowa tests of basic skills.* Boston: Houghton-Mifflin Co.

Holden, M. H., and MacGinitie, W. H. (1972). Children's conceptions of word boundaries in speech and print. *Journal of Educational Psychology, 63,* 551-557.

Huttenlacher, J. (1964). Children's language: Word-phrase relationship. *Science, 143,* 264-265.

Karpova, S. N. (1966). Abstracted in English by D. I. Slobin, Abstract of Soviet studies of child language. In F. Smith and S. A. Miller (Eds.), *The genesis of language.* Cambridge, MA: MIT Press.

Kavanagh, J. F., and Mattingly, I. G. (1972). *Language by ear and by eye.* Cambridge, MA: MIT Press.

LaPray, M., and Ross, R. (1972). San Diego quick assessment. In LaPray, M. (Ed.), *Teaching children to become independent readers*. New York: The Center for Applied Research in Education.

Liberman, A. M., Cooper, F. S., Shankweiler, D., and Studdert-Kennedy, M. (1967). Perception of the speech code. *Psychological Review, 74,* 431–461.

Liberman, I. (1973). Segmentation of the spoken word and reading acquisition. *Bulletin of the Orton Society, 23,* 65–77.

Liberman, I., Shankweiler, D., Fischer, F. W., and Carter, B. (1974). Explicit phoneme and syllable segmentation in the young child. *Journal of Experimental Psychology, 18,* 201–212.

MacGinitie, W. (1975). Research on children's understanding of linguistic units. Paper presented at the Twentieth Annual Convention of the International Reading Association, May, 1975.

Madden R., Gardner, E. F., Rudman, H. C., Karlsen, B., and Merwin, J. C. (1973). *Stanford achievement test.* New York: Harcourt Brace Jovanovich.

Mattingly, I. G. (1972). Reading, the linguistic process and linguistic awareness. In J. F. Kavanagh and I. G. Mattingly (Eds.), *Language by ear and by eye.* Cambridge, MA: MIT Press.

Papandropoulou, E., and Sinclair, H. (1974). What is a word? Experimental study of children's ideas on grammar. *Human Development, 17,* 241–258.

Reid, J. F. (1966). Learning to think about reading. *Educational Research, 9,* 56–62.

Rosner, J. (1973). *Auditory motor program in perceptual skills curriculum.* New York: Walker Educational Book Company.

Rosner, J., and Simon, D. (1971). The auditory analysis test: An initial report. *Journal of Hearing Disabilities, 4,* 384–392.

Roswell, F. G., and Chall, J. S. (1963). *Roswell-Chall auditory blending test.* New York: Essay Press.

Savin H. B. (1972). What the child knows about speech when he starts to learn to read. In J. F. Kavanagh and I. G. Mattingly (Eds.), *Language by ear and by eye.* Cambridge, MA: MIT Press.

Sawyer, D. J. (1975). *Auditory segmenting abilities and reading skill development among first grade boys.* Syracuse, NY: Syracuse University, Reading and Language Arts Center.

Sawyer, D. J., (1983). Observed patterns in the refinement of phonemic segmenting abilities among first grade boys. *Reading-Canada-Lecture.*

Sawyer, D. J. (1983). *Sawyer test of auditory segmentation (Level I and II).* Syracuse, NY: Syracuse University, Reading and Language Arts Center.

Sawyer, D. J. (1981). The relationship between selected auditory abilities and beginning reading achievement. *Language, Speech and Hearing Services in the Schools,* April, pp. 95–99.

Shelly, M. (in preparation). *The concept of a "critical period of prediction" in the measurement of reading acquisition.* Syracuse, NY: Syracuse University, Reading and Language Arts Center.

Silvaroli J. (1976). *Classroom reading inventory* (3rd Ed.). Dubuque, IA: Wm. C. Brown Co.

Spaanenburg, L. (1982). *The effects of sound manipulation training on auditory segmentation and word recognition tasks.* Syracuse, NY: unpublished doctoral dissertation, Syracuse University.

Stanovich, K. E. (1982). Individual differences in the cognitive processes of reading. I. Word decoding. *Journal of Learning Disabilities, 14* (8), 485–493.

Templeton, S., and Spivey, E. (1980). The concept of word in young children as a function of level of cognitive development. *Research in the Teaching of English, 14,* 265–278.

APPENDIX 12-1

TASKS TO ASSESS CHILDREN'S AWARENESS OF UNITS OF SPOKEN AND WRITTEN LANGUAGE: INDICES OF READINESS FOR BEGINNING READING INSTRUCTION

Question	Activity	Observation/Conclusion
I. Can each child recognize individual words in a spoken sentence when every word is picturable? Relevance for reading instruction: Some instruction seeks to teach children to recognize (to name) units teachers call words. Children need to have a concept of "word" as part of a message to respond adequately to teaching that forces focus on individual words.	Teacher seats a small group of children around him or her on the floor. Say "I'm going to say a sentence. You say it again after me and clap your hands once for each word you hear." Practice one or two sentences, such as "Mary ran home." "Dan looks sad." Then try three more sentences, such as "Cookies taste good." "John laughed." "My toe hurts."	Watch the children carefully to see (a) who performs confidently? (b) who is only imitating others—looking at others and lagging behind? (c) who is clapping but not matching each clap with one of the words? Conclusions: (1) confident performers should go on to testing for question 2. (2) children who imitate or do not name (b and c above) should be tested individually. If individual testing shows they do not consistently identify *each* word in a spoken sentence engage them in activities described for the *word awareness* group (see text).

Appendix 12-1. Continued

Question	Activity	Observation/Conclusion
II. Can each child recognize individual words in a spoken sentence when some words are not picturable? Relevance for reading instruction: Many of the first words children are taught as whole words serve grammatical function but are devoid of meaning: "the," "is," "for," "and." Children must recognize such words as being entities apart from the content words these usually join ("the apple," "is happy," etc.) if they are to understand the focus of sight word instruction.	Same procedure as above. Use examples such as "John ran to the car." "I fell in the mud." Use test sentences, such as "Play in the yard." "Mother went to the store."	Watch the children carefully to see: (a) who performs confidently (b) who is imitating others (c) who is clapping but not naming; who is naming but not clapping. (d) who groups "in the" with "yard" as one unit or "to the" with "store"? Conclusions: (1) Confident performers may be ready to learn whole words as sight words. (2) Confident performers may be ready for testing at the next level—recognizing word boundaries in printed sentences. (3) Children who are unsure (b to d above) should be tested individually. If individual testing confirms that they do not recognize grammatical function words as separate from adjoining content words, engage them in related activities described for the *word awareness* group (see text).

Appendix 12-1. Continued

Question	Activity	Observation/Conclusion
III. Can each child locate individual words in a printed sentence? Relevance for reading instruction: Children must be able to recognize where a word begins and ends if instruction focused on the names of whole words is to be grasped. This is especially important if basal texts used to teach reading are not routinely supplemented with language experience stories.	Print a sentence on the chalk board. Read it aloud. Have each child come up and put his or her hands around one target word. For example, "I can jump." Read the sentence and point to each word as it is read. Ask one child to come up and put his or her hands around "I" and remind him or her that "I" is the first word. Continue for the second or middle word and the last word. Be sure each child has a turn finding words in different parts of sentences. Three to five word sentences are a reasonable length for kindergartners.	If any child has difficulty with this task, help him or her find the correct word. Remind all children that spaces separate words. Provide many opportunities for such children to learn that spaces mark the boundaries between words.
IV. Can children blend separate sounds into a recognized whole word? Relevance for reading instruction: Children must understand that separate sounds may be joined together to make a new sound that is recognized as a real word. This awareness is the foundation of applying sound-symbol knowledge to decoding words not recognized at sight.	Gather together four or five children near you. Tell them you will say parts of a real word and they are to listen and try to decide what word the parts go together to make. Begin with two part words such as m - e (me), s - e (see), s - a (say), ta - ble (table). Be sure that some group and some individual responses are given. Go on to three and four part words such as s - a - t (sat), b - ō - t (boat), d -an- ce (dance), el - e- phan - t (elephant). Pronounce each part with at least one second between each part.	(a) Children who can blend parts into recognizable whole words have the prerequisite ability to apply subsequent knowledge of the sound-symbol system to the process of decoding. (b) Children who have difficulty blending parts into whole words are likely to be most successful if beginning reading instruction focuses on learning whole words rather than sound-symbol correspondences. Experiences with blending syllables and sounds to whole words should be provided.

Appendix 12-1. Continued

Question	Activity	Observation/Conclusion
V. Can children recognize the parts of rhyming words that are alike and the parts that are different? Relevance for reading instruction: Recognizing the part of rhyming words that are alike and where the words are different signals the onset of phoneme segmentation and suggests readiness for decoding activities that focus on phonogram patterns and initial consonant substitution.	Gather a few children together. Tell them you are going to say two words. They are to listen and tell you if the two words have parts that sound alike. Say "hat," "sat." Ask, "Does 'hat' have a part that sounds like 'sat'?" When children say "yes," ask, "What part of 'hat' sounds like 'sat'?" If children cannot say "at," tell them and write the two words on the board. Say each again and underline "at" in each. Next ask, "Where are 'hat' and 'sat' different?" Help children to say that "hat" and "sat" are different at the beginning but are alike at the end. Go on with additional word pairs such as "kick" - "stick," "will" - "pill," "hop" - "top," as well as "hit" - "top" or "hat" - "up."	(a) Note those children who quickly grasp the task and perform easily whether or not the word pairs rhyme. These children are beginning to be aware of sounds in words and a *word family* approach to decoding can be joined with learning whole words. (b) Note those children who appear confused and miss this item frequently. These children have not yet become aware of sounds as parts of words. Reading instruction should focus on learning to recognize whole words. Supplement that with hearing rhyming stories, completing rhyming couplets, and so forth, to foster growth in their awareness of parts within whole words.

Appendix 12–1. Tasks to Assess Children's Awareness of Units of Spoken and Written Language: Indices of Readiness for Beginning Reading Instruction—Continued

Question	Activity	Observation/Conclusion
VI. Can children segment one-syllable words into component phonemes? Relevance for reading instruction: Children must be personally aware that words are composed of isolatable sounds before a phonics approach to decoding can be personally and independently applied.	Gather together a small group of children. Tell them you are going to say a word. Ask them to listen for the sounds in that word. Say, "me." Ask them to say "me" and to think about just the first part. Ask, "Who can say just the first part of 'me'" (exaggerate the m-m sound)?" If one or more respond, go on to ask who can say the other sound in "me" (exaggerate both m-m and ē-ē sounds). If no one can say the "m" sound in isolation, say "In 'me' I hear 'm-m' at the beginning; I hear 'ē-ē' at the end—'m-m' - 'ē-ē,' 'me.'" Give other examples such as "see," "tōē," and "ate." When you believe at least some children understand what the task requires, go on to give about six test items, such as "say" (s-ā), "no" (n - o), "ache" (ā - k), "made" (m - ā - d), "hat" (h - ă - t), "pit" (p - ĭ - t), "seat" (s - ē - t).	(a) Children who respond with the correct separate sounds for most of the two and three phoneme words (whether long or short vowel sounds are used) show that they are personally aware of separate sounds that make up words. These children are probably ready to learn and apply phonics as an approach to decoding. (b) Children who cannot isolate the sounds in two and three phoneme words (even when long vowel sounds are used) with some degree of confidence and consistency are probably not ready to profit from phonics instruction. These children might benefit from activities such as those provided at levels F through H of the *Auditory Motor Program* (Rosner, 1973) as a supplement to reading instruction that focuses on whole word learning and some "word family" learning.

TRANSITIONAL NOTE

Chapters 11 and 12 focus on methods the educator and clinician can use to evaluate reading skills. Operating on the principle that reading is a language-based skill, the authors have provided comprehensive and specific probes. Reading, as an overlay behavior, demands that a student has a basic command of the linguistic code, an understanding of the purposes why that linguistic code is used for communication, and metalinguistic skills that permit reflecting upon the code. Similar skills are needed for becoming a proficient writer.

"Writing is a late-acquired activity that follows speech phylogenetically, developmentally, and structurally. . . . It follows considerable cognitive and linguistic development in the psychological history of each individual; and it is built on preexisting structures of cognition and language, recoding and extending them beyond their previous limits" (Litowitz, 1981, p. 73). Litowitz suggests that knowledge about a student's written language skills can be best ascertained by an analysis of what the student brings to the task as well as the nature of writing and the specific writing task itself.

In Chapter 13, Isaacson presents a model for the assessment of written language that considers the purpose, the process and the product of writing. Like Litowitz, cited above, Isaacson looks at the gestalt of the writing task; it begins with what the individual brings to it and ends with the refinements that education and publication require.

Litowitz, B. E. (1981). Developmental issues in written language. *Topics in Language Disorders,* *1* (2), 73–90.

CHAPTER 13

Assessing Written Language Skills

Stephen Isaacson

The written language skills of American students is currently a topic of concern. National studies have shown that student language–verbal scores have declined since the mid-1960s (Brown, 1981). Both educators and editors of popular periodicals have called attention to the "writing crisis" in public education and the vital need to reemphasize writing skills in the schools.

A written language problem is often one of the first signals to the classroom teacher that a child has a serious learning problem. In fact, the definition of learning disability includes a disorder in "using spoken or written language" (National Advisory Committee on Handicapped Children, 1968, p. 34). However, writing is an overlooked area in many special education classes. In one survey, only about 37% of IEPs written for learning disabled students had objectives in language arts skills, whereas over 60% had objectives in reading (Schenck, 1981).

The problem for special education teachers is knowing where the focus of remedial instruction should be placed. The first step in setting appropriate written language objectives is accurately assessing the specific deficiencies. A profile of a student's strengths and weaknesses enables the teacher to identify the instructional need.

METHODS OF ASSESSMENT

Writing abilities can be assessed directly by both *holistic* and *atomistic* measures, and indirectly by *norm-referenced* (or standardized) tests. Holistic evaluation is a guided procedure for scoring or ranking written compositions based on subjective rater judgments, usually of several language factors taken together (Cooper, 1977). Evaluators make overall judgments of quality by assigning a numerical score on a graded scale of 1 to 5 or 1 to 10. Atomistic scoring, on the other hand, takes into account discrete countable features of the written product, such as number of words per sentence or letters per word, to assess writing skill (Lloyd-Jones, 1977). Norm-referenced tests are indirect in that, with few exceptions, they require recognition—not production—of correct writing conventions, usually in a multiple-choice format. The language subtests of almost all standardized achievement tests, such as the Stanford Achievement Test or the Comprehensive Tests of Basic Skills, are indirect tests of written language.

In the mid-1950s holistic scoring, widely used at the time, came under attack when its reliability was brought into serious question (Mishler and Hogan, 1982). Indirect measures are thought to be more objective than the subjective holistic scales since scorers are not called upon to make personal judgments (Stiggins, 1981); answers are either right or wrong. Indirect measures have another advantage in that they can be machine scored. The major limitation of indirect measures is the difficulty, if not impossibility, of measuring several aspects of composition by multiple-choice responses (an issue of validity). In other words, multiple-choice tests measure the student's ability to recognize standard English usage but not actual composition skills.

Because of the perceived shortcomings of indirect tests, there has been a renewed interest in tests that require a sample of student writing. Holistic scoring, in new and varied forms, is again the focus of interest among educators (Cooper, 1977; Mishler and Hogan, 1982). The reliability of holistic measures can be increased by (1) elaborating the scale into several items that focus the rater's attention on specific relevant features, and (2) careful training of raters.

Several educational researchers have proposed specific, countable indicators of underlying composition factors (Cartwright, 1969; Christensen, 1968; Deno, Marston, and Mirkin, 1982; Finn, 1977; Hunt, 1965; Marcus, 1977). These direct measures have the advantages of objectivity, which holistic measures do not have, and direct sampling of student writing, which indirect measures do not have.

A MODEL FOR ASSESSMENT

The lack of teacher knowledge about written language and its assessment can be attributed to a lack of good theoretical models. Many ideas about written language are taken from theories of oral language. Vygotsky (1962), however, stressed that writing is a separate linguistic function, differing in both the structure and mode of functioning. Written language has a higher level of abstraction than oral language and requires greater detachment on the part of the sender. Correlational studies, too, such as Spearritt's (1979), have found no support for a single "expressive communication skill" (speaking and writing); these two components are separate factors.

Only in recent years have theories of written language, as a domain separate from oral language, been discussed. The three facets of written expression that should be included in a theoretical model of writing are the *purpose* for writing, the *process* of writing, and the *product* of writing.

Purpose for Writing

The first facet of written language teachers must take into account is purpose. Very young children view labeling as *the* function of writing, integrating written graphics within their drawings (Dyson, 1982). Other children write to initiate and maintain social contacts. Their "letters" do not communicate any particular message so much as create a form around which to organize a social event. Purpose is equally important among older writers. Britton (1978) pointed out that able writers produce great variations in product measures such as syntactic complexity in relation to the differentiated functions of writing.

Britton (1978) also proposed three functions of writing: expressive, poetic, and transactive. Expressive is language close to the self, verbalizing the speaker's consciousness, and is relatively unstructured. Poetic writing is a patterned verbalization of the writer's feelings and ideas and is not restricted to poems. Transactional discourse is language to get things done; it performs, persuades, and instructs. Awareness of purpose pervades all decisions the writer makes at both the global and the sentence level, impacting propositional and lexical planning.

Process of Writing

In addition to the purpose for writing, a theoretical model should consider the process of writing. Most authors consider the writing process to have three parts (Nold, 1981):

1. *Planning:* The thinking process before and during writing.

2. *Transcribing:* The translation of thoughts to graphic representation.

3. *Reviewing:* Backward movements to read and assess what has been written.

The relationship among these three subprocesses is shown in Figure 13-1.

Humes (1983) proposed a fourth subprocess: *revising*—changes made to the text after the draft is completed. Nold (1981), on the other hand, stated that it is incorrect to assume that revision is a one-time process that occurs only at the end of the writing session. Rather, it is a continual process of reviewing what has been written and then making the necessary changes, at either the planning or the transcribing stage (Figure 13-1). Good writers tend to be slower and do more revising, stopping more often to reread (Petty, 1978).

The writing process is complex. Subprocesses have been identified by Humes, 1983; Nold, 1981; Phelps-Gunn and Phelps-Terasaki, 1982; and Scardamalia, 1981, who have described the mechanical, cognitive, and attentional demands required by the complexity of the task. The mechanical aspects of the task require that a variety of visual and motor systems function well individually and that they also combine and integrate efficiently (Phelps-Gunn and Phelps-Terasaki, 1982). A child's development in writing, as in other cognitive abilities, is also based on the ability to take progressively more content variables into account during single acts of judgment: ideas, related events, different points of view, and so forth (Scardamalia, 1981). In addition, each subprocess involves focal attention and is constrained by the limits of short-term memory (Nold, 1981). The three subprocesses described by Nold (1981) and illustrated in Figure 13-1 cannot operate simultaneously and, if the task is moderately difficult, even one subprocess may overload. Thus, a skilled writer must employ strategies to handle the overload on attention. Each subprocess relies on knowledge, beliefs, and other constructs in long-term memory; the richness and accuracy of these constructs affect the ease and quality of the writing.

Product of Writing

Several authors have posited theories on the product components of written expression, the third facet of the model. Myklebust (1965) suggested just three components: productivity, meaning, and syntax (which referred to word usage and punctuation rather than the grammatical structure of the sentence). Later authors (Cartwright, 1969; Cooper, 1977; Polloway and Smith, 1982) made the distinction between fluency, (the number of words or sentence length) and sentence complexity, which is a better predictor of written language maturity as judged by holistic measures. Myklebust also overlooked vocabulary, a component other authors (Cartwright, 1969; Straw, 1981) have identified as an important factor.

When different theories of language are compared side by side, five principal components seem to emerge:

1. *Fluency:* The generation of simple sentences and elaboration into compositions of gradually increasing length.

Figure 13-1. The writing process. From Nold, E. W. (1981). Revising. In Frederiksen, C. H., and Dominic, J. F. (Eds.), *Writing: The nature, development, and teaching of written communication (Vol. 2.)* **(pp. 67-79). Hillsdale, NJ: Erlbaum. Reprinted with permission.**

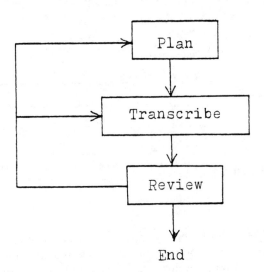

2. *Syntactic Maturity:* The production of sentences of increasing complexity.

3. *Vocabulary:* Fewer repetitions of favored words and the use of more sophisticated words.

4. *Content:* Attention to organization of thought, originality, and style.

5. *Conventions:* The mechanical aspects of writing, such as margins, grammar, spelling and punctuation.

The component of fluency comprises a *translating* aspect (the transcription of thought to graphic representation), (Humes, 1983), and a *motor* aspect, (the fine motor skills that permit legible transcription).

Integration of Purpose, Process, and Product

Figure 13-2 presents a model of written language that integrates all three dimensions: purpose, process, and product. In addition to these three dimensions, Scardamalia and Bereiter (1983) described a metacognitive function they called *executive control,* which refers to the writer's ability to monitor the overall process of writing, allocating resources to the various subprocesses and switching from one subprocess to another when

Figure 13–2. Model of written language.

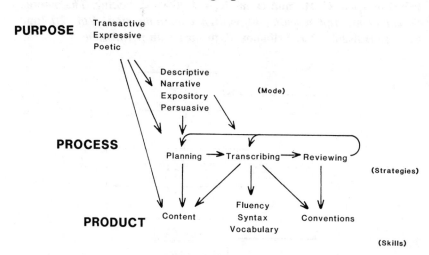

appropriate. The authors' key assumption was that by providing children with an executive control routine, more cognitive and attentional resources could be directed toward evaluative, tactical, and production decisions.

While each facet of the model is equally important to the writing outcome, the directional nature of the model suggests examination of the written product to be the most efficient way for teachers to evaluate writing. The purpose of writing is usually set by the teacher. When it is not, the teacher can assess the student's purpose directly ("What kind of composition are you going to write?"). However, most often teachers assess purpose indirectly—i.e., by the content of the written product. It is usually clear in the composition whether the student intended to narrate a first-person story, explain how something works, or express himself or herself poetically.

Similarly, much about the writing process can be assessed indirectly through evaluation of the written product. Cooper and Matsuhashi (1983) pointed out the interdependence of process and product. By studying text features and structure, researchers identify the composing problems writers must solve and decisions they must make. The best process studies move back and forth between observations of the writing process and examination of writing produced by the process. Product features are one form of objective evidence by which insights regarding the process are corroborated. Scores on conventions, for example, demonstrate the success with which the student reviewed and edited his or her work.

From the perspective of overall merit, the quality of the product is the primary facet to be considered because writing is valuable or useful only as its product is read and appreciated by the reader. The purpose or process of writing matters because each of these is reflected in the product. Although examination of purpose and process give valuable pedagogical information to the teacher of writing, in the end it is only the product that interests the intended audience.

Simple direct measures are ideally suited to teachers who need to monitor student progress. A teacher does not have to gather data on every skill in each of the language factors. After an initial diagnostic assessment, the teacher can select objectives from just one or two factors that are appropriate for the student. Simple direct measures can be taken frequently and, in doing so, the teacher has important data from which instructional decisions can be made.

Direct measures give current information for reporting student progress in five areas. A teacher can program specifically to the areas of fluency, syntactic maturity, vocabulary, content, and writing conventions. Teachers do not have to rely on standardized achievement scores obtained only twice a year. Reported information can be as current as the previous day.

Finally, direct measures provide a useful means of giving students feedback on their performance. Countable measures can be easily charted or graphed to indicate performance trends. Polloway and Smith (1982) recommend a technique of selective checking, whereby the teacher avoids excessive correction by selecting one or, perhaps, two particular skills to monitor.

FIVE PRINCIPAL COMPONENTS TO BE ASSESSED

Fluency

Assessing fluency requires measuring the degree to which the student becomes more proficient at writing down words and sentences into compositions of gradually increasing length.

Method. Count the total number of words written.

Corresponding Objective. The student will write original compositions of _____ words or more (within _____ minutes).

Suggested Criteria (Deno, Mirkin, and Wesson, 1984)

Grade	(To increase) Multiply baseline by	(Mastery level) Average number of words
1	2.6	15
2	1.6	28
3	1.2	37
4	1.1	41
5	1.1	49
6	1.1	53

The multiplier (middle column above) represents the average rate of progress over a nine month period from a national sample of over 500 students. Deno, Mirkin, and Wesson (1984) recommend that if the product of the multiplier times the total number of words is larger than the suggested mastery level (column on right), use the average number of words as the student's long-range goal. Otherwise, add the product to the mastery level average and divide by 2 to set the criterion. Deno and co-workers also suggest using averages from your own school or district.

Example: A 2nd grade student writes three compositions of 8, 13, and 10 words, respectively. The teacher will use the median score (10) as the baseline (or pretest) score.

1. The multiplier for grade 2 is 1.6.
   The product of 10 (baseline) times 1.6 (multiplier) is 16.
2. The product (16) is less than the grade level average (28); therefore, the product and grade level score will be averaged to set the goal.
   16 + 28 = 44
   44 ÷ 2 = 22

The student's fluency goal will be a composition of 22 words.

Syntactic Maturity

Assessing syntactic maturity requires measuring the degree to which a student uses expanded, more complex sentences. There are several methods suggested in the literature. Here are two:

Method 1. Count the number of sentences that fall into each of the following categories (Polloway and Smith, 1982, p. 343):

Fragment: My dog with the sore foot.
Simple: I am riding a bike.
Compound: She was going to school and she saw a police car.

Complex: After he saw her, she went away laughing.
Example: (Fragment)
     This morning while I was coming to school.
     I was riding my bike and I saw Sherry and she
                         (Compound)   (Simple)
     was playing with her brother. I said hi.

Fragments: 1
Simple: 1
Compound: 1 (run-on)
Complex: 0

An appropriate goal for this student would be to decrease the use of fragments and run-on sentences by learning to embed these clauses within other sentences, thereby making complex sentences.

For example: This morning, while I was coming to school on my bike, I saw Sherry.

Corresponding Objective. The student will write complex forms in _____% of his or her composition sentences.

Suggested Criterion. No available norms.

Method 2. Calculate the average T-unit length (Hunt, 1965; 1977). A T-unit is the minimal group of words that stands on its own as a sentence, with nothing left over. It may have one or more subordinate clauses attached to or embedded within it.

For example: I like bananas.   (1 T-unit)
     Although I prefer bananas,
     I also like apples.   (1 T-unit)

A compound sentence, however, is composed of two or more T-units, since either part can stand alone as a sentence.

For example: I prefer bananas, but I like apples.
     I prefer bananas   = 1 T-unit
     I like apples   = 1 T-unit
     _____
     Total per sentence   = 2 T-units

To calculate T-unit length:
1. Count the total number of words.
2. Count the total number of T-units.
3. Divide the number of words by the number of T-units.
Example:
          I was riding my bike/and I saw
          Sherry/and she was playing with
          her brother./I said hi./
                              (4 T-units)
     19 (words) ÷ 4 (T-units) = 4.8 words/T-unit

Corresponding Objective. The student will increase sentence complexity to an average of _____ words per T-unit in original compositions.

Suggested Criteria (extrapolated from means reported by Perron, 1974, p. 29)

Grade	Average Words per T-unit
3	7
4	8
5	9
6	10

T-unit length is the direct measure that has received the most attention by researchers since it was suggested by Hunt in 1965. T-unit length is highly correlated not only with holistic measures of written expression but also with reading comprehension (Hunt, 1977). Other measures of syntactic complexity used by researchers include proportion of words in free (or unrestricted) modifiers (Christensen, 1968) and the number of embedding transformations per T-unit (Heil, 1976).

Vocabulary

A teacher can assess a student's written vocabulary by judging the uniqueness or maturity of the words used in the composition. There are several suggested methods:

Method 1. Count the number of unusual words, subjectively selected—i.e., those words the student has not used before (Polloway and Smith, 1982, p. 345).
Example:

> It's hard to describe my dog. He's big. (My mom says he's enormous.) He eats a lot but not too much. He doesn't have long hair and he doesn't have short hair. He's just kind of average.

Unusual words: enormous, average

Corresponding Objective. The student will use new words in his or her compositions at a rate of _____ new words per week.

Suggested Criterion. No available norms.

Method 2. Calculate the proportion of *mature words,* by using a list of *frequently used* words as a reference (Finn, 1977).

1. Count the number of words in the composition not on the list of frequently used words.

2. Divide by total number of words.

3. Multiply by 100 for percentage of mature words used.

Example (using previous paragraph):

Words *not* on Finn's list of undistinguished words (1977):

describe	hair
dog	short
mom	kind
enormous	average
eats	

Number of mature words = 9

Total number of words = 37

$$\frac{9}{37} = .24$$

The proportion of mature words in the paragraph is 24%.

Corresponding Objective. The student will increase his or her written vocabulary to a proportion of _____ mature words per composition.

Suggested Criteria (extrapolated from means reported by Churchman, 1983, and Deno, Marston, and Mirkin, 1982)

Grade	Average
3	20%
4	25%
5	30%
6	35%

Method 3. Calculate the Type Token Ratio (TTR), or the proportion of unrepeated words in a composition (Cartwright, 1969):

1. Count the number of repetitions.

2. Subtract from the total number of words.

3. Divide by the total number of words.

4. Multiply by 100 for percentage.

Example (using the same paragraph):

Repeated words:

my

he's (repeated twice)

he (repeated twice)

doesn't   Number of repeated words = 8

have   37 (total words) − 8 = 29 original words

hair

$$\frac{29}{37} = .78 \text{ (Type Token Ratio)}$$

The proportion of original words is 78%.

Corresponding Objective. The student will avoid repeating favored words in his or her composition, using a proportion of at least _____ original words.

Suggested Criterion. No available norms.

Although TTR was intended as a measure of vocabulary, it may in fact be a multiple-factor measure. In pilot studies with academically gifted students, TTR is highly correlated with fluency and syntactic maturity.

Another measure of vocabulary used by Deno and associates (1982) is number of large words. Large words are defined as those containing seven or more letters.

Content

Cooper and Matsuhashi (1983) have proposed the only atomistic measure of content. They assessed the degree of *cohesion* in a composition by identifying seven kinds of referents to key concepts introduced in the first sentence of the passage. However, this assessment requires a more careful and time-consuming analysis than teachers usually have time to do. To assess content, therefore, we turn to the use of holistic scoring.

Method. Rate the student on aspects of content using an analytic scale (Cooper, 1977).

Items on the scale will vary according to the mode of composition— e.g., narrative, descriptive, persuasive, and so forth. In Table 13-1 are three examples of analytic scales related to particular modes of expression.
Example: Table 13-1 contains three analytical scales, each reflecting a different mode of written expression. An example of how a teacher may score a student composition using this kind of scale is given later in the chapter.

Suggested Objective. The student will improve the __(e.g., shape and sequence)__ content of his or her compositions, achieving an average rating of _____ or better (scale of 5).

Suggested Criterion. 4.

Conventions

Important as fluency, syntax, vocabulary, and content are to written expression, it is also important that students can write a composition in a form that is presentable to others. Studies of teacher ratings of student compositions demonstrate that teachers are more strongly influenced by the formal, mechanical aspects of writing than by other factors (Moran,

Table 13-1. Evaluation of Content

Narrative Mode	Low				High
Background: Well detailed	1	2	3	4	5
Shape and Sequence: Clear beginning and end	1	2	3	4	5
Characterization: Central figure "real"	1	2	3	4	5
Imagination: Novelty and humor	1	2	3	4	5
Total Score (add four scores above):					
Expository Mode					
Ideas: Depth and relevance	1	2	3	4	5
Development: Clear direction and purpose	1	2	3	4	5
Coherence: Transitions, logic, and unity	1	2	3	4	5
Variety, originality, and imagination	1	2	3	4	5
Total Score (add four scores above):					
Descriptive Mode					
Topic: Interesting, relevant	1	2	3	4	5
Perception: Sensitive, thorough analysis, unique perspective	1	2	3	4	5
Style: Appropriate voice, originality, sense of audience	1	2	3	4	5
Coherence: Relevant examples, logical development	1	2	3	4	5
Total Score (add four scores above):					

1982). It is important, therefore, that the teacher weigh conventions equally with the other language factors.

Method. Count errors in writing conventions using a checklist (Fig. 13-3).

Suggested Objective. The student will use correct ___(e.g., spelling and punctuation)___ in his or her composition with 90% accuracy.

Example: Figure 13-3 shows a paragraph scoring card used by one resource room teacher to assess writing conventions. Subtracting errors from a total possible score of 40 lets the student attain a positive score, whereas counting only errors focuses on the child's mistakes. Use of the scoring sheet for evaluation will be demonstrated later in the chapter.

Figure 13–3. Evaluating writing conventions.

PARAGRAPH SCORING

Words   10 minus #errors

Word usage   (subject–verb/noun–pronoun agreement)
Spelling

Margins   10 minus #errors

Left margin, right margin, name, date, skip line,

title centered, indent

Punctuation   10 minus #errors

Capitals, periods, question marks, commas,

quotation marks, etc.

Handwriting   10 minus #errors

Touching lines, legible, formed correctly

TOTAL SCORE   40 possible

(90% criterion = 36)

Multiple-Factor Measures

Multiple-factor measures are measures that reflect more than one aspect of written language. Type Token Ratio was described previously as being a multiple-factor measure, having high correlations with both fluency and syntactic maturity. Here are two other methods of assessment that cross the boundaries drawn between components of written language.

Method 1. Count the correct word sequences (Videen, Deno, and Marston, 1982). Correct word sequences (CWS) are two adjacent, correctly spelled words that are acceptable within the context of the phrase. CWS is highly correlated with total number of words (fluency), words spelled correctly, holistic composition ratings, and word scores weighted according to developmental level.

    1. Place a caret (∧) over every correct sequence and an inverted caret (∨) under every incorrect sequence. (The first sequence is BLANK to first word; the last is last word to BLANK.)

    2. Include inverted carets before *and* after misspelled words.

Example:

       ^My^dog ͮchasd ͮthe^ball.^

       ^The^ball ͮhigh^in^the ͮaire. ͮ

    Score: 8 CWS (5 incorrect)

Suggested Objective. The student will increase the quality and fluency of his or her writing by using _____ correct word sequences (per _____ minutes) in original compositions.

Suggested Criteria (extrapolated from means reported in Videen et al., 1982)

Grade	Number of Correct Word Sequences
3	25
4	35
5	45
6	55

Method 2. Use Fry's Readability Graph extended through the preprimer level to determine complexity of sentence structure and sophistication of vocabulary used (Marcus, 1977, pp. 258–259). Fry's readability formula (Fry, 1968) is based on a sample of 100 words. However, anything *per 100* is a percentage. Therefore, if the child's composition is less than 100 words long, calculate the proportion of sentences and syllables by the following steps:

1. Count the number of words.
2. Calculate the proportion of sentences per words:
(Number of sentences ÷ number of words) × 100.
3. Calculate the proportion of syllables to words:
(Number of syllables ÷ number of words) × 100.
4. Use the Maginnis (1969) adaptation of Fry's graph (extended through preprimer level) to estimate approximate grade level (Fig. 13-4).

An Example

To illustrate the application of these assessment techniques, five measures have been applied in the analysis of a student writing sample. This sample appears in Figure 13-5 and the analysis-scoring appears in Figure 13-6. The paragraph was written by Eldon, a fourth grade resource room student, to the topic "Things I Like to Do."

Fluency. Total number of words = 34. Eldon's score fell short of what the average fourth grade student can produce. To set a long-term goal, the teacher multiplied 34 by the appropriate multiplier (1.1) to achieve a product of 37.4. The product then was averaged with the fourth grade norm (41) for a long-term goal of 39 words.

Syntactic Maturity. There are six T-units in the passage, each divided by a slash mark (/). The compound sentence was divided into two T-units. Dividing six T-units by the number of words (34) gives an average T-unit length of 5.7, which falls short of the expected fourth grade average (8). Using a procedure similar to the one for fluency, the teacher set a long-term goal of 7 words per T-unit.

Vocabulary. The high-frequency words from Finn's list of undistinguished words (1977) are marked with a line under the first letter of the word. The mature words are those *not* marked, and there are 16. The proportion is computed by dividing 16 by the total number of words (34), which equals .47 or 47%. This is a good score; no objective for vocabulary will be set.

Content. An analytical scale for descriptive compositions was used to evaluate Eldon's passage. Below are the categories and the rating given each by Eldon's teacher:

Topic:	4	The topic was relevant to the assigned theme, but was not unique.
Perception:	2	Eldon made only the most general remarks about the show.
Style:	3	Eldon began with a personal voice, but soon drifted into an impersonal, general style, beginning each T-unit with *he*.

Coherence: 4   Eldon stuck to the topic, but there was no apparent order to his descriptions of Matthew Star.

Conventions. The scoring guide in Figure 13–4 was used to evaluate Eldon's conformity to the formal conventions of written expression. Here are the scores he received:

	No. of Errors	Points	Error
Words	-2	8	grammar: *me* as subject spelling: "favrite"
Margins	0	10	
Punctuation	0	10	
Handwriting	-2	8	vertical strokes "sticking together" (Circled in Fig. 13–5)
Total Score	-4	36	(90% criterion)

Eldon met the criterion for conventions.

Figure 13–4. Fry's readability graph, extended through preprimer level. From G. H. Maginnis (1969), The readability graph and informal reading inventories. *The Reading Teacher,* **22, 516–518. Used by permission of the publisher.**

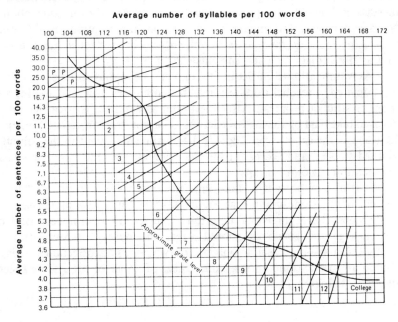

Figure 13–5. Eldon's composition.

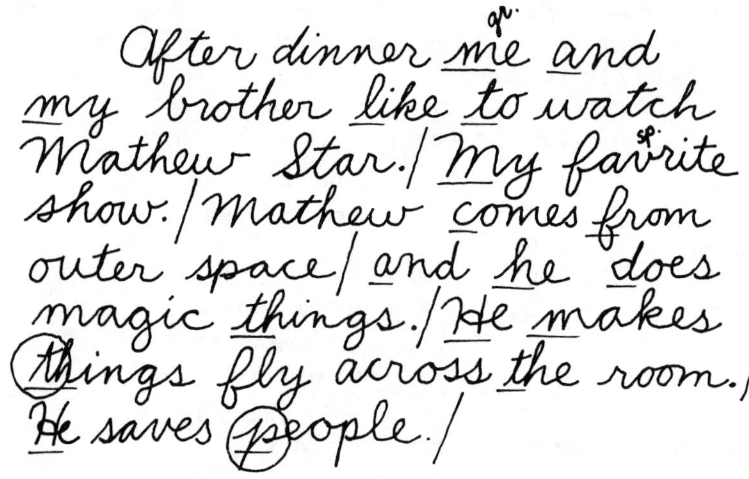

> After dinner *me* and my brother like to watch Mathew Star./ My favrite show./ Mathew comes from outer space/ and he does magic things./ He makes things fly across the room./ He saves people./

The teacher set goals for Eldon in fluency (criterion of 39 words) and syntactic maturity (criterion of 7 words per T-unit). A goal in content was not set because (1) three goals are too many, and (2) it is possible that an increase in fluency will improve the quality of content. Writing *more* about Matthew Star may have enhanced Eldon's score in perception. In addition, the teacher may add *favorite* to Eldon's spelling list and teach him the use of *I* as the subject of a sentence instead of *me*.

As was mentioned earlier in the chapter, once a diagnostic assessment is completed, a teacher does not need to score every aspect of writing to monitor student progress. After the initial assessment, the teacher only needs to take data on the factors relevant to the student's objective(s). Figure 13-6 shows the scores from Eldon's diagnostic assessment in the column marked "PRE" and scores for his fluency and syntactic maturity goals on subsequent compositions.

It is also important to note that marking a paper given back to a student in the same manner as Figure 13-5 is not a wise practice. It is recommended that analytical notations be made on a xerox copy of the student's paper. Feedback should stress the positive aspects of the composition and limit itself to only one or two points of correction. Scoring should always be done on a separate sheet of paper or on a score sheet like that in Figure 13-6.

Figure 13-6. Composition score sheet.

Student Name: Eldon

Composition Score Sheet

if relevant to objective(s)	Factor	Measure	PRE	1	2	3	4	5	6	7	8	POST
		Date:	3/1	3/7	3/14	3/27	4/4	4/12				
	Type of Composition	D = Descriptive N = Narrative E = Expository P = Persuasive	D	D	N	D	P	E				
✓	Fluency	Total # words Criterion: 39	34	30	35	36	29	38				
✓	Syntactic Maturity	T-unit length Criterion: 7 wds/T	5.7	5.8	5.5	5.7	6.0	5.8				
	Vocabulary	# mature words Criterion: 25%	47%									
	Content	Interesting Topic	4									
	1 = poor 5 = very good	Sensitive Perception	2									
		Appropriate Style	3									
		Coherence/Logic	4									
		Total Content Score (Add all four above)	13									
	Conventions # errors	Grammar usage	-1	me as subject								
		Punctuation	0									
		Spelling	-1									
		Handwriting	-2	t, p								
		Margins	0									
		Total Conventions Criterion: -4/36	-4									

SUMMARY AND CONCLUSIONS

Because learning disabled children characteristically have problems with written expression, as with other language skills, special education teachers must know how to accurately assess a student's written language skills and write corresponding instructional objectives. Although holistic scoring and standardized tests have traditionally been used to evaluate written language abilities, they are not as useful to a classroom teacher as simple, direct measures using samples of the student's writing.

The model of written language proposed in this chapter has three facets: *purpose, process,* and *product.* Since a writing purpose and process always result in a written product, the latter is the most appropriate and efficient means to evaluate all three. Simple direct measures can be used with each of the five product components: *fluency, syntactic maturity, vocabulary, content,* and *conventions.*

An overriding problem in the field of written language evaluation is the lack of research; there is weak empirical support for most models of written expression and the assessment techniques related to them. T-unit is one unit of measure which has support from many studies and large numbers of students. Although other techniques have proved useful in research, they have yet to be validated by classroom use. Teachers, therefore, must become classroom researchers, testing the methods as they use them and comparing the usefulness of one with another. The techniques described in this chapter were chosen with the belief that they are among the most useful methods for a teacher. Trying them out in various combinations should result in an assessment battery individually appropriate to any teacher's given purpose or classroom.

REFERENCES

Britton, J. (1978). The composing processes and the functions of writing. In C. R. Cooper, and L. Odell (Eds.), *Research on composing: Points of departure* (pp. 13-28). Urbana, IL: National Council of Teachers of English.

Brown, R. (1981). National assessment of writing ability. In C. H. Frederiksen and J. F. Dominic (Eds.), *Writing: The nature, development, and teaching of written communication* (Vol. 2. *Process, development, and communication)* (pp. 31-38). Hillsdale, NJ: Erlbaum.

Cartwright, G. P. (1969). Written expression and spelling. In R. M. Smith (Ed.), *Teacher diagnosis of educational difficulties* (pp. 95-117). Columbus, OH: Charles Merrill.

Christensen, F. (1968). The problem of defining a mature style. *English Journal, 57,* 572-579.

Churchman, K. M. (1983). *Comparison of seven measures of writing products by intermediate students in learning disability and regular classrooms* (unpublished master's thesis). Tempe, AZ: Arizona State University.

Cooper, C. R. (1977). Holistic evaluation of writing. In C. R. Cooper and L. Odell (Eds.), *Evaluating writing: Describing, measuring, judging* (pp. 3–31). Buffalo, NY: National Council of Teachers of English.

Cooper, C. R., and Matsuhashi, A. (1983). A theory of the writing process. In M. Martlew (Ed.), *The psychology of written language: Developmental and educational perspectives* (pp. 3–39). Chichester, England: John Wiley & Sons.

Deno, S., Marston, D., and Mirkin, P. (1982). Valid measurement procedures for continuous evaluation of written expression. *Exceptional Children, 48,* 368–371.

Deno, S. L., Mirkin, P. K., and Wesson, C. (1984). How to write effective data-based IEP's. *Teaching Exceptional Children, 16,* 99–104.

Dyson, A. H. (1982). Talking with young children writing. *Childhood Education, 59,* 30–35.

Finn, P. A. (1977). Computer-aided description of mature word choices in writing. In C. R. Cooper and L. Odell (Eds.), *Evaluating writing: Describing, measuring, judging.* Buffalo, NY: National Council of Teachers of English.

Fry, E. (1968). A readability formula that saves time. *Journal of Reading, 11,* 513–516, 575–578.

Heil, H. F. (1976). *The relationship of certain written language variables to measures of reading comprehension in the primary grades* (unpublished report). Hofstra University (ERIC Document Reproduction Service No. ED 145 457).

Humes, A. (1983). Research on the composing process. *Review of Educational Research, 53,* 201–216.

Hunt, K. W. (1965). *Grammatical structures written at three grade levels.* NCTE Research Report No. 3. Urbana, IL: National Council of Teachers of English (ERIC Document Reproduction Service No. ED 113 735).

Hunt, K. W. (1977). Early blooming and late blooming syntactic structures. In C. R. Cooper and L. Odell (Eds.), *Evaluating writing: Describing, measuring, judging* (pp. 91–104). Buffalo, NY: National Council of Teachers of English.

Lloyd-Jones, R. (1977). Primary trait scoring. In C. R. Cooper and L. Odell (Eds.), *Evaluating writing: Describing, measuring, judging* (pp. 33–66). Buffalo, NY: National Council of Teachers of English.

Maginnis, G. H. (1969). The readability graph and informal reading inventories. *The Reading Teacher, 22,* 516–518.

Marcus, M. (1977). *Diagnostic teaching of the language arts.* New York: John Wiley & Sons.

Mishler, C. and Hogan, T. P. (1982). Holistic scoring of essays: Remedy for evaluating the third R. *Diagnostique, 8,* 4–16.

Moran, M. R. (1982). Analytical evaluation of formal written language skills as a diagnostic procedure. *Diagnostique, 8,* 17–31.

Myklebust, H. (1965). *Development and disorders of written language: Picture story language test.* New York: Grune & Stratton.

National Advisory Committee on Handicapped Children. (1968). *First annual report: Special education for handicapped children.* Washington, DC: US Office of Education.

Nold, E. W. (1981). Revising. In C. H. Frederiksen and J. F. Dominic (Eds.), *Writing: The nature, development, and teaching of written communication* (Vol. 2. *Process, development and communication)* (pp. 67–79). Hillsdale, NJ: Erlbaum.

Perron, J. D. (1974). *An exploratory approach to extending the syntactic development of fourth-grade students through the use of sentence-combining methods* (unpublished doctoral dissertation). Bloomington, IN: Indiana University.

Petty, W. (1978). The writing of young children. In C. R. Cooper and L. Odell, (Eds.), *Research on composing: Points of departure* (pp. 73–83). Urbana, IL: National Council of Teachers of English.

Phelps-Gunn, T., and Phelps-Terasaki, D. (1982). *Written language instruction: Theory and remediation.* Rockville, MD: Aspen Systems.

Polloway, E. A. and Smith, J. E., Jr. (1982). *Teaching language skills to exceptional learners.* Denver, CO: Love.

Scardamalia, M. (1981). How children cope with the cognitive demands of writing. In C. H. Frederiksen and J. F. Dominic (Eds.), *Writing: The nature, development, and teaching of written communication* (Vol. 2. *Process, development, and communication)* (pp. 81-104). Hillsdale, NJ: Erlbaum.

Scardamalia, M., and Bereiter, C. (1983). The development of evaluative, diagnostic, and remedial capabilities in children's composing. In M. Martlew (Ed.), *The psychology of written language: Developmental and educational perspectives* (pp. 67-95). Chichester, England: John Wiley & Sons.

Schenck, S. J. (1981). An analysis of IEP's for LD youngsters. *Journal of Learning Disabilities, 14,* 221-223.

Spearritt, D. (July, 1979). *Relationships among the four communication skills during the primary school years.* Paper presented at the Conference on Developing Oral Communication Competence in Children, Armidale, Australia (ERIC Document Reproduction Service No. ED 180 025).

Stiggins, R. J. (1981). *A guide to published tests of writing proficiency.* Portland, OR: Clearinghouse for Applied Performance Testing, Northwest Regional Educational Laboratory.

Straw, S. B. (1981). Grammar and the teaching of writing: Analysis versus synthesis. In V. Froese and S. B. Straw (Eds.), *Research in the language arts: Language and schooling.* (pp. 147-161). Baltimore: University Park Press.

Videen, J., Deno, S., and Marston, D. (1982). *Correct word sequences: A valid indicator of proficiency in written expression* (Research Report No. 84). Minneapolis: University of Minnesota, Institute for Research on Learning Disabilities.

Vygotsky, L. S. (1962). *Thought and language.* Cambridge, MA: MIT Press.